Register Now for Online Access to Your Book!

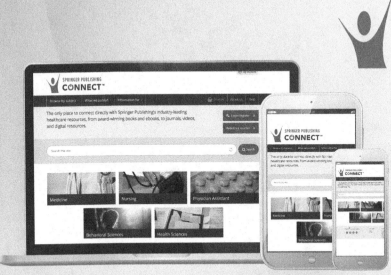

SPRINGER PUBLISHING
C⏻NNECT™

Your print purchase of *Palliative and Hospice Care Nursing Guidelines,* **includes online access to the contents of your book**—increasing accessibility, portability, and searchability!

Access today at:
http://connect.springerpub.com/content/reference-book/978-0-8261-4448-5
or scan the QR code at the right with your smartphone. Log in or register, then click "Redeem a voucher" and use the code below.

VH84W0VU

Scan here for
quick access.

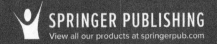

SPRINGER PUBLISHING
View all our products at springerpub.com

PALLIATIVE AND HOSPICE
CARE NURSING GUIDELINES

Patricia Moyle Wright, PhD, MBA, MSN, CRNP, ACNS-BC, CHPN, CNE, FPCN, is a professor of nursing, and an affiliated faculty member in the Department of Health Administration and Human Resources at The University of Scranton in Scranton, Pennsylvania, where she teaches in the undergraduate and graduate programs. Dr. Wright brings more than 25 years of experience in the field of hospice and palliative care to her teaching and truly loves to inspire students to provide the best possible care to those facing their last moments. She also continues to provide direct care to patients who are terminally ill through her work as a per diem hospice nurse practitioner. Outside of the classroom and clinical settings, Dr. Wright shares her love of end-of-life nursing care with others through her writing. She is the author of numerous articles and book chapters on issues related to end-of-life care. She is co-editor of the award-winning text *Perinatal and Pediatric Bereavement in Nursing and Other Health Professions* (Springer Publishing), which was chosen as the 2016 AJN Book of the Year in the category of Palliative Care and Hospice. She is also the author of a ready reference text for nurses entitled *Fast Facts for the Hospice Nurse: A Concise Guide to End-of-Life Care*, as well as *Certified Hospice and Palliative Nurse (CHPN) Exam Review: A Study Guide With Review Questions*, which was a 2020 AJN Book of the Year award-winner in the category of Palliative Care and Hospice.

PALLIATIVE AND HOSPICE CARE NURSING GUIDELINES

Patricia Moyle Wright,
PhD, MBA, MSN, CRNP, ACNS-BC, CHPN, CNE, FPCN

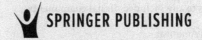

SPRINGER PUBLISHING

Springer Publishing Company, LLC
www.springerpub.com
connect.springerpub.com

Acquisitions Editor: John Zaphyr
Compositor: Diacritech

ISBN: 978-0-8261-4449-2
ebook ISBN: 978-0-8261-4451-5
DOI: 10.1891/9780826144515

Printed by BnT

The author and the publisher of this Work have made every effort to use sources believed to be reliable to provide information that is accurate and compatible with the standards generally accepted at the time of publication. Because medical science is continually advancing, our knowledge base continues to expand. Therefore, as new information becomes available, changes in procedures become necessary. We recommend that the reader always consult current research and specific institutional policies before performing any clinical procedure or delivering any medication. The author and publisher shall not be liable for any special, consequential, or exemplary damages resulting, in whole or in part, from the readers' use of, or reliance on, the information contained in this book. The publisher has no responsibility for the persistence or accuracy of URLs for external or third-party internet websites referred to in this publication and does not guarantee that any content on such websites is, or will remain, accurate or appropriate.

Library of Congress Cataloging-in-Publication Data

LCCN: 2023940156

Contact sales@springerpub.com to receive discount rates on bulk purchases.

Publisher's Note: **New and used products purchased from third-party sellers are not guaranteed for quality, authenticity, or access to any included digital components.**

Printed in the United States of America.

This book is dedicated to all of the nurses who touch the lives of patients and families facing end-of-life issues each day. You have chosen to work in the most sacred of spaces, the nexus of life and death. May your work be a shining light in the darkest of times and may you inspire others through your care and professionalism.

—Patricia Moyle Wright

CONTENTS

APPENDICES

PREFACE

This book is offered to support the work of palliative and hospice nurses who care for the most vulnerable among us. This comprehensive resource is intended to be a reference guide for clinicians in primary care, palliative care, hospice care, long-term care, and home care. With a dual focus on evaluation and intervention, these guidelines provide the information that palliative and hospice nurses need in a concise and organized manner. *Palliative and Hospice Care Nursing Guidelines* is organized by body system, and each system reviews common diagnoses encountered in palliative and hospice care. For each individual diagnosis, a definition is provided along with the incidence and prevalence, etiology, pathophysiology of the disease, predisposing factors, subjective and objective data, diagnostic tests, differential diagnoses, potential complications, disease-modifying treatments, palliative interventions/symptom management, prognosis, and nursing interventions.

In Section I, the opening chapter of the text introduces palliative care, reviews referral guidelines for serious illness, and offers a sample palliative care referral tool. In the second chapter, general and disease-specific hospice care admission guidelines are presented. Section I then closes with an overview of disease trajectories for common chronic illnesses, general indicators of poor prognosis, prognostic tools, and approaches to establishing and documenting goals of care.

Section II offers guidelines for approaching the care of patients who have a diagnosis of end-stage cancer. Chapters 5 to 8 in this section thoroughly address cancers of the head and neck, chest and abdomen, reproductive system, and blood, skin, and bone. An advantage of this text is the inclusion of both common and uncommon cancer types, featuring a thorough explanation of each. In addition to a careful review of numerous cancer diagnoses, each chapter features valuable information such as guidelines for staging various types of cancer, physical assessment techniques, disease-specific treatments, management of symptoms, and signs of disease progression.

Section III continues the detail-oriented discussion of serious illness but focuses on noncancer diagnoses such as cardiac disease, dementia, hepatic disorders, immunologic disorders, infectious diseases (including COVID-19), neurological disorders, neurovascular disorders, pulmonary disorders, and renal disorders. Chapters 9 to 17 feature information on interventions for various noncancer diagnoses, staging and classification guidelines for each diagnosis, system-specific assessment techniques, differentiation of manifestations of diagnoses, and disease sequelae.

In addition to conveying guidelines for palliative care, this book also includes numerous resources for clinicians such as comprehensive tables of diagnostic tests, disease-specific palliative interventions, prognostic and screening tools, patient teaching resources, clinician resources, and guides to symptom management, pain management, and wound care. The intent of this book was to create a resource for nurses seeking an overview of common diagnoses encountered in palliative and hospice care, disease manifestations, typical trajectories of illness, and recommendations for nursing care. It is my sincere hope that this text provides foundational information to support excellent end-of-life and palliative nursing care.

Patricia Moyle Wright

ACKNOWLEDGMENTS

I gratefully acknowledge my family's unwavering support for my determination to write about, teach, and practice end-of-life care. Most especially, I thank my parents, John and Patricia Moyle, for the selfless love and support you have offered me throughout my life. No one could ask for more loving, more giving, or more encouraging parents. I am also grateful to my husband, David, for supporting me and loving me through every twist and turn of the past 30+ years. You are a true gift. And, finally, to my adult children, thank you for being the shining lights in my life. May you find fulfillment, love, and blessings in your life and work and may all of your dreams come true.

I am also grateful for the support of my colleagues, some of whom have been my friends for over 20 years. You inspire me to be a better nurse, a better teacher, and a better person year by year. I would especially like to thank my friend and mentor, Cheryl Fuller, PhD, CRNP, for your friendship, love, and support throughout the years.

I would also like to gratefully acknowledge the editorial staff of Springer Publishing Company for their outstanding professionalism and dedication to the nursing profession. I am especially grateful to Elizabeth Nieginski who has worked with me for many years on many projects. I so appreciate your encouragement, guidance, and patience. Special thanks is also due to John Zaphyr, Senior Acquisitions Editor, Nursing, for immense support in finishing final edits to this book.

INTRODUCTION TO HOSPICE AND PALLIATIVE CARE

CHAPTER 1

INTRODUCTION TO PALLIATIVE CARE

PALLIATIVE CARE

DEFINITION/CHARACTERISTICS

A. Care for seriously ill patients with complex health needs.

B. Life expectancy is not a factor in eligibility for care (as it is hospice care).

C. Ideally involves care from an interdisciplinary team (see Table 1.1).

D. Emphasis of care is on symptom management.

E. The patient may continue curative/disease-modifying interventions.

F. Care may be provided in various settings (home, hospital, etc.).

G. Services may or not be covered by Medicare or other third-party payers.

GENERAL PALLIATIVE CARE REFERRAL GUIDELINES

A. Referral may be made to palliative care if any of the following are present, despite optimal medical treatment:

1. Newly diagnosed life-limiting illness requiring management of physical or emotional symptoms.

2. Conflict or uncertainty regarding prognosis, appropriate treatment options, do not resuscitate (DNR) status, and/or requests from patient or family for futile care.

3. Patient has had two or more recent hospitalizations for serious illness or is admitted from a long-term care facility or assisted living.

4. Patient's condition is declining as evidenced by unintentional weight loss, increasing reliance on others for completion of activities of daily living (ADLs) or progressive decline in medical status.

B. Patient has a serious illness and limited or nonexistent family or social support networks.

1. Patient and/or family require(s) psychological, spiritual, or emotional support during the course of the serious illness.

2. Patient, family, or provider requests a consult to determine hospice appropriateness (Center to Advance Palliative Care, 2020; SPICT, 2021).

PALLIATIVE CARE REFERRAL GUIDELINES FOR CANCER

A. Initiate palliative care if any factors in General Palliative Care Referral Guidelines (Table 1.2) are present and:

1. Cancer metastasizes or advances despite treatment.

2. Karnofsky Performance Scale (KPS) score is <50% or Eastern Cooperative Oncology Group score is >3 (see Appendices A-2 and A-4).

3. Patient has brain metastasis, spinal cord compression, or neoplastic meningitis.

4. Malignant hypercalcemia occurs

B. Progressive pleural/peritoneal or pleural effusions are present or worsen.

PALLIATIVE CARE REFERRAL GUIDELINES FOR CARDIAC DISEASE

A. Initiate palliative care if any factors in General Palliative Care Referral Guidelines (Table 1.2) are present, and the patient has:

1. Extensive and advanced cardiac disease.

2. Recurrent symptoms (i.e., dyspnea, angina, edema) despite optimal treatment.

3. Exacerbation of symptoms with minimal exertion.

PALLIATIVE CARE REFERRAL GUIDELINES FOR DEMENTIA

A. Initiate palliative care if any factors in General Palliative Care Referral Guidelines (Table 1.2) are present, and the patient has:

1. Inability to carry out ADL without assistance.

2. Decreased intake secondary to dysphagia or poor appetite.

3. Recurrent infections.

4. Incontinence.

5. Increasing isolation related to impaired communication.

6. Frequent falls or unsteady gait.

PALLIATIVE CARE REFERRAL GUIDELINES FOR KIDNEY DISEASE

A. Initiate palliative care if any factors in General Palliative Care Referral Guidelines (Table 1.2) are present, and the patient:

1. Has stage 4 or 5 kidney disease.

2. Exhibits diminishing functional status.

3. Chooses to forego dialysis.

PALLIATIVE CARE REFERRAL GUIDELINES FOR LIVER DISEASE

A. Initiate palliative care if any factors in General Palliative Care Referral Guidelines (Table 1.2) are present, and the patient has:

▶

TABLE 1.1   ROLES OF INTERDISCIPLINARY TEAM MEMBERS

ROLE	DESCRIPTION
Certified Nurses' Aide	Provides personal care as well as light household services, as needed. Supervised by the RN.
Bereavement Care Team/ Bereavement Counselor	Provides counseling and support to family/significant others after the death of the patient.
Chaplain	Provides emotional and spiritual care to patients and families. May serve as a liaison to local clergy and/or coordinate needed spiritual support services for patients and families in distress.
LPN/LVN	A licensed nurse who completes an accredited, state-approved program of study focused on the care of patients in a variety of healthcare settings. The LPN/LVN administers medications, treatments, and interventions tailored to the individual needs of patients and families. Supervised by the RN.
NP	An RN with extensive postgraduate training who provides advanced assessment of the patient's physical, mental, psychological, and spiritual needs. Works with the interdisciplinary team to develop appropriate plans of care. Treats patients' underlying conditions and symptoms pharmacologically and/or non-pharmacologically. Scope of practice is established by individual state Boards of Nursing and varies from state to state.
Pharmacist	A healthcare professional with extensive postgraduate education who works with the interdisciplinary team to determine and recommend pharmacological approaches to disease treatment and symptom management. Provides teaching regarding the safe use of medications, drug interactions, side effects, and safe storage and disposal of medications. Dispenses and/or compounds prescription medications to specifically meet the needs of the patient.
Physician	Treats patient's underlying illness and symptoms pharmacologically and/or non-pharmacologically. Verifies patient's diagnosis and terminality, if appropriate. Collaborates with other members of the interdisciplinary team and medical specialists to provide seamless care transitions.
Rehabilitation Services	Plans and implements interventions for symptom control and maintenance of basic functional skills.
RN	A licensed nurse who provides and coordinates care for patients and families in all care settings including hospitals, long-term care facilities, and in the community. Scope of practice is established by individual state Boards of Nursing and may vary from state to state.
Social Services	Identifies social, emotional, financial, and family needs related to the patient's serious illness. Provides individual and family support and connects patient and family to community support services as needed.

LPN, licensed practical nurse; LVN, licensed vocational nurse; NP, nurse practitioner.

Sources: American Psychological Association. (2022). *APA dictionary of psychology.* https://dictionary.apa.org/; Centers for Medicare & Medicaid Services. (2021). *Medicare benefit policy manual.* https://www.cms.gov/Regulations-and-Guidance/Guidance/Manuals/Downloads/bp102c09.pdf; Healthcare Chaplains Ministry Association. (2020). *What is a chaplain?* https://www.hcmachaplains.org/what-is-a-chaplain/; U.S. Bureau of Labor Statistics. (2021). *Occupational outlook handbook.* https://www.bls.gov/ooh/healthcare/pharmacists.htm.

TABLE 1.2 GENERAL PALLIATIVE CARE REFERRAL GUIDELINES

A REFERRAL FOR PALLIATIVE SERVICES IS REQUESTED FOR (PLEASE CHECK ALL THAT APPLY):

Medical status:
- ☐ Uncontrolled symptoms
- ☐ Complex or persistent symptoms despite optimal treatment
- ☐ Complex medical needs requiring ongoing coordination of health services
- ☐ Decline in medical, nutritional, or functional status despite optimal treatment

Advance care planning needs:
- ☐ No advance directive is in place and patient has life-limiting illness
- ☐ Disagreement regarding plan of care
- ☐ Guidance needed regarding life-sustaining or disease-modifying treatments

Interdisciplinary care:
- ☐ Patient/family would benefit from the coordinated support and interventions of the palliative care team (e.g., medical, nursing, medical social services, chaplain)

Prognostication:
- ☐ Patient's life expectancy is likely 12 months or less

Other:

1. Cirrhosis with one or more of the following during the previous 12-month period:
   a. Refractory ascites.
   b. Hepatic encephalopathy.
   c. Hepatorenal syndrome.
   d. Bacterial peritonitis.
   e. Recurrent variceal bleeding.

2. And liver transplant is not an option or patient chooses to forego.

PALLIATIVE CARE REFERRAL GUIDELINES FOR NEUROLOGICAL DISEASE

A. Initiate palliative care if any factors in General Palliative Care Referral Guidelines (Table 1.2) are present and:

1. Patient has a Folstein Mini Mental Score <20 (see https://www.parinc.com).

2. Patient or family considering artificial nutrition or mechanical ventilation.

3. Status epilepticus is present for greater than 24 hours.

4. Patient has advanced disease and is dependent for all ADLs.

PALLIATIVE CARE REFERRAL GUIDELINES FOR RESPIRATORY DISEASE

A. Initiate palliative care if any factors in General Palliative Care Referral Guidelines (Table 1.2) are present, and patient has:

1. Severe or very severe lung disease (forced expiratory volume [FEV]$_1$ ≤50% of predicted value).

2. Dyspnea at rest or with minimal exertion.

3. Hypoxia at rest or with minimal exertion.

4. Reliance on supplemental oxygen.

5. History of mechanical ventilation or mechanical ventilation is contraindicated.

PALLIATIVE CARE REFERRAL GUIDELINES FOR VASCULAR DISEASE

A. Initiate palliative care if any factors in General Palliative Care Referral Guidelines (Table 1.2) are present and:

1. Advancing vascular disease is noted despite optimal treatment.

2. Surgical intervention is contraindicated.

3. Worsening or nonhealing lower extremity wounds (Center to Advance Palliative Care, 2020; U.S. Centers for Medicare & Medicaid Services, 2019).

REFERENCES

American Psychological Association. (2022). *APA dictionary of psychology.* https://dictionary.apa.org/

Center to Advance Palliative Care. (2020). *Palliative care referral criteria.* https://www.capc.org/documents/286/

Centers for Medicare & Medicaid Services. (2021). *Medicare benefit policy manual.* https://www.cms.gov/Regulations-and-Guidance/Guidance/Manuals/Downloads/bp102c09.pdf

Healthcare Chaplains Ministry Association. (2020). *What is a chaplain?* https://www.hcmachaplains.org/what-is-a-chaplain/

SPICT. (2021). *Supportive & palliative care indicators tool (SPICT).* https://www.spict.org.uk/

U.S. Bureau of Labor Statistics. (2021). *Occupational outlook handbook.* https://www.bls.gov/ooh/healthcare/pharmacists.htm

U.S. Centers for Medicare & Medicaid Services. (2019). *Local coverage determination (LCD): Hospice determining terminal status (L33393).* https://www.cms.gov/medicare-coveragedatabase/details

CHAPTER 2

INTRODUCTION TO HOSPICE CARE

HOSPICE CARE

DEFINITION/CHARACTERISTICS

A. Reserved for patients with a life expectancy of about 6 months.

B. Utilizes a holistic team approach to care (see Table 1.1 in Chapter 1).

C. Emphasis is on symptom management rather than curative care.

D. Patient no longer desires curative/disease-modifying interventions (see Figure 2.1).

E. Care is typically provided in the home but can be provided in other settings.

F. Bereavement services are provided for up to 1 year after patient death.

G. Services covered by the hospice Medicare benefit and other third-party payers.

H. Eligibility for hospice care is supported by general and disease-specific guidelines (see Tables 2.1 and 2.2).

GENERAL HOSPICE ELIGIBILITY GUIDELINES

A. General indicators of poor prognosis.
  1. Recurrent or intractable infection.
  2. Diminished nutritional status, as evidenced by:
    a. Unintentional weight loss/decreasing body mass index (BMI; see Appendix A-1).
    b. Decreasing mid-arm circumference (MAC) (see Appendix A-1).
    c. Decreasing abdominal girth.
    d. Decreasing albumin levels.
  3. Dysphagia that leads to inadequate oral intake or to aspiration.
  4. Scores of <70% on the Karnofsky Performance Scale (KPS) or the Palliative Performance Scale (PPS; see Appendices A-2 and A-3).
  5. Functional Assessment Staging Tool (FAST) scale score of ≥7a (see Appendix A-5).
  6. Frequent need for medical care or frequent hospitalizations.
  7. New-onset pressure ulcers or worsening of existing pressure ulcers despite optimal care.
  8. Dependence for two or more activities of daily living (ADLs).

AMYOTROPHIC LATERAL SCLEROSIS HOSPICE CRITERIA

A. Impaired respiration as evidenced by dyspnea or vital capacity <30%, if available.

B. Patient foregoes mechanical ventilation.

C. Rapid disease progression over the course of the past 12 months with life-threatening disease complications.

CANCER HOSPICE CRITERIA

A. Diagnosis of cancer with distant metastasis.

B. Disease progression despite treatments.

C. Chooses to forego disease-modifying treatments.

CARDIAC DISEASE HOSPICE CRITERIA

A. Patient is symptomatic despite optimal treatment.

B. Patient is not a candidate for surgical intervention or chooses to forego surgery.

C. Patient's heart disease meets New York Heart Association, class IV criteria (see Appendix A-8).

D. Supportive factors include:
  1. Treatment-resistant arrhythmias.
  2. History of cardiac arrest or resuscitation.
  3. Unexplained syncope.
  4. Brain embolism of cardiac origin.
  5. Concomitant HIV disease.

DEMENTIA HOSPICE CRITERIA

A. FAST scale score of 7 or higher (see Appendix A-5).

B. Patient is unable to:
  1. Ambulate.
  2. Dress self.
  3. Bathe without assistance.

C. Patient exhibits:
  1. Urinary and fecal incontinence.
  2. Lack of meaningful speech (uses ≤ six words).

D. Patient has experienced at least one of the following within the previous 12 months:
  1. Aspiration pneumonia.
  2. Septicemia.
  3. Pyelonephritis or other upper urinary tract infection.
  4. Recurrent infections despite antibiotic treatment.
  5. Multiple stage 3 to 4 decubiti (see Appendix F-2).
  6. Inability to maintain nutritional status exhibited by:
    a. A 10% weight loss in the past 6 months.
    b. Decreasing serum albumin.

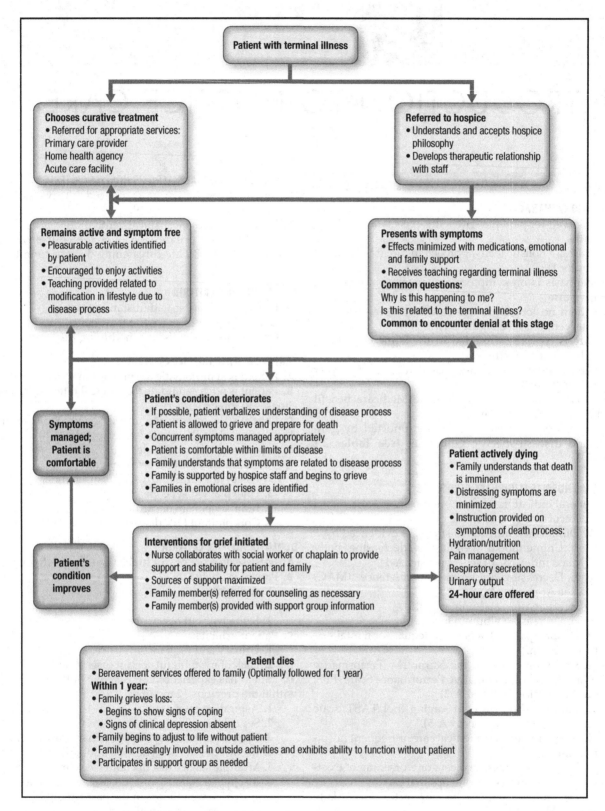

FIGURE 2.1 Critical pathway for terminal care.

Source: Adapted from Wright, P. M. (2001). A critical pathway for interdisciplinary hospice care. *American Journal of Hospice and Palliative Medicine, 18*(1), 31–34. https://doi.org/10.1177/1049909101018001

TABLE 2.1   GENERAL HOSPICE ELIGIBILITY GUIDELINES

Types of disease trajectory	• Rapid decline: short period of steady decline (e.g., cancer) • Saw-toothed decline: episodes of exacerbations, never back to previous baseline (e.g., COPD) • Slow insidious decline: prolonged dwindling (e.g., dementia, frailty)
Key questions to ponder 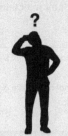	**Pain and symptom management** • What are the symptoms we are managing? What does it take to keep them under control? • How often are these symptoms escalating or the patient is having a crisis? **Disease progression/change in quality of life** • What evidence of decline are we seeing, reading, observing (e.g., food intake, weight, physical assessment, arm circumference, mental status, change in medications/O_2)? • What is the patient/family telling us about decline (as evidenced by, e.g., stamina, ADLs, sleep/rest, social engagement, activities, symptoms, pain, psychospiritual issues)? **LCD criteria** • Does the patient still meet LCD guidelines? • Does the disease trajectory (pattern and momentum of decline) still reflect a terminal condition? **Instability** • Is the patient relatively stable? What would happen if hospice services were removed? • Will the improvement be sustained? What is the course of care and caregiver challenge?

Clinical status guidelines (use if there are no LCD-specific disease guidelines)	• Intractable serious infections: pneumonia, pyelonephritis, septicemia, recurrent fevers
	• Progressive inanition (exhaustion, lethargy) evidenced by:
	  ■ > ↓ 10% weight in the past 6 months or BMI <22 kg/m² (not due to depression/diuretics)
	  ■ ↓ MAC (acromion [shoulder] to olecranon [elbow]) or abdominal girth
	  ■ ↓ skin turgor, ill-fitting clothes, increasing skin folds if weight not documented
	  ■ Laboratory: albumin <25; ↓ cholesterol
	  ■ Dysphagia with measured aspiration (e.g., history of choking/gagging with feeding) or ↓ intake as evidence by decreasing cups of food consumed
	• Symptoms (intractable/poorly responsive): dyspnea with ↑ respiratory rate; cough; nausea/vomiting; diarrhea; pain requiring ↑ doses of major analgesics
	• Signs: ↓ systolic blood pressure >90 mmHg or ↑ postural hypotension; ascites; edema; venous, arterial, lymphatic obstruction; weakness; ↓ level of consciousness
	• Laboratory: ↑ PCO_2 or ↓ PO_2/Sao_2; ↑ calcium, creatinine, or liver function; ↑↓ serum Na⁺ or ↑ K⁺
	• ↓ PPS due to disease progression
	• ↓ FAST: 7a >6 words; 7b ~1 word; unable to: walk-7c, sit up-7d, smile-7e, hold head up-7f
	• ↓ ADLs: ambulation, bathing, continence, dressing, feeding, transfer
	• Progressive stage 3–4 pressure ulcers despite optimal care
	• ↑ ED visits, hospitalization, physician visits related to first diagnosis prior to election of hospice

Baseline to use with specific disease guidelines 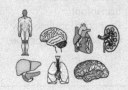	• Documented clinical progression of disease: multiple ED visits, hospitalizations, home visits • PPS <70% (PPS for stroke or HIV <50%) • Partial/full dependence for 2+ ADLs: ambulation, bathing, continence, dressing, feeding, transfer • Significant comorbidities, e.g., congestive heart failure, COPD, DM, ischemic heart, renal, liver, HIV, dementia, neurological (cerebrovascular accident, amyotrophic lateral sclerosis, Parkinson disease), autoimmune (lupus, rheumatoid arthritis) • Receiving supportive, palliative, comfort care or treatment to comfort/improve functional level (e.g., intravenous fluids, nasogastric tubes, transfusions, palliative chemotherapy, or radiation therapy)

(continued)

TABLE 2.1   GENERAL HOSPICE ELIGIBILITY GUIDELINES (*CONTINUED*)

Additional guidelines for neuromuscular diseases, multiple sclerosis, Parkinson disease	• Rapid disease progression or complications in the last 12 months • Independent ADLs ↓ to assistance/dependency, e.g., walker, wheelchair, bedbound • Clear speech ↓ to unintelligible • Critical nutritional impairment: ↓ progression eating > pureed; ↓ intake fluids/food to sustain life; continuing weight loss; dehydration; without artificial feeding methods • ↓ breathing capacity, dyspnea/O₂ at rest, declines ventilator • Signs and symptoms of infection: upper urinary tract infection (kidney infection); sepsis; recurrent aspiration pneumonia or fevers after antibiotics • Stage 3/4 decubitus

ADLs, activities of daily living; COPD, chronic obstructive pulmonary disease; DM, diabetes mellitus; FAST, Functional Assessment Staging Tool; LCD, local coverage determination; PPS, Palliative Performance Scale; BMI, body mass index; MAC, mid-arm circumference.

Source: Adapted from Jones, M. Harrington, T., & Mueller, G. (2013). Hospice admission eligibility: A staff education project. *Journal of Hospice & Palliative Nursing, 15*(2), 114–122.

TABLE 2.2   DISEASE-SPECIFIC HOSPICE ELIGIBILITY GUIDELINES

DISEASE	ALL OF THESE CRITERIA	AT LEAST ONE OF THESE CRITERIA	SUPPORTIVE FACTORS
ALS	Disease progression in the last 12 months by one of following: • ↓ to wheelchair/bed • ↓ ~unintelligible speech • ↓ ~pureed diet • ↓ most ADLs	• Vital capacity <30% or <60% with two symptoms (dyspnea at rest, unable to lie supine, use of accessory muscles, weak cough, sleep-disordered breathing) + declines ventilator • ↓ nutrition within the last 12 months: intake < sustain life, ↓ weight, dehydration, no TF	See also "At least one of these criteria" for dementia
Cancer	Disease with distant metastases or CA with poor prognosis (e.g., pancreatic)	• Continued decline on therapy • Declines further therapy	
Dementia	• FAST score 7 • ↓ communicate 7a, 7b • ADLs with assistance • Walk with assistance • ↑ incontinent urine/stool	• Aspiration pneumonia, UTI • Food/fluids < sustain life • Not a candidate for TF • Weight loss >10% • Fever recurrent on antibiotics • Stage 3–4 decubitus • Laboratory: albumin <2.5	
Heart	New York Heart Association class IV: symptomatic at rest on diuretics and vasodilators	• Ejection fraction <20% • Refractory angina	• Symptomatic arrhythmias • Not a candidate for transplant • Past cardiopulmonary resuscitation, syncope, HIV

(continued)

TABLE 2.2 DISEASE-SPECIFIC HOSPICE ELIGIBILITY GUIDELINES (*CONTINUED*)

DISEASE	ALL OF THESE CRITERIA	AT LEAST ONE OF THESE CRITERIA	SUPPORTIVE FACTORS
HIV	PPS <50% Laboratory: CD4 <25 cells/µL or > 100,000 copies/mL	• Central nervous system/ systemic lymphoma • Loss of >10% body mass • *Mycobacterium avium* complex bacterium • Refractory cryptosporidium, Kaposi, toxoplasmosis • Encephalopathy, ↓ renal	• Persistent diarrhea ~1 year • Laboratory: albumin <2.5 • Age >50 years • Active substance abuse • No AIDS prescription • ↓ CHF, ↓ liver, ↓ AIDS dementia
Kidney	• No dialysis • No renal transplant	Laboratory: creatinine clearance • <10 mL/min • <15 mL/min DM or CHF • <20 mL/min DM + CHF Laboratory: serum creatinine • >8.0 mg/dL • >6.0 mg/dL, diabetes	Acute renal failure • Comorbidities: heart, lung, AIDS, disseminated intravascular coagulation, sepsis, ventilator • Laboratory: albumin <3.5 • Laboratory: platelets <25,000 Chronic renal failure: uremia, oliguria, K⁺ >7.0, pericarditis, fluid overload
Liver	Laboratory: International Normalized Ratio >1.5 Laboratory: albumin <2.5	• Ascites • History: peritonitis • History: variceal bleeding • Hepatic encephalopathy • Laboratory: ↑ blood urea nitrogen, ↑ creatinine urine: Na <10 mEq/L, <400 mL/d	• Progressive malnutrition • ↓ muscle, ↓ strength, ↓ endurance • Active alcoholism >80 g/d • Liver cancer • Hepatitis B and C (refractory to interferon)
Pulmonary	• Dyspnea at rest = bed to chair, cough fatigue • ↑ ED/hospital for upper respiratory tract infection • Room air saturation <88%		• Right heart failure (cor pulmonale) • Weight loss >10% over 6 months • Resting tachycardia >100/min
Stroke	• PPS <40% • Acute >3 d: coma or obtunded and myoclonus • Chronic: FAST score 7, KPS and PPS <50%, no ADLs, weight loss >10%, albumin <2.5	Coma: any three of the following on day 3 of coma: • Abnormal brainstem response • Abnormal/no verbal response • Absent withdrawal from pain • Laboratory: creatinine >1.5 mg/dL	

Note: Adapted for educational purposes only using local coverage determination for hospice-determining terminal status, NHIC, Corp, 2009.

ᵃPlus PPS <70%, partial/full dependence for 2+ ADLs and significant comorbidities.

ADLs, activities of daily living; ALS, amyotrophic lateral sclerosis; CA, cancer; CHF, congestive heart failure; COPD, chronic obstructive pulmonary disease; DM, diabetes mellitus; FAST, Functional Assessment Staging Tool; KPS, Karnofsky Performance Scale; PPS, Palliative Performance Scale; TF, tube feeding; UTI, urinary tract infection.

Source: Adapted from Jones, M. Harrington, T. & Mueller, G. (2013). Hospice admission eligibility: A staff education project. *Journal of Hospice & Palliative Nursing, 15*(2), 114–122.

HUMAN IMMUNODEFICIENCY VIRUS DISEASE HOSPICE CRITERIA

A. CD4+ count of 100,000 copies/mL and one of the following despite treatment:

1. Central nervous system (CNS) lymphoma.
2. Unintentional loss of at least 10% lean body mass.
3. Mycobacterium avium complex (MAC) bacteremia.
4. Progressive multifocal leukoencephalopathy.
5. Systemic lymphoma.
6. Visceral Kaposi sarcoma.
7. Renal failure in the absence of dialysis.
8. Cryptosporidium infection.
9. Toxoplasmosis.

B. KPS ≤50% (see Appendix A-2).

C. Supportive factors include:

1. Chronic, persistent diarrhea (>1 year).
2. Persistent serum albumin of <2.5.
3. Active substance abuse.
4. Age >50 years.
5. Absence of or ineffective HIV drug therapy.
6. Advanced AIDS dementia complex.
7. Congestive heart failure with symptoms at rest.
8. Advanced liver disease.

ACUTE RENAL FAILURE HOSPICE CRITERIA

A. Patient is not receiving or seeking dialysis or kidney transplant.

B. Creatinine clearance is:

1. <10 mL/min (<15 mL/min in diabetics).
2. Serum creatinine >8.0 mg/dL (>6.0 for diabetics).

A. Supportive factors include:

1. Comorbid conditions.
2. Mechanical ventilation.
3. Malignancy.
4. Chronic lung disease.
5. Advanced cardiac disease.
6. Advanced liver disease.
7. Sepsis.
8. Immunosuppression/AIDS.
9. Platelet count <25,000.
10. Disseminated intravascular coagulation.
11. Gastrointestinal bleeding.

CHRONIC RENAL FAILURE HOSPICE CRITERIA

A. Patient is not receiving or seeking dialysis or kidney transplant.

B. Creatinine clearance is:

1. <10 mL/min (<15 mL/min in diabetics).
2. Serum creatinine >8.0 mg/dl (>6.0 for diabetics).

C. Supportive factors include:

1. Uremia.
2. Oliguria.
3. Intractable hyperkalemia (>7.0).
4. Uremic pericarditis.
5. Hepatorenal syndrome.
6. Intractable fluid overload.

LIVER DISEASE HOSPICE CRITERIA

A. Prolonged prothrombin time (5 seconds over control or International Normalized Ratio [INR] of >1.5).

B. Serum albumin < 2.5 g/dL.

C. End-stage liver disease present.

D. Patient has *at least one* of the following:

1. Refractory ascites.
2. Spontaneous bacterial peritonitis.
3. Hepatorenal syndrome.
4. Hepatic encephalopathy.
5. Recurrent esophageal bleeding despite intensive therapy.

E. Supportive factors include:

1. Progressive malnutrition.
2. Muscle wasting.
3. Decreasing endurance.
4. Active alcoholism (>80 g ethanol/day).
5. Hepatocellular carcinoma.
6. HBsAG (hepatitis B)-positive status.
7. Refractory hepatitis C.

F. Patients awaiting liver transplant and who meet the criteria for hospice may be admitted but should be discharged if a donor organ is procured.

PULMONARY DISEASE HOSPICE CRITERIA

A. Disabling dyspnea at rest that is:

1. Poorly responsive to bronchodilators.
2. Results in decreased functional capacity.

B. Progression of pulmonary disease as evidenced by:

1. Increased need for medical care.
2. Frequent hospitalization for respiratory infection or respiratory failure.

C. Serial decrease in forced expiratory volume (FEV).

1. FEV >40 mL is objective evidence that supports disease progression.
2. It is not necessary to obtain FEV if not already documented.

D. Hypoxemia at rest on room air as evidenced by:

1. Partial pressure of oxygen (PO_2) ≤55 mmHg or oxygen saturation of ≤88%.
2. Hypercapnia as evidenced by partial pressure of carbon dioxide (PCO_2) ≥50 mmHg.

E. Supportive factors include:

1. Right heart failure secondary to pulmonary disease.
2. Unintentional weight loss >10% of body weight during the previous 6 months.
3. Resting tachycardia (>100 beats/minute).

STROKE HOSPICE CRITERIA

A. KPS or PPS <40% (see Appendices A-2 and A-3).

B. Inability to maintain hydration and nutrition as evidenced by:

1. Weight loss of >10% in the past 6 months or >7.5% in the past 3 months.
2. Low serum albumin.

▶

3. Severe dysphagia that prevents proper caloric intake.

4. Aspiration pneumonia not responsive to speech therapy interventions.

C. Diagnostics indicating poor prognosis following stroke.

D. Supportive factors include:

1. Aspiration pneumonia.
2. Upper airway infection.
3. Sepsis.
4. Refractory stage 3–4 decubiti (see Appendix F-3).
5. Recurrent fever despite treatment with antibiotics.

COMA HOSPICE CRITERIA

A. Patient has any three of the following on day 3 of the coma:

1. Abnormal brainstem response.
2. Absent verbal response.
3. No withdrawal response to painful stimuli.
4. Serum creatinine >1.5 mg/dL.

B. Supportive factors include:

1. Aspiration pneumonia and upper airway infection.
2. Sepsis and refractory stage 3–4 decubiti (see Appendix F-3).
3. Recurrent fever despite treatment with antibiotics (Centers for Medicare & Medicaid Services, 2019).

REFERENCE

Centers for Medicare & Medicaid Services. (2019). *Local coverage determination (LCD): Hospice, determining terminal status.* https://www.cms.gov/medicare-coverage-database/view/lcd.aspx?LCDId=33393&

CHAPTER 3

PROGNOSTICATION AND PROGNOSTIC TOOLS

TYPES OF DISEASE TRAJECTORIES

DEFINITION/CHARACTERISTICS
A. Sudden death (see Appendix C-1).
   1. Death is unexpected and swift (e.g., accident, stroke, acute illness).
   2. Typically occurs in otherwise healthy people.
   3. Can occur in those with chronic illness if from an unrelated cause.
B. Short period of decline (see Appendix C-1).
   1. Time from diagnosis to death is about 6 months without intervention.
   2. Typical trajectory for patients who have cancer.
C. Lengthy declinatory trajectory with periodic exacerbations (see Appendix C-1).
   1. Time from diagnosis to death is about 2 to 5 years or more.
   2. Associated with chronic illness such as heart failure or obstructive lung disease.
D. Prolonged period of decline (see Appendix C-1).
   1. Time from diagnosis to death is typically 6 to 8 years or more.
   2. Associated with dementia, frailty, and debility.
E. Catastrophic event (see Appendix C-1).
   1. Involves a sudden change in health event (e.g., stroke, aneurysm).
   2. Time from diagnosis to death varies.
   3. Some patients may require life-sustaining interventions for months or years (Ballentine, 2018; Comstock & Scherer, 2016; Murray et al., 2005).

GENERAL INDICATORS OF POOR PROGNOSIS
A. Recurrent or intractable infection.
B. Diminished nutritional status as evidenced by:
   1. Unintentional weight loss.
   2. Decreasing mid-arm circumference (MAC; see Appendix A-1).
   3. Body mass index (BMI; see Appendix A-1).
   4. Decreasing abdominal girth.
   5. Deceasing albumin levels.
C. Dysphagia that leads to inadequate oral intake or aspiration.

D. Scores of <70% on the Karnofsky Performance Scale (KPS) or the Palliative Performance Scale (PPS; see Appendices A-1 andA-2).
E. Functional Assessment Staging Tool (FAST) scale score of ≥7a (see Appendix A-5).
F. Frequent need for medical care or frequent hospitalizations.
G. New-onset pressure ulcers or worsening of existing pressure ulcers despite optimal care.
H. Dependence for two or more activities of daily living (ADLs; Center to Advance Palliative Care, 2020; SPICT, 2021; U.S. Centers for Medicare & Medicaid Services, 2019).

GENERAL PROGNOSTIC TOOLS
A. KPS (see Appendix A-2).
   1. Initially developed to monitor functional status throughout treatment for cancer.
   2. Reliable and valid tool for determining functional status.
   3. Scores range from 0% to 100%, with higher scores indicating greater functional ability and lower scores indicating poor medical prognosis (Karnofsky & Burchenal, 1949).
B. PPS (see Appendix A-3).
   1. Based on the KPS.
   2. Scores range from 0% to 100%, with lower scores indicating poorer prognosis.
   3. A score of ≤70% generally supports hospice eligibility; for diagnosis of cerebrovascular accident (CVA) or HIV, a score of ≤50% supports hospice admission (Victoria Hospice, 2021).
C. Walter index.
   1. A simple point-based scale used to evaluate risk of mortality (high, intermediate, low) within 1 year of hospitalization in patients aged 70 or older.
   2. Factors used to calculate prognosis include functional status, renal function, patient's sex, and the clinician's estimate of prognosis.
   3. The electronic tool can be accessed at https://eprognosis.ucsf.edu/walter.php (Walter et al., 2001). ▶

D. ePrognosis (n.d.).

1. This website offers numerous prognostic calculators for clinicians to access.

2. Cancer screening guidelines and communication guidelines are also available.

3. Decision-making tools available for patient use are available at https://eprognosis.ucsf.edu/decision_aids.php.

4. Screening tools for clinician use are available at https://eprognosis.ucsf.edu/.

CONDITION-SPECIFIC PROGNOSTIC TOOLS

A. Brain metastasis.

1. The Graded Prognostic Assessment (GPA) tool has been developed and tested for over a decade.

2. The GPA provides a mean survival time based on various factors such as the primary cancer site, patient's age, KPS score, and other variables (Sperduto, Berkey et al., 2008, Sperduto, Watanabe et al., 2008).

3. The GPA is available at https://brainmetgpa.com/.

4. A downloadable app (App store and Google Play for this tool is available at https://qxmd.com/calculate/calculator_357/brain-metastases-prognostic-index).

B. Cancer.

1. The Eastern Cooperative Oncology Group (ECOG; see Appendix A-4) performance scale was originally developed to assess the status of oncology patients over time.

2. Used to measure disease progression.

C. Dementia.

1. The FAST (see Appendix A-5) is used to evaluate functional status in patients with dementia.

a. Scores range from 1 (no impairment) to 7 (severe impairment).

b. A score of 6 to 7 is associated with increased mortality.

c. A score of ≥ 7 indicates hospice eligibility (Reisberg et al., 1988; Sampson et al., 2013).

D. Frailty.

1. The Clinical Frailty Scale (CFS; see Appendix A-6) is used to determine level of frailty in older adults as compared with others of the same age.

2. Frailty is a risk factor for morbidity and mortality.

3. The CFS, when used in a hospital setting, is an independent predictor of mortality.

4. Scores range from 1 (very fit) to 9 (terminally ill).

5. A training module on use of the CFS is available at: https://rise.articulate.com/share/deb4rT02lvONbq4AfcMNRUudcd6QMts3#/.

6. A downloadable app (App store and Google Play) for this tool is available at https://www.acutefrailtynetwork.org.uk/Clinical-Frailty-Scale/Clinical-Frailty-Scale-App (Rockwood & Theou, 2020; Wallis et al., 2015).

E. Renal disease.

1. Thamer Risk Score (see Appendix A-7).

a. Used to inform patient–clinician discussions regarding short-term dialysis survivor likelihood.

b. Useful for predicting 3- and 6-month mortality after initiating dialysis.

c. Takes the following patient factors into account:

i. Age.

ii. Albumin level.

iii. Dependence for ADLs.

iv. Residence in a long-term care facility.

v. Cancer status.

vi. Heart failure status.

vii. Recent hospitalizations (Thamer et al., 2015).

REFERENCES

Ballentine, J. M. (2018). *The five trajectories: Supporting patients during serious illness.* https://csupalliativecare.org/wp-content/uploads/Five-Trajectories-eBook-02.21.2018.pdf

Center to Advance Palliative Care. (2020). *Palliative care referral criteria.* https://www.capc.org/documents/286/

Comstock, P., & Scherer, J. S. (2016). *Fast facts and concepts #326: Illness trajectories: Description and clinical use.* https://www.mypcnow.org/fast-facts/

ePrognosis. (n.d.). *What would you like to do?* https://eprognosis.ucsf.edu/index.php

Karnofsky, D. A., & Burchenal, J. H. (1949). *The clinical evaluation of chemotherapeutic agents.* Columbia University Press.

Murray, S. A., Kendall, M., Boyd, K., & Sheikh, A. (2005). Illness trajectories and palliative care. *BMJ, 330*(7498), 1007–1011. https://doi.org/10.1136/bmj.330.7498.1007

Reisberg, B. (1988). Functional assessment staging (FAST). *Psychopharmacology Bulletin, 24*(4), 653–659 https://medworks-media.com/journals/psychopharmacology-bulletin/

Rockwood, K., & Theou, O. (2020). Using the clinical frailty scale in allocating scarce health care resources. *Canadian Geriatrics Journal, 23*(3), 254–259. https://doi.org/10.5770/cgj.23.463

Sampson, E. L., Leurent, B., Blanchard, M. R., Jones, L., & King, M. (2013). Survival of people with dementia after unplanned acute hospital admission: A prospective cohort study. *International Journal of Geriatric Psychiatry, 28*(10), 1015–1022. https://doi.org/10.1002/gps.3919

Sperduto, C. M., Watanabe, Y., Mullan, J., Hood, T., Dyste, G., Watts, C., Bender, G.P., & Sperduto, P. (2008). A validation study of a new prognostic index for patients with brain metastases: The Graded Prognostic Assessment. *Journal of Neurosurgery, 109*(Supplement), 87–89. https://doi.org/10.3171/JNS/2008/109/12/S14

Sperduto, P. W., Berkey, B., Gaspar, L. E., Mehta, M., & Curran, W. (2008). A new prognostic index and comparison to three other indices for patients with brain metastases: An analysis of 1,960 patients in the RTOG database. *International Journal of Radiation Oncology Biology Physics, 70*(2), 510–514. https://doi.org/10.1016/j.ijrobp.2007.06.074

SPICT. (2021). *Supportive & Palliative Care Indicators Tool (SPICT).* https://www.spict.org.uk/

Thamer, M., Kaufman, J. S., Zhang, Y., Zhang, Q., Cotter, D. J., & Bang, H. (2015). Predicting early death among elderly dialysis patients: Development and validation of a risk score to assist shared decision making for dialysis initiation. *American Journal of Kidney Diseases, 66*(6), 1024–1032. https://doi.org/10.1053/j.ajkd.2015.05.014

U.S. Centers for Medicare & Medicaid Services. (2019). *Local coverage determination (LCD): Hospice—determining terminal status (L33393)*. https://www.cms.gov/medicare-coveragedatabase/details/lcddetails.aspx

Victoria Hospice. (2021). *Clinical tools for professionals*. https://victoriahospice.org/how-we-can-help/clinical-tools/

Wallis, S. J., Wall, J. B. R. W. S., Biram, R. W. S., & Romero-Ortuno, R. (2015). Association of the clinical frailty scale with hospital outcomes. *QJM: An International Journal of Medicine, 108*(12), 943–949. https://doi.org/10.1093/qjmed/hcv066

Walter, L. C., Brand, R. J., Counsell, S. R., Palmer, R. M., Landefeld, C. S., Fortinsky, R. H., & Covinsky, K. E. (2001). Development and validation of a prognostic index for 1-year mortality in older adults after hospitalization. *JAMA, 285*:2987–2994.

CHAPTER 4

ESTABLISHING GOALS OF CARE

ESTABLISHING GOALS OF CARE

APPROACHES TO SERIOUS CONVERSATIONS

A. Address the patient holistically.
  1. Establish rapport.
  2. Acknowledge support persons.
  3. Inquire about concerns—not just diagnosis.
  4. Address emotions and quality of life.
B. Use a conversation guide, such as:
  1. The Serious Illness Conversation Guide (see Appendix C-2) to guide:
    a. Setting up the conversation.
    b. Assessing understanding and preferences.
    c. Sharing prognosis.
    d. Exploring key topics.
    e. Closing the conversation.
    f. Documenting the conversation.
  2. Breaking the compassion wall (see Appendix C-3) to guide:
    a. Validating emotions.
    b. Sharing decision-making.
    c. Answering patient and family questions.
    d. Help patients stay connected.
  3. SPIKES model (see Appendix C-4) to structure:
    a. Setting.
    b. Perceptions.
    c. Invitation.
    d. Knowledge sharing.
    e. Emotions.
    f. Strategy and summary.
C. Refrain from persuasive argumentation.
D. Center yourself before and after (Ariande Labs, 2015; Baile et al., 2000; Murphy, 2020; Patterson, 2018).

DOCUMENTING PATIENT WISHES

A. Advance directives (see Figure 4.1) are legal documents outlining medical wishes.
B. There are several forms available:
  1. Custom-designed by patient, sometimes with legal assistance.

▶

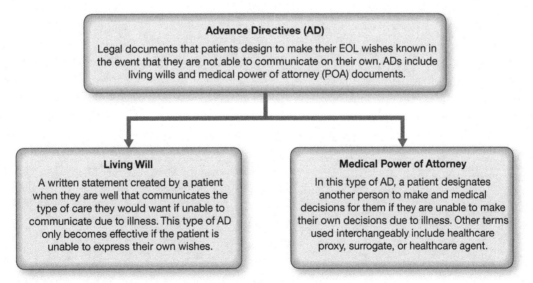

Advance Directives (AD)

Legal documents that patients design to make their EOL wishes known in the event that they are not able to communicate on their own. ADs include living wills and medical power of attorney (POA) documents.

Living Will

A written statement created by a patient when they are well that communicates the type of care they would want if unable to communicate due to illness. This type of AD only becomes effective if the patient is unable to express their own wishes.

Medical Power of Attorney

In this type of AD, a patient designates another person to make and medical decisions for them if they are unable to make their own decisions due to illness. Other terms used interchangeably include healthcare proxy, surrogate, or healthcare agent.

FIGURE 4.1 Advance directives.

Source: Adapted from National Institute on Aging. (2019). *Advance care planning: Healthcare directives.* https://www.nia.nih.gov/health/advance-care-planning-healthcare-directives

2. Five Wishes.
  a. Legally valid in most states (see www.five wishes.org/).
  b. Available in multiple languages.
3. POLST (see Appendices B-2, B-3, B-4, C-5, and C-6).
  a. Name differs by state (see https://polst.org/program-names/).
  b. Portable medical order that specifies patient's wishes.
  c. Used with patients at risk for life-threatening medical events.
  d. Completed during a conversation with a healthcare provider.
  e. After completing form, advise patient to:
      i. Keep form on refrigerator or in medicine cabinet.
      ii. Carry with them if traveling or being admitted to a facility.
  f. Requires signature of healthcare provider.
  g. Print on brightly colored paper, if possible.
  h. Forms may vary from state to state (see www.polst.org/map).
      i. A national POLST form is available at https://polst.org.national-form/ (Five Wishes, 2020; National POLST, 2021).

REFERENCES

Ariande Labs. (2015). *Serious illness conversation guide.* http://www.instituteforhumancaring.org/documents/Providers/Serious-Illness-Guide-old.pdf

Baile, W. F., Buckman, R., Lenzl, R., Global, G., Beale, E. A., & Kudelka, A. P. (2000). SPIKES: A six-step protocol for delivering bad news: Application to the patient with cancer. *The Oncologist, 5*(4), 302–311. https://doi.org/10.1634/theoncologist:5-4-302. http://theoncologist.alphamedpress.org/

Five Wishes. (2020). *Advance care planning for you and your loved ones.* https://fivewishes.org/five-wishes/individuals-families/individuals-and-families

Murphy, R. (2020, April 24). *Breaking down the compassion wall.* https://accelerate.uofuhealth.utah.edu/connect/breaking-dow-the-compassion-wall

National POLST. (2021). *About POLST.* https://polst.org/about/

Patterson, P. (2018, January 4). *Five ways to have a serious conversation.* https://accelerate.uofuhealth.utah.edu/connect/paige-patterson-five-ways-to-have-a-serious-conversation

SECTION

GUIDELINES FOR END-STAGE CANCER

CHAPTER 5

CANCERS OF THE HEAD AND NECK

BRAIN CANCER

DEFINITION/CHARACTERISTICS
A. Intracranial growth of malignant cells.
B. Tumors arising from brain (glia) cells are called gliomas.
C. Brain tumors can be classified as:
   1. Astrocytomas.
   2. Glioblastoma multiforme.
   3. Meningiomas.
   4. Medulloblastomas.
   5. Oligodendrogliomas and ependymomas.
   6. Neuronal tumors (American Association of Neurological Surgeons, 2021; Laws et al., 2018).

INCIDENCE AND PREVALENCE
A. The overall risk of developing brain cancer is < 1%.
B. About 25,000 individuals are diagnosed annually.
C. More males affected than females (American Cancer Society, 2021).

ETIOLOGY
A. The exact etiology is unknown (Cancer Treatment Centers of America, 2021).

PATHOPHYSIOLOGY
A. Primary tumors arise within brain tissue.
B. Secondary tumors originate elsewhere and metastasize to the brain.
C. Malignant intracranial tumors metastasize quickly.
D. Brain tumors develop their own blood supply.
E. These new vessels can bleed or become occluded, causing stroke-like symptoms.
F. Brain tumors can also compress or invade surrounding brain tissue causing:
   1. Increased intracranial pressure.
   2. Cerebral edema.
   3. Obstruction of the sinuses.
   4. Obstruction of arterial flow.
   5. Obstruction of cerebral spinal fluid drainage (American Association of Neurological Surgeons, 2021; Merck Sharp & Dohme, 2021).

PREDISPOSING FACTORS
A. Age (more common in children and older adults).
B. Sex (more common in males).
C. Environmental exposure (chemicals, pesticides, etc.).
D. Genetic predisposition, particularly TP_{52} genetic mutations.
E. Exposure to Epstein–Barr virus or cytomegalovirus.
F. Exposure to electromagnetic fields.
G. Exposure to therapeutic X-irradiation.
H. Race and ethnicity (Whites more likely to develop gliomas).
I. Dietary intake of nitrates (American Society of Clinical Oncology, 2020).

SUBJECTIVE DATA
A. Headache.
B. Visual changes.
C. Changes in sense of smell.
D. Nausea.
E. Drowsiness and/or fatigue.
F. Memory changes.
G. Loss of balance.
H. Emotional lability.
I. Personality changes (American Association of Neurological Surgeons, 2021; American Society of Clinical Oncology, 2020, Roth et al., 2021).

OBJECTIVE DATA
A. Gait dysfunction.
B. Facial drooping.
C. Paralysis.
D. Seizures.
E. Mental status changes.
F. Hearing loss.
G. Dysphagia.
H. Changes in critical thinking ability.
I. Vomiting.
J. Neuropsychiatric symptoms (aggression, mania, psychosis, violent behavior).
K. Decreased muscle control and/or lack of coordination (American Association of Neurological Surgeons, 2021; American Brain Tumor Association, 2021).

DIAGNOSTIC TESTS
A. See Appendix Table 5A.1 for listing of common diagnostic tests.
B. For grading of brain tumors, see Figure 5.1.

DIFFERENTIAL DIAGNOSES
A. Abscess.
B. Aneurysm.

▶

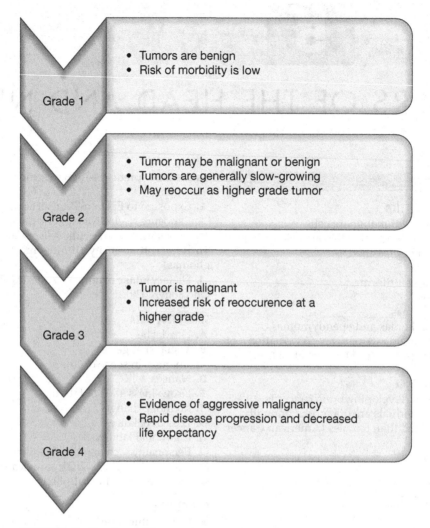

FIGURE 5.1 Grading of brain tumors.

Source: Adapted from Gupta, A. & Dwivedi, T. (2017). A simplified overview of World Health Organization classification update of central nervous system tumors 2016. *Journal of Neurosciences in Rural Practice, 8*(4), 629. https://doi.org/10.4103/jnrp.jnrp_168_17

C. Cerebrovascular accident.
D. Dementia.
E. Drug use.
F. Fungal brain disease.
G. Intracranial hemorrhage.
H. Meningitis.
I. Multiple sclerosis.
J. Subarachnoid hemorrhage.
K. Subdural hematoma (Collins, 2018; Seller & Symons, 2018).

POTENTIAL COMPLICATIONS

A. Acute complications of advanced cancer (see Appendix C-7).
B. Seizures.

C. Cognitive impairment.
D. Venous thromboembolism.
E. Ischemic stroke (Roth et al., 2021).

DISEASE-MODIFYING TREATMENTS

A. Surgical interventions.
B. Chemotherapy (see Figure 5.2).
C. Radiation.
D. Stereotactic radiation therapy.
E. Proton therapy.
F. Tumor-treating fields.
G. Immunotherapy.
H. Immunovirotherapy (American Brain Tumor Association, 2021; Bernstock et al., 2021).
I. See Figure 5.2 for principles of cytotoxic chemotherapy.

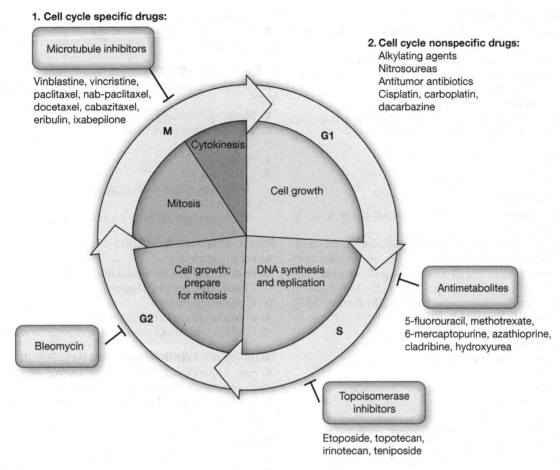

1. Cell cycle specific drugs:

Microtubule inhibitors

Vinblastine, vincristine, paclitaxel, nab-paclitaxel, docetaxel, cabazitaxel, eribulin, ixabepilone

2. Cell cycle nonspecific drugs:
Alkylating agents
Nitrosoureas
Antitumor antibiotics
Cisplatin, carboplatin, dacarbazine

M
Cytokinesis
Mitosis
G1
Cell growth
Cell growth; prepare for mitosis
DNA synthesis and replication
G2
S

Bleomycin

Antimetabolites

5-fluorouracil, methotrexate, 6-mercaptopurine, azathioprine, cladribine, hydroxyurea

Topoisomerase inhibitors

Etoposide, topotecan, irinotecan, teniposide

FIGURE 5.2 Principles of cytotoxic chemotherapy.

PALLIATIVE INTERVENTIONS/SYMPTOM MANAGEMENT
A. See Appendix Table 5A.2 for listing of palliative interventions and symptom management.
B. See Appendix D-3 for overview of common symptoms.

PROGNOSIS
A. Prognosis varies according to the type of tumor.
B. The 5-year prognosis in metastatic disease is 36%.
C. The 10-year prognosis in metastatic disease is 31%.
D. Survival rate decreases with age (American Cancer Society, 2021).

NURSING INTERVENTIONS
A. Monitor for signs of disease progression.
B. Ensure proper symptom management related to increased intracranial pressure.
C. Address emotional needs, such as depression and anxiety.
D. Provide spiritual support.
E. Monitor caregiver stress (see Appendix B-5).
F. Implement interventions for pain and symptom management (see Appendix B-1).

G. Educate patient to take all medications as prescribed.
H. Educate patient and family regarding disease trajectory.
I. Encourage completion of advance directives.
J. Educate patient and family regarding availability of palliative care.
K. Educate patient and family regarding availability of hospice care (when appropriate).

ESOPHAGEAL CANCER

DEFINITION/CHARACTERISTICS
A. Malignancy affecting tissues of or the lining of the esophagus.
B. There are two types of esophageal cancer:
   1. Squamous cell (occurs within the flat cell lining of the esophagus).
   2. Adenocarcinoma (occurs within mucus-producing cells in the esophagus; National Cancer Institute, 2021b).

INCIDENCE AND PREVALENCE

A. Approximately 19,200 new cases are diagnosed annually.
B. Significantly more men than women affected.
C. Esophageal cancer represents 1% of cancers in the United States each year.
D. More common outside of the United States.
E. Sixth leading cause of death globally (American Cancer Society, 2021; Yang et al., 2016).

ETIOLOGY

A. Exact etiology is unknown.

PATHOPHYSIOLOGY

A. Chronic inflammation of esophageal tissue leads to malignancy.
B. Arises within the squamous epithelia of the middle and lower thirds of the esophagus or the islands of columnar cells near the gastroesophageal junction.
C. Esophageal cancer can spread rapidly to lungs and liver through the lymphatic system (McCance, 2019; Sommers, 2019; Yang et al., 2016).

PREDISPOSING FACTORS

A. Smoking tobacco products.
B. Alcohol use.
C. Gastroesophageal reflux disease (GERD).
D. Barrett esophagus.
E. Helicobacter pylori infection.
F. Exposure to dietary carcinogens such as nitrosamines and polyaromatic hydrocarbons.
G. Occupational exposure to perchloroethylene.
H. Genetic predisposition.
I. Possible link to herpes papillomaviruses 16 and 18 (Sommers, 2019; Yang et al., 2016).

SUBJECTIVE DATA

A. Odynophagia (painful swallowing).
B. Dysphagia and/or aspiration.
C. Pain.
D. Generalized weakness (Sommers, 2019).

OBJECTIVE DATA

A. Weight loss.
B. Coughing and/or hemoptysis.
C. Weakness of extremities.
D. Vocal changes.
E. Hoarseness (American Cancer Society, 2021; Sommers, 2019).

DIAGNOSTIC TESTS

A. See Appendix Table 5A.1 for listing of common diagnostic tests.

DIFFERENTIAL DIAGNOSES

A. Esophagitis.
B. Barrett esophagus.
C. Esophageal candidiasis.
D. Disseminated sclerosis of the esophagus (Seller & Symons, 2018).

POTENTIAL COMPLICATIONS

A. Acute complications of advanced cancer (see Appendix C-7).
B. Bleeding esophageal varices.
C. Tracheoesophageal fistulas.
D. Anemia.
E. Pneumonia.
F. Metastasis to:
   1. Retroperitoneal or celiac lymph nodes.
   2. Liver.
   3. Lungs (Wright, 2019; Xu et al., 2019; Xu et al., 2020).

DISEASE-MODIFYING TREATMENTS

A. Esophagectomy.
B. Endoscopic mucosal resection (EMR)
C. Chemotherapy (see Figure 5.2).
D. Radiation therapy.
E. Immune checkpoint inhibitors.
F. HER2 inhibitors (American Cancer Society, 2021).

PALLIATIVE INTERVENTIONS/SYMPTOM MANAGEMENT

A. See Appendix Table 5A.2 for listing of palliative interventions and symptom management.
B. See Appendix D-3 for overview of common symptoms.

PROGNOSIS

A. The 5-year survival rate is 20%.
B. Survival rates are higher if cancer is detected early (American Cancer Society, 2021).

NURSING INTERVENTIONS

A. Teach patient to take all medications as prescribed.
B. Educate patient and family on disease trajectory (see Appendix B-1).
C. Adjust consistency of diet as needed for dysphagia.
D. Administer medications in crushed or liquid form, if needed.
E. Use high-calorie, high-protein supplements as needed.
F. Monitor for signs of respiratory infection.
G. Keep red towels at home in case esophageal varices begin to bleed (to reduce visual impact of the bleeding).
H. Address emotional needs, such as depression and anxiety.
I. Encourage smoking cessation (see Appendices B-10 and C-9).
J. Teach patient to avoid alcohol use (see Appendix B-6).
K. Provide spiritual support.
L. Monitor caregiver stress (see Appendix B-5).
M. Encourage completion of advance directives.   ▶

N. Educate patient and family regarding availability of palliative care.

O. Educate patient and family regarding availability of hospice care (when appropriate).

ORAL CANCER

DEFINITION/CHARACTERISTICS

A. Malignancy that affects the tissues of the oral cavity, including the:

1. Mucosal lip.
2. Buccal mucosa.
3. Lower alveolar ridge.
4. Upper alveolar ridge.
5. Retromolar gingiva.
6. Floor of the mouth.
7. The anterior two-thirds of the tongue (Laws et al., 2018).

INCIDENCE AND PREVALENCE

A. Approximately 54,000 new cases annually.

B. Males are roughly twice as likely as females to be affected.

C. There are more than 11,000 deaths each year from oral cancer (American Cancer Society, 2022a).

ETIOLOGY

A. The cause is multifactorial, likely related to lifestyle choices such as:

1. Tobacco use.
2. Alcohol use.
3. Diet (Sim, 2021; Vyas et al., 2019).

PATHOPHYSIOLOGY

A. Cell mutations caused by carcinogens disrupt cell growth and cell signaling.

B. Multistep process of carcinogenesis involves:

1. Hyperplasia.
2. Dysplasia to in situ and invasive carcinomas.

C. Progression is attributable to loss of heterozygosity within particular chromosomes (Ernani & Saba, 2015; Sim, 2021).

PREDISPOSING FACTORS

A. Use of tobacco products (smoking and smokeless).

B. Alcohol use.

C. Betel quid with tobacco.

D. Betel quid without tobacco.

E. Possible link to herpes papillomavirus 16.

F. Previous head or neck cancer (Hinkle & Cheever, 2022; McCance, 2019).

SUBJECTIVE DATA

A. Few or no symptoms early in the disease process.

B. As the disease progresses, symptoms may appear, such as:

1. Pharyngitis.
2. Otalgia.
3. Dysphagia.
4. Dysarthria.
5. Paresthesias.

OBJECTIVE DATA

A. Visible, bleeding, nonhealing sore(s) in mouth.

B. Cervical lymphadenopathy.

C. Blood-tinged sputum.

D. Weight loss.

E. Trismus (American Cancer Society, 2022b; Ernani & Saba, 2015).

DIAGNOSTIC TESTS

A. See Appendix Table 5A.1 for listing of common diagnostic tests.

DIFFERENTIAL DIAGNOSES

A. Actinic keratosis.

B. Erythroplasia.

C. Lichen planus.

D. Lichenoid lesions.

E. Mucosal candidiasis (Sim, 2021).

POTENTIAL COMPLICATIONS

A. Acute complications of advanced cancer (see Appendix C-7).

B. Mucositis.

C. Infection.

D. Salivary changes.

E. Neurosensory changes.

F. Disfigurement.

G. Metastasis to:

1. Mandible.
2. Cervical lymph nodes.
3. Lungs (Epstein et al., 2012; Tomioka et al., 2021).

DISEASE-MODIFYING TREATMENTS

A. Surgical interventions such as:

1. Hemiglossectomy (removal of half of the tongue).
2. Total glossectomy (removal of the tongue).

B. Chemotherapy (see Figure 5.2).

C. Radiation therapy (American Cancer Society, 2022b; Hinkle & Cheever, 2022).

PALLIATIVE INTERVENTIONS/SYMPTOM MANAGEMENT

A. See Appendix Table 5A.2 for listing of palliative interventions and symptom management.

B. See Appendix D-3 for overview of common symptoms.

PROGNOSIS

A. Prognosis worsens as tumor thickens and metastasizes.

B. The American Joint Committee on Cancer recommends use of performance tools such as the Eastern Cooperative Oncology Group (ECOG; Appendix A-4) and Karnofsky Performance Scale (KPS; Appendix A-2) to predict survival.

C. The 5-year relative survival rate is 67% (American Cancer Society, 2022a; Laws et al., 2018).

NURSING INTERVENTIONS

A. Teach patient to take all medications as prescribed.

B. Educate patient and family on disease trajectory (see Appendix B-1).

C. Adjust consistency of diet as needed for dysphagia.

D. Administer medications in crushed or liquid form, if needed.

E. Use high-calorie, high-protein supplements as needed.

F. Monitor for signs of respiratory infection.

G. Arrange for speech therapy as needed.

H. Encourage lifestyle modifications such as:
  1. Smoking cessation (see Appendices B-10 and C-9).
  2. Reducing or stopping alcohol use (see Appendix B-6).
  3. Proper diet and exercise.
  4. Good sleep hygiene.

I. Address emotional needs, such as depression and anxiety.

J. Ensure proper airway management and arrange for needed supplies such as suctioning equipment.

K. Encourage patient to verbalize concerns about body image.

L. Provide spiritual support.

M. Monitor caregiver stress (see Appendix B-5).

N. Encourage completion of advance directives.

O. Educate patient and family regarding availability of palliative care.

P. Educate patient and family regarding availability of hospice care (when appropriate).

THYROID CANCER

DEFINITION/CHARACTERISTICS

A. Metastatic disease that arises from within the thyroid gland.

B. The four main types of thyroid cancer are:
  1. Papillary.
  2. Follicular.
  3. Medullary.
  4. Anaplastic (National Cancer Institute, 2021b).

INCIDENCE AND PREVALENCE

A. Approximately 44,200 new cases are diagnosed annually.

B. Thyroid cancer affects about 1.2% of men and women (National Cancer Institute, 2021a).

ETIOLOGY

A. Exact cause is unknown but related factors include:
  1. Exposure to radiation.
  2. Genetic predisposition (American Cancer Society, 2021).

PATHOPHYSIOLOGY

A. Characterized by rapid proliferation of thyroid cells.

B. Enlargement of thyroid gland leads to:
  1. Dysphagia.
  2. Hoarseness.
  3. Dyspnea.

C. Most common sites of metastasizes are:
  1. Lymph nodes.
  2. Lung(s).
  3. Bone (Mayo Clinic, 2021; Sommers, 2019; Wright, 2019).

PREDISPOSING FACTORS

A. Radiation to the head and neck.

B. Prolonged secretion of thyroid-stimulating hormone.

C. Genetic predisposition.

D. Female sex.

E. Asian heritage (Mayo Clinic, 2021; Sommers, 2019).

SUBJECTIVE DATA

A. Often asymptomatic in the early stages of disease.

B. Pain in the front of the neck, sometimes radiating to ears.

C. Dyspnea.

D. Dysphagia.

E. Chronic cough (American Cancer Society, 2021; Sommers, 2019).

OBJECTIVE DATA

A. Palpable thyroid nodule (see Figure 5.3).

B. Hoarseness (American Cancer Society, 2021; Sommers, 2019).

DIAGNOSTIC TESTS

A. See Appendix Table 5A.1 for listing of common diagnostic tests.

DIFFERENTIAL DIAGNOSES

A. Colloid nodule.

B. Thyroid adenoma or hyperplastic nodule, single (solid or complex).

C. Nontoxic multinodular goiter.

D. Toxic adenoma, single.

E. Toxic multinodular goiter.

F. Cystic mass.

G. Infection.

H. Congenital anomalies.

I. Trauma.

J. Graves disease (Pynnonen et al., 2017).

POTENTIAL COMPLICATIONS

A. Acute complications of advanced cancer (see Appendix C-7).

B. Hypocalcemia.

C. Laryngeal nerve palsy.

D. Enlargement of thyroid gland may lead to:
  1. Dysphagia.
  2. Vocal changes.
  3. Dyspnea.

▶

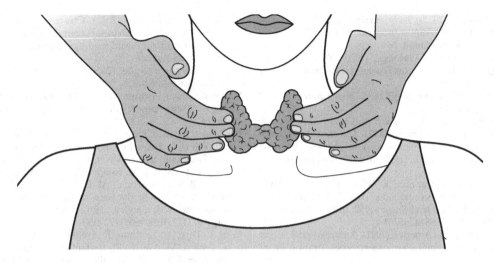

FIGURE 5.3   Palpation of the thyroid gland.

E. Metastasis to:
  1. Lymph nodes.
  2. Lungs.
  3. Bone (Wright, 2019).

DISEASE-MODIFYING TREATMENTS
A. Lobectomy.
B. Thyroidectomy.
C. Lymph node removal.
D. Radioactive iodine (radioiodine) therapy.
E. External beam radiation.
F. Chemotherapy (see Figure 5.2).
G. Kinase inhibitors.
H. Multikinase inhibitors.
I. RET inhibitors.
J. Neurotrophic tyrosine receptor kinase (NTRK) inhibitors
K. V-raf murine sarcoma viral oncogene homolog B1 (BRAF) and mitogen-activated protein kinase kinase (MEK) inhibitors (American Cancer Society, 2021).

PALLIATIVE INTERVENTIONS/SYMPTOM MANAGEMENT
A. See Appendix Table 5A.2 for listing of palliative interventions and symptom management.
B. See Appendix D-3 for overview of common symptoms.

PROGNOSIS
A. Overall, the 5-year survival rate is 98%.
B. Survival is based on the type and stage of cancer.
  1. For localized papillary, follicular, and medullary thyroid cancers, 5-year survival rate is nearly 100%.
  2. For localized anaplastic thyroid cancer, the 5-year survival rate is 31%.
  3. The 5-year survival rate for metastatic anaplastic thyroid cancer is 3% (American Society of Clinical Oncology, 2021).

NURSING INTERVENTIONS
A. Monitor for signs and symptoms of disease progression.
B. Assess quality of life.
C. Educate patient and family on disease trajectory.
D. Teach patient to take all medications as prescribed.
E. Adjust consistency of diet as needed for dysphagia.
F. Provide moving air and/or supplemental oxygen for dyspnea.
G. Utilize pharmacological and non-pharmacological interventions to address anxiety.
H. Encourage smoking cessation (see Appendices B-10 and C-9).
I. Address emotional needs.
J. Provide spiritual support.
K. Monitor caregiver stress (see Appendix B-5).
L. Encourage completion of advance directives.
M. Educate patient and family regarding availability of palliative care.
N. Educate patient and family regarding availability of hospice (when appropriate).

REFERENCES
Alvarenga, A., Campos, M., Dias, M., Melão, L., & Estevão-Costa, J. (2017). BOTOX-A injection of salivary glands for drooling. *Journal of Pediatric Surgery*, *52*(8), 1283–1286. https://doi.org/10.1016/j.jpedsurg.2016.09.074

American Association of Neurological Surgeons. (2021). *Brain tumors.* https://www.aans.org/en/Patients/Neurosurgical-Conditions-and-Treatments/Brain-Tumors

American Brain Tumor Association. (2021). *Cancer A to Z.* https://www.cancer.org/cancer.html

American Cancer Society. (2021). *Melanoma skin cancer.* https://www.cancer.org/cancer/melanoma-skin-cancer.html

American Cancer Society. (2022a). *Cancer facts and figures.* https://www.cancer.org/content/dam/cancer-org/research/cancer-facts-and-statistics/annual-cancer-facts-and-figures/2022/2022-cancer-facts-and-figures.pdf

American Cancer Society. (2022b). *Early detection, diagnosis, and staging.* https://www.cancer.org/cancer/liver-cancer/detection-diagnosis-staging/how-diagnosed.html

American Society of Clinical Oncology. (2020). *Brain tumor risk factors.* https://www.cancer.net/cancer-types/brain-tumor/risk-factors

American Society of Clinical Oncology (2021). *Types of cancer.* https://www.cancer.net/cancer-types

Bernstock, J. D., Hoffman, S. E., Chen, J. A., Gupta, S., Kappel, A. D., Smith, T. R., & Chiocca, E. A. (2021). The current landscape of oncolytic herpes simplex viruses as novel therapies for brain malignancies. *Viruses, 13*(6), 1158. https://doi.org/10.3390/v13061158

Buchmann, L., Ashby, S., Cannon, R. B., & Hunt, J. P. (2015). Psychosocial distress in patients with thyroid cancer. *Otolaryngology--Head and Neck Surgery, 152*(4), 644–649. https://doi.org/10.1177/0194599814565761

Cancer Treatment Centers of America. (2021). *Brain cancer risk factors.* https://www.cancercenter.com/cancer-types/brain-cancer/risk-factors

Collins, D. C. (2018). *Differential diagnosis and treatment in primary care.* Wolters Kluwer Health.

Epstein, J. B., Thariat, J., Bensadoun, R. J., Barasch, A., Murphy, B. A., Kolnick, L., Popplewell, L., & Maghami, E. (2012). Oral complications of cancer and cancer therapy: From cancer treatment to survivorship. *CA: A Cancer Journal for Clinicians, 62*(6), 400–422. https://doi.org/10.3322/caac.21157

Ernani, V., & Saba, N. F. (2015). Oral cavity cancer: Risk factors, pathology, and management. *Oncology, 89*(4), 187–195. https://doi.org/10.1159/000398801

Fusco, F. (2021). Mouth care. In E. Bruera, I. J. Higginson, C. F. von Gunten, & T. Morita (Eds.), *Textbook of palliative medicine and supportive care.* Taylor & Francis Group.

Guyer, D. L., Almhanna, K., & McKee, K. Y. (2020). Palliative care for patients with esophageal cancer: A narrative review. *Annals of Translational Medicine, 8*(17). https://doi.org/10.21037/atm-20-3676

Hinkle, J. L., & Cheever, K. H. (2022). *Textbook of medical-surgical nursing.* Wolters Kluwer.

Kluger, B. M., Ney, D. E., Bagley, S. J., Mohile, N., Taylor, L. P., Walbert, T., & Jones, C. A. (2020). Top ten tips palliative care clinicians should know when caring for patients with brain cancer. *Journal of Palliative Medicine, 23*(3), 415–421. https://doi.org/10.1089/jpm.2019.0507

Laws, E. R., Curran, W. J., Bondy, M. L., Brat, D. J., Brem, H., Chang, S. M., Colen, R. R., Lopes, M. B., Louis, D. N., Pradas, M. D., Schiff, D., Vallerand, T. M., Wen, P. Y., & Werner-Wasik, M. (2018). Brain and spinal cord. In M. B. Amin, S. B. Edge, F. L. Greene, D. R. Byrd, R. K. Brookland, M. K. Washington, J. E. Gershenwald, C. C. Compton, K. R. Hess, D. C. Sullivan, J. M. Jessup, J. D. Brierley, L. E. Gaspar, R. L. Schilsky, C. M. Balch, D. P. Winchester, E. A. Asare, M. Madera, D. M. Gress & L. R. Meyer (Eds.), *AJCC Cancer Staging Manual* (8th ed.). Springer International Publishing.

Mayo Clinic. (2021). *Thyroid cancer.* https://www.mayoclinic.org/diseases-conditions/thyroid-cancer/symptoms-causes/syc-20354161

McCance, K. L. (2019). Cancer epidemiology. In K. L. McCance & S. E. Huether (Eds.), *Pathophysiology: The biologic basis for disease in adults and children* (8th ed.). Elsevier-Mosby.

McGeachan, A. J., & Mcdermott, C. J. (2017). Management of oral secretions in neurological disease. *Practical Neurology, 17*(2), 96–103. https://doi.org/10.1136/practneurol-2016-001515

Merck Sharp & Dohme. (2021). *Overview of intracranial tumors.* https://www.merckmanuals.com/professional/neurologic-disorders/intracranial-and-spinal-tumors/overview-of-intracranial-tumors

National Cancer Institute. (2021a). *Cancer statistics.* https://seer.cancer.gov/statistics/

National Cancer Institute. (2021b). *NCI dictionary of cancer terms.* https://www.cancer.gov/publications/dictionaries/cancer-terms

Pynnonen, M. A., Gillespie, M. B., Roman, B., Rosenfeld, R. M., Tunkel, D. E., Bontempo, L., Brook, I., Chick, D. A., Colandrea, M., Finestone, S. A., Fowler, J. C., Griffith, C. C., Henson, Z., Levine, C., Mehta, V., Salama, A., Scharpf, J., Shatzkes, D. R., Stern, W. B. . . . Corrigan, M. D. (2017). Clinical practice guideline: Evaluation of the neck mass in adults. *Otolaryngology–Head and Neck Surgery, 157*(2_suppl), S1–S30. https://doi.org/10.1177/0194599817722550

Roth, P., Pace, A., Le Rhun, E., Weller, M., Ay, C., Moyal, E. C. J., Coomans, M., Giusti, R., Jordan, K., Nishikawa, R., Winkler, F., Hong, J. T., Ruda, R., Villà, S., Taphoorn, M. J. B., Wick, W., Preusser, M., on behalf of the EANO Executive Board, ., & ESMO Guidelines Committee. (2021). Neurological and vascular complications of primary and secondary brain tumours: EANO-ESMO Clinical Practice Guidelines for prophylaxis, diagnosis, treatment and follow-up. *Annals of Oncology, 32*(2), 171–182. https://doi.org/10.1016/j.annonc.2020.11.003

Seller, R. H., & Symons, A. B. (2018). *Differential diagnosis of common complaints.* Elsevier.

Sim, C. Q. (2021, May 5). *Cancers of the oral mucosa.* https://emedicine.medscape.com/article/1075729-overview#a4

Sommers, M. S. (2019). *Davis's diseases and disorders: A nursing therapeutics manual* (6th ed.). F.A. Davis Co.

Tomioka, H., Yamagata, Y., Oikawa, Y., Ohsako, T., Kugimoto, T., Kuroshima, T., Hirai, H., Shimamoto, H., & Harada, H. (2021). Risk factors for distant metastasis in locoregionally controlled oral squamous cell carcinoma: A retrospective study. *Scientific Reports, 11*(1), 1–6. https://www.nature.com/articles/s41598-021-84704-w

Vyas, T., Kuthiala, P., & Vishnoi, P. (2019). Oral cancer: Etiology and its diagnostic aids. *International Journal of Drug Research and Dental Science, 1*(2), 13–18. https://doi.org/10.36437/ijdrd.2019.1.2.G

Walker, P. W. (2016). Other symptoms: Xerostomia, hiccups, pruritus, pressure ulcers and wounds care, lymphedema, and myoclonus. In S. Yennuraajalingam & E. Bruera (Eds.), *Oxford handbook of hospice and palliative medicine and supportive care* (2nd ed.). Oxford University Press.

Wright, P. M. (2019). *Certified hospice and palliative nurse (CHPN®) exam review.* Springer Publishing Company.

Xu, Q. L., Li, H., Zhu, Y. J., & Xu, G. (2020). The treatments and postoperative complications of esophageal cancer: A review. *Journal of Cardiothoracic Surgery, 15*(1), 1–10. https://cardiothoracicsurgery.biomedcentral.com/articles/10.1186/s13019-020-01202-2

Xu, Z. G., Zhao, Y. B., Yu, J., Bai, J. Y., Liu, E., Tang, B., & Yang, S. M. (2019). Novel endoscopic treatment strategy for early esophageal cancer in cirrhotic patients with esophageal varices. *Oncology Letters, 18*(3), 2560–2567. https://doi.org/10.3892/ol.2019.10532

Yang, C. S., Chen, X., & Tu, S. (2016). Etiology and prevention of esophageal cancer. *Gastrointestinal Tumors, 3*(1), 3–16. https://www.karger.com/Article/FullText/443155

APPENDIX

TABLE 5A.1 DIAGNOSTIC TESTS FOR CANCERS OF THE HEAD AND NECK

TYPE	NOTES
Physical examination	• Thorough neurological examination (brain) • Physical examination with focused oral assessment to include use of vital staining (Toluidine Blue or Lugol's iodine) or Vizilite (oral) • Thorough physical exam, including palpation of thyroid gland (thyroid; see Figure 5.3) • Thorough physical exam, including gastrointestinal symptoms (esophageal)
Imaging	• CT (or CAT scan)—brain, esophageal, oral, thyroid • MRI—brain, esophageal, oral, thyroid • PET scan; detects recurring tumors—brain, esophageal, oral, thyroid • Dynamic CT or dynamic MRI (brain) • MRS angiography and MRA—brain • Barium swallow test, endoscopy and endoscopic ultrasound, bronchoscopy, thoracoscopy, laparoscopy (esophageal) • Ultrasound of thyroid, radioiodine scan, chest x-ray (thyroid)
Laboratory tests	• Complete blood count • Lumbar puncture to analyze cerebral spinal fluid, hormone levels to determine involvement of endocrine system (brain) • Biomarkers and tumor testing (brain, esophageal) • Genetic testing (esophageal) • Liver function studies, calcium level, serum ferritin level, alpha-antitrypsin level, alpha-antiglycoprotein level (oral) • TSH, T3 and T4 (thyroid hormones)—thyroid, thyroglobulin, calcitonin, CEA—thyroid
Pathology	• Biopsy (needle, stereotactic, or open biopsy) • Brain tumor grading (see Figure 5.1) • Tumor grading (TNM; see Appendix C-8) • Genetic testing (brain) • Photodiagnosis, gene therapy, proliferation index, silver staining of nucleolar organizer region-associated proteins (AgNOR analysis)—oral

CEA, carcinoembryonic antigen; MRA, magnetic resonance angiography; MRS, magnetic resonance spectroscopy; TNM, tumor, node, metastasis;TSH, thyroid-stimulating hormone.

Sources: American Association of Neurological Surgeons. (2021). *Brain tumors.* https://www.aans.org/en/Patients/Neurosurgical-Conditions-and-Treatments/Brain-Tumors; American Brain Tumor Association. (2021). *Cancer A to Z.* https://www.cancer.org/cancer.html; American Cancer Society. (2021). *Melanoma skin cancer.* https://www.cancer.org/cancer/melanoma-skin-cancer.html; American Cancer Society. (2022b). *Early detection, diagnosis, and staging.* https://www.cancer.org/cancer/liver-cancer/detection-diagnosis-staging/how-diagnosed.html; Ernani, V., & Saba, N. F. (2015). Oral cavity cancer: Risk factors, pathology, and management. *Oncology, 89*(4), 187–195. https://doi.org/10.1159/000398801; Sim, C. Q. (2021, May 5). Cancers of the oral mucosa. https://emedicine.medscape.com/article/1075729-overview#a4; Vyas, T., Kuthiala, P., & Vishnoi, P. (2019). Oral cancer: Etiology and its diagnostic aids. *International Journal of Drug Research and Dental Science, 1*(2), 13–18. https://doi.org/10.36437/ijdrd.2019.1.2.G

TABLE 5A.2   PALLIATIVE INTERVENTIONS/SYMPTOM MANAGEMENT FOR CANCERS OF THE HEAD AND NECK

SYMPTOM	INTERVENTION
Anorexia	• Use of appetite stimulants (see Appendix D-1) • Offer small, frequent meals and snacks. Offer nutritional supplements
Anxiety and depression (see Appendix D)	• Antidepressants, anxiolytics, or benzodiazepines as indicated by patient's condition, age, and life expectancy • Non-pharmacological interventions
Caregiver burden	• Support of interdisciplinary hospice or palliative team • Non-pharmacological interventions for caregivers (see Appendix D)
Drooling (oral)	• Use of anticholinergic medications (see Appendix D-1) • Injection of botulinum toxin A into salivary glands • Skin care to prevent excoriation from saliva
Dysphagia (esophageal cancer, oral cancer, thyroid cancer)	• Debulking of tumor(s) to address dysphagia • Stent placement for dilation of esophagus • Dietary modification (puree, thickened liquids, etc.) • Crush medications or use liquid formulations when possible
Dyspnea (thyroid)	• Corticosteroids for reducing inflammation (see Appendix D-1) • Bronchodilators for opening airways (mechanism of action of relaxation of muscular bands that surround bronchi, thus widening the airway; see Appendix D-1) • Diuretics to reduce systemic congestion (see Appendix D-1) • Anticholinergics to reduce secretions, especially at the end of life (see Appendix D-1) • Use of fans • Lower temperature in room
Fatigue and somnolence	• Psychostimulants (see Appendix D)
Gastrointestinal symptoms (esophageal, oral; see Appendix D-1)	• Antacids • Antiemetics • Promotility agents • Laxatives • Antidiarrheals

Intracranial swelling (brain)	• Corticosteroids (see Appendix D-1)
	 • Dexamethasone most frequently used
	    ▪ Lowest possible dose should be used
	    ▪ Monitor for effects of long-terms steroid use
	    ▪ In certain cases of steroid dependency, bevacizumab may be considered as a palliative care intervention to reduce steroid dose

Nausea and vomiting	• Antiemetics (see Appendix D-1) • Non-pharmacological interventions (see Appendix D-2)
Neuropathies	• Antidepressants (see Appendix D-1) • Anticonvulsants (i.e., gabapentin) • Anesthetics (i.e., ketamine) • Opioids
Pain management	• See Appendix E

(continued)

TABLE 5A.2 PALLIATIVE INTERVENTIONS/SYMPTOM MANAGEMENT FOR CANCERS OF THE HEAD AND NECK (*CONTINUED*)

SYMPTOM	INTERVENTION
Pathological fractures	• Treatment of localized pain • Joint stabilization • For lower extremity compression fractures, surgical stabilization with or without joint replacement, if patient's condition and prognosis are favorable • For vertebral compression fractures, VP or BKP may be considered, depending on patient's condition and prognosis
Psychosocial distress/body image changes	• Antidepressants • Non-pharmacological interventions (see Appendix D-2)
Seizures (brain)	• Antiepileptic medications (see Appendix D-1) • Most commonly used is levetiracetam • If patient is unable to swallow, intranasal midazolam, rectal diazepam, or buccal clonazepam may be used
Stomatitis (oral)	• Treat underlying cause, if possible (e.g., candidiasis, viral infections) • Use of amifostine, if indicated • Offer the patient ice chips or sips of water as tolerated • Oral topical anesthetics
Xerostomia (oral)	• Ensure adequate fluid intake; provide sips of water or ice chips as tolerated • Discontinue medications that cause xerostomia, if possible • If supplemental oxygen is in use, add humidification • Use salivary supplements or stimulants (e.g., pilocarpine) • Offer patient sugar-free gum, if able to chew without pain • Provide moist, soft foods at mealtimes • Non-pharmacological interventions (see Appendix D-2)

BKP, balloon kyphoplasty; VP, vertebroplasty.

Sources: Alvarenga, A., Campos, M., Dias, M., Melão, L., & Estevão-Costa, J. (2017). BOTOX-A injection of salivary glands for drooling. *Journal of Pediatric Surgery, 52*(8), 1283–1286. https://doi.org/10.1016/j.jpedsurg.2016.09.074; Buchmann, L., Ashby, S., Cannon, R. B., & Hunt, J. P. (2015). Psychosocial distress in patients with thyroid cancer. *Otolaryngology—Head and Neck Surgery, 152*(4), 644–649. https://doi.org/10.1177/01945998 14565761; Fusco, F. (2021). Mouth care. In E. Bruera, I. J. Higginson, C. F. von Gunten, & T. Morita (Eds.), *Textbook of palliative medicine and supportive care.* Taylor & Francis Group; Guyer, D. L., Almhanna, K., & McKee, K. Y. (2020). Palliative care for patients with esophageal cancer: A narrative review. *Annals of Translational Medicine, 8*(17). https://doi.org/10.21037/atm-20-3676; Kluger, B. M., Ney, D. E., Bagley, S. J., Mohile, N., Taylor, L. P., Walbert, T., & Jones, C. A. (2020). Top ten tips palliative care clinicians should know when caring for patients with brain cancer. *Journal of Palliative Medicine, 23*(3), 415–421. https://doi.org/10.1089/jpm.2019.0507; McGeachan, A. J., & Mcdermott, C. J. (2017). Management of oral secretions in neurological disease. *Practical Neurology, 17*(2), 96–103. https://doi.org/10.1136/practneurol-2016-001515; Walker, P. W. (2016). Other symptoms: Xerostomia, hiccups, pruritus, pressure ulcers and wounds care, lymphedema, and myoclonus. In S. Yennuraajalingam & E. Bruera (Eds.), *Oxford handbook of hospice and palliative medicine and supportive care* (2nd ed.). Oxford University Press.

CHAPTER 6

CANCERS OF THE CHEST AND ABDOMEN

BREAST CANCER

DEFINITION/CHARACTERISTICS
A. Malignancy that originates in breast tissue.
B. Most breast cancers originate in the milk ducts.
C. There are several specific types of breast cancer:
   1. Ductal carcinoma in situ (DCIS).
   2. Inflammatory breast cancer.
   3. Invasive lobular carcinoma.
   4. Lobular carcinoma in situ (LCIS).
   5. Male breast cancer.
   6. Paget disease of the breast.
   7. Recurrent breast cancer.

INCIDENCE AND PREVALENCE
A. Most common cancer among American women, with the exception of skin cancer.
B. Women have a 13% chance of developing breast cancer at some point in their lives.
C. About 282,000 new cases of invasive breast cancer are diagnosed annually.
D. About 49,000 new cases of DCIS are diagnosed annually (American Cancer Society, 2021b).

ETIOLOGY
A. Exact cause is unknown but related factors include:
   1. Exposure to radiation.
   2. Genetic predisposition (American Cancer Society, 2021b).

PATHOPHYSIOLOGY
A. Abnormal cells proliferate and congeal into a mass that can be visualized on x-ray, mammography, or ultrasound.
B. Most common sites of metastasis include the:
   1. Lung(s).
   2. Pleura.
   3. Liver.
   4. Brain (American Cancer Society, 2021b; Wright, 2019).

PREDISPOSING FACTORS
A. Personal history of breast cancer.
B. First-degree relative with breast cancer (mother, daughter, sister).
C. Genetic predisposition (BRCA1 or BRCA2).
D. Early or late menarche.
E. Radiation therapy to breast or chest.
F. Alcohol abuse.
G. Obesity.
H. Advanced maternal age at birth of first child or nulliparity.
I. Dense breast tissue (on mammography; Mayo Clinic, 2023; Wright, 2019).

SUBJECTIVE DATA
A. The majority of women are asymptomatic.
B. Masses are often incidental findings or discovered through screening (American Society of Clinical Oncology, 2021).

OBJECTIVE DATA
A. Lump or thickening in the breast or axilla.
B. Change in breast size or shape.
C. New-onset inverted nipple.
D. Discharge from nipple.
E. Scaly, red, swollen skin around areola (Paget disease).
F. Dimpling of skin of breast that looks like the skin of an orange (peau d'orange; see Figure 6.1; Seller & Symons, 2018; Wright, 2019).

DIAGNOSTIC TESTS
A. See Appendix Table 6A.1 for listing of common diagnostic tests.

DIFFERENTIAL DIAGNOSES
A. Benign mass such as:
   1. Papillomas.
   2. Sclerosing adenosis.
   3. Duct ectasia.
   4. Lobular neoplasia.
   5. Apocrine metaplasia.
B. Gynecomastia.
C. Ductal ectasia.
D. Mondor disease.
E. Sporadic puerperal mastitis (Seller & Symons, 2018).

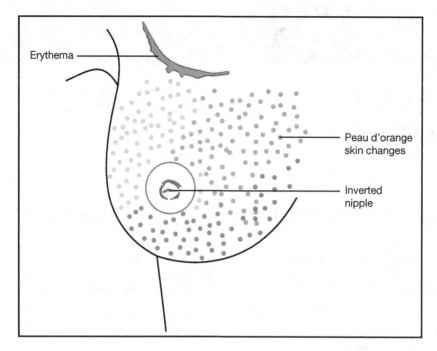

FIGURE 6.1   Signs of inflammatory breast cancer.

POTENTIAL COMPLICATIONS

A. Acute complications of advanced cancer (see Appendix C-7).

B. Metastasis to the:

    1. Lungs.

    2. Pleura.

    3. Liver.

    4. Brain.

C. Bone pain.

D. Pathological fractures.

E. Spinal cord compression.

F. Neurological pain.

G. Hypercalcemia.

H. Lymphedema.

I. Psychosocial changes.

J. Altered body image (Watson et al., 2019; Wright, 2019).

DISEASE-MODIFYING TREATMENTS

A. Noninvasive breast cancer:

    1. Mastectomy or lumpectomy.

    2. Radiation may or may not be indicated.

B. Early stage:

    1. Mastectomy or lumpectomy.

    2. Radiation.

    3. Chemotherapy (see Figure 5.2 in Chapter 5).

    4. Endocrine therapy.

    5. Adjuvant trastuzumab.

    6. Neoadjuvant therapy.

C. Locally advanced:

    1. Neoadjuvant therapy.

    2. Chemotherapy (see Figure 5.2 in Chapter 5).

    3. Hormonal therapy.

D. Metastatic disease:

    1. Endocrine therapy.

    2. Chemotherapy (see Figure 5.2 in Chapter 5).

    3. Radiation.

    4. Osteoclast inhibition (American Cancer Society, 2021b; Watson et al., 2019).

PALLIATIVE INTERVENTIONS/SYMPTOM MANAGEMENT

A. See Appendix Table 6A.2 for listing of palliative interventions and symptom management.

B. See Appendix D-3 for overview of common symptoms.

PROGNOSIS

A. The chance of dying from breast cancer is 1 in 39 (2.6%).

B. The 5-year survival rate for noninvasive breast cancer is about 90%.

C. The 10-year survival rate is about 84%.

D. The 5-year survival rate when breast cancer is confined to the breast is about 99%.

E. The 5-year survival rate when breast cancer has metastasized to regional lymph nodes is 86%.

F. The 5-year survival rate when distant metastasis has occurred is 28%.

G. Survival rates in Black women are 9% to 10% lower than those for White women (see Figure 6.2; American Cancer Society, 2021b; American Society of Clinical Oncology, 2021).

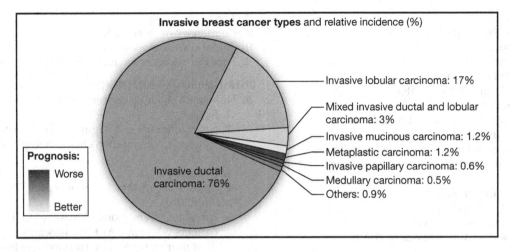

FIGURE 6.2 Breast cancer prognoses.

Source: Adapted from Häggströmm, M. (2019). *Pie chart of histopathologic types of invasive breast cancer.* Author.

NURSING INTERVENTIONS

A. Encourage patient to take medications as prescribed.
B. Review common symptoms related to diagnosis and encourage patient to report symptoms quickly (see Appendix B-1).
C. Provide information regarding community support groups and reputable online groups and/or resources.
D. Assess body image distortion (postmastectomy, hair loss, etc.) and provide resources as needed.
E. Discuss prognosis and survivorship.
F. Encourage smoking cessation (see Appendices B-10 and C-9).
G. Encourage lifestyle modification, as needed (see Appendix B-6).
H. Encourage completion of advance directives.
I. Educate patient and family regarding availability of palliative care services.
J. Educate patient and family regarding availability of hospice care (when appropriate).
K. Monitor caregiver stress (see Appendix B-5).

LUNG CANCER

DEFINITION/CHARACTERISTICS

A. Malignancy that originates in lung tissue or lung structures such as the:
    1. Bronchi.
    2. Bronchioles.
    3. Alveoli.
B. There are four types of lung cancer:
    1. Non-small cell.
    2. Small cell.
    3. Pleuropulmonary blastoma.
    4. Tracheobronchial tumor (National Cancer Institute, 2021b).

INCIDENCE AND PREVALENCE

A. Most common cancer in the United States.
B. Most common cause of cancer death in the United States.
C. Most common types are non-small cell lung cancer and small cell lung cancer.
D. Each year, more than 235,700 new cases are diagnosed.
E. There are approximately 132,000 deaths annually (National Cancer Institute, 2021a).

ETIOLOGY

A. The leading cause of small cell and non-small cell lung cancer is smoking tobacco products.
B. Up to 80% of small cell and non-small cell lung cancer cases are related to smoking and/or exposure to secondhand smoke.
C. Causes of lung cancer in nonsmokers may include exposure to:
    1. Radon.
    2. Air pollution.
    3. Asbestos.
    4. Diesel exhaust.
    5. Industrial chemicals or dusts.
D. When lung cancer occurs in nonsmokers, it is usually diagnosed at a younger age and may be genetically linked.
E. Pleuropulmonary blastoma and tracheobronchial tumors are rare forms of lung cancer that occur in children. The exact etiology is not known, but there may be a genetic predisposition (National Cancer Institute, 2023a; National Organization for Rare Disorders, 2021).

PATHOPHYSIOLOGY

A. The exact pathophysiology is not fully understood.
B. It is believed that repeated exposure to carcinogens causes genetic changes that promote carcinogenesis (Siddiqui & Siddiqui, 2020).

PREDISPOSING FACTORS

A. Smoking tobacco products (cigarettes and cigars). ▶

B. Exposure to:
1. Secondhand smoke.
2. Radon.
3. Asbestos.
4. Inhaled chemicals.
5. Arsenic in drinking water.
6. Air pollution.
7. Beta-carotene dietary supplements.
8. Previous radiation to lungs.
9. Personal or family history of lung cancer.

C. Factors currently under investigation include exposure to:
1. Marijuana smoking.
2. Use of e-cigarettes.
3. Use of talc or talcum powders.

D. HIV (American Cancer Society, 2021b).

SUBJECTIVE DATA
A. Dyspnea.
B. Cough (productive or nonproductive).
C. Shortness of breath.
D. Chest or shoulder pain.
E. Fatigue.
F. Loss of appetite (American Society of Clinical Oncology, 2021; Siddiqui & Siddiqui, 2020).

OBJECTIVE DATA
A. Hemoptysis.
B. Hoarseness.
C. Unintentional weight loss (American Society of Clinical Oncology, 2021; Siddiqui & Siddiqui, 2020).

DIAGNOSTIC TESTS
A. See Appendix Table 6A.1 for listing of common diagnostic tests.

DIFFERENTIAL DIAGNOSES
A. Pneumonia.
B. Bronchitis.
C. Tracheobronchitis.
D. Chronic obstructive pulmonary disease.
E. Diffuse interstitial lung disease.
F. Laryngitis.
G. Lung abscess.
H. Pericarditis.
I. Tuberculosis (Robertson, 2021).

POTENTIAL COMPLICATIONS
A. Acute complications of advanced cancer (see Appendix C-7).
B. Metastasis to the:
1. Opposite lung.
2. Adrenal gland.
3. Bone.
4. Brain.
5. Liver.

C. Malignant pleural effusion.
D. Hypercalcemia.
E. Malignant pericardial effusion.
F. Thromboembolism.
G. Pulmonary hemorrhage.
H. Spinal cord compression.
I. Superior vena cava syndrome (Eldridge, 2020).

DISEASE-MODIFYING TREATMENTS
A. Non-small cell lung cancer treatments:
1. Surgery.
2. Chemotherapy (see Figure 5.2 in Chapter 5).
3. Cytotoxic combination chemotherapy (see Figure 5.2).
4. Radiation.
5. Epidermal growth factor receptor (EGFR) tyrosine inhibitors.
6. Anaplastic lymphoma kinase (ALK) inhibitors for patients who have ALK translocations.
7. v-raf murine sarcoma viral oncogene homolog B1 (BRAF) V600E and mitogen-activated protein kinase kinase (MEK) inhibitors for patients who have BRAF V600E mutations.
8. ROS1 inhibitors for patients who have ROS1 rearrangements.
9. Neurotrophic tyrosine receptor kinase (NTRK) inhibitors for patients who have NTRK fusions.
10. Rearranged during transfection (RET) proto-oncogene inhibitors for patients who have RET fusions.
11. Immune checkpoint inhibitors with or without chemotherapy.
12. Everolimus.
13. Immunotherapy.

B. Small cell lung cancer treatments:
1. Surgery.
2. Chemotherapy (see Figure 5.2 in Chapter 5).
3. Radiation.
4. Prophylactic cranial radiation.
5. Immune checkpoint modulation and combination chemotherapy.

C. Childhood pleuropulmonary blastoma treatments:
1. Surgery.
2. Adjuvant chemotherapy (see Figure 5.2 in Chapter 5).

D. Childhood tracheobronchial tumors treatments:
1. Conservative pulmonary resection.
2. Chemotherapy and radiation are indicated only if:
   a. Metastasis is present.
   b. Tumor is the rhabdomyosarcoma histologic type (National Cancer Institute, 2023a).

PALLIATIVE INTERVENTIONS/SYMPTOM MANAGEMENT
A. See Appendix Table 6A.2 for listing of palliative interventions and symptom management.
B. See Appendix D-3 for overview of common symptoms.

PROGNOSIS
A. The 5-year survival rate for cancer of the lung or bronchus is 21.7%.
B. Survival rate increases if cancer is detected in earlier stages.

▶

C. About 50% to 89% of children with pleuropulmonary blastoma are successfully treated.

D. Outcomes depend on type of pleuropulmonary blastoma and other individual factors.

E. The prognosis for most children with tracheobronchial tumors is very good after surgical resection.

F. Rhabdomyosarcoma carries a higher risk of morbidity and mortality (American Society of Clinical Oncology, 2021; National Cancer Institute, 2023a).

NURSING INTERVENTIONS

A. Teach patient to avoid smoking or secondhand smoke.

B. Encourage smoking cessation (see Appendices B-10 and C-9).

C. Provide teaching regarding symptom management (e.g., dyspnea, pain; see Appendix B-1).

D. Provide teaching regarding proper use of supplemental oxygen.

E. Encourage periods alternating rest and activity.

F. Provide information regarding community support groups and reputable online groups and/or resources.

G. Discuss prognosis and survivorship.

H. Encourage completion of advance directives.

I. Educate patient and family regarding availability of palliative care.

J. Educate patient and family regarding availability of hospice care (when appropriate).

K. See Table 6.1 and Figure 6.3 for lung cancer staging.

L. Monitor caregiver stress (see Appendix B-5).

LIVER CANCER

DEFINITION/CHARACTERISTICS

A. Malignancy that originates in the tissue of the liver or bile duct (National Cancer Institute, 2023b).

INCIDENCE AND PREVALENCE

A. There are about 42,200 new cases annually.

B. Liver cancer represents 2.2% of all new cancer cases.

C. The most common type of primary tumor is hepatocellular carcinoma.

D. Because symptoms may be vague, liver cancer is often initially diagnosed at a late stage (Hubert & VanMeter, 2018; National Cancer Institute, 2023b).

ETIOLOGY

A. The exact etiology is unknown, but the most common risk factor is chronic hepatitis B or C infection.

B. Tumors result from prolonged exposure to carcinogens, which cause mutations in liver cells (Hubert & VanMeter, 2018; National Cancer Institute, 2023b).

PATHOPHYSIOLOGY

A. Liver cancer progresses in stages and may result from damage to liver tissue caused by cirrhosis, other chronic liver diseases, and/or chronic viral infections.

B. It is believed that toll-like receptor (TLR) activation plays a role in the development and progression of inflammation-associated liver cancer (see Figure 6.4; American Liver Foundation, 2017; Kiziltas, 2016).

Stage	Description
TABLE 6.1	**STAGING OF NON-SMALL CELL LUNG CANCER**
0	Cancer cells are detectable in the lining of the bronchus. No metastasis.
IA	Tumor size up to 3 cm. No metastasis.
IB	Tumor size is between 3 and 4 cm. No metastasis.
IIA	Tumor size is 4 to 5 cm and is contained within the chest cavity. No metastasis.
IIB	Tumor size is up to 5 cm and has spread to nearby lymph nodes but no further.
IIIA	Tumor size is up to 5 cm and has spread to mediastinal lymph nodes but has not spread to other locations.
IIIB	Tumor size is up to 5 cm and has spread to mediastinal or clavicular lymph nodes but has not spread to other locations.
IIIC	Tumor size greater than 5 cm and has spread to mediastinal or clavicular lymph nodes but has not spread to other locations.
IVA	Tumor of any size and has invaded lymph nodes and structures within the chest cavity.
IVB	Tumor of any size that has spread outside of the chest cavity.

Source: Adapted from Lababede, O., & Meziane, M. A. (2018). The eighth edition of TNM staging of lung cancer: Reference chart and diagrams. *The Oncologist, 23*(7), 844. https://theoncologist.onlinelibrary.wiley.com/doi/pdfdirect/10.1634/theoncologist.2017-0659

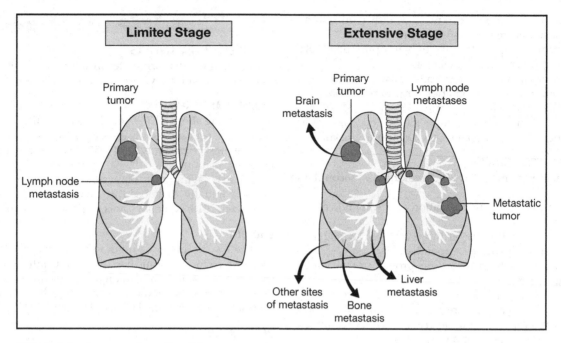

FIGURE 6.3 Staging of small cell lung cancer.

Source: Adapted from Tecentriq. (n.d.). *Learning about small cell lung cancer.* https://www.tecentriq.com/sclc/about.html?c=pdl16 d97f901de&gclid=CjwKCAiAzrWOBhBjEiwAq85QZ4m80VQaFvTlEKTvlFYh7BklF8RALbZRVabLswoDd_-ASnAW-bnKhoCs4gQAvD_ BwE&gclsrc=aw.ds

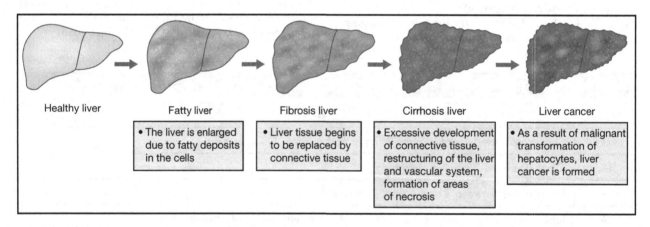

FIGURE 6.4 Progression of liver disease.

Source: Hripliva, T. M. (2022). *Progression of liver disease.* https://www.dreamstime.com/illustration-stages-liver-damage-such-as-fatty-fibrosis-cirrhosis-cancer-image200794923

PREDISPOSING FACTORS

A. Gender (more common in males).
B. Race and ethnicity (Asian Americans and Pacific Islanders are at highest risk).
C. Chronic viral hepatitis (B or C).
D. Cirrhosis.
E. Nonalcoholic fatty liver disease.
F. Primary biliary cirrhosis.
G. Inherited metabolic diseases.
H. Alcohol overuse.
I. Tobacco use.
J. Obesity.
K. Type 2 diabetes.
L. Certain rare cancers.
M. Tyrosinemia.
N. Alpha-1-antitrypsin deficiency.
O. Porphyria cutanea tarda.
P. Glycogen storage diseases.
Q. Wilson disease.
R. Aflatoxins.
S. Vinyl chloride and thorium dioxide (Thorotrast) exposure.
T. Anabolic steroids (American Cancer Society, 2021b).

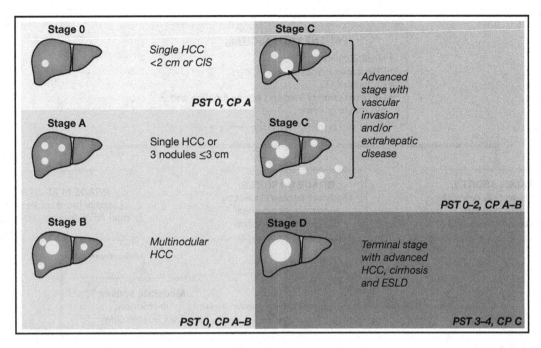

FIGURE 6.5 The Barcelona Clinic Liver Cancer system.

Source: Lurje, I., Czigany, Z., Bednarsch, J., Roderburg, C., Isfort, P., Neumann, U. P., & Lurje, G. (2019). *HCC stages according to BCLC.* https://commons.wikimedia.org/wiki/File:HCC_stages_according_to_BCLC.png

TABLE 6.2 CANCER OF THE LIVER ITALIAN PROGRAM SCORING SYSTEM AND PROGNOSTICATION VALUES

CLIP Scoring System Liver cancer			
	Scores		
Variables	0	1	2
Child–Pugh stage	A	B	C
Tumor morphology	Uninodular *and* extension ≤50%	Multinodular *and* extension ≤50%	Massive *or* extension >50%
AFP (ng/dL)	<400	≥400	
Portal vein thrombosis	No	Yes	

The CLIP score for a patient with hepatocellular carcinoma is calculated by assigning a score (0, 1, or 2) to each of four clinical factors: (a) Child–Pugh stage, (b) number of tumor nodules and whether the tumor extends through ≤50% or >50% of the liver, (c) AFP, and (d) portal vein thrombosis.

These scores are added together to yield a CLIP score of 0 to 6, with median survival by CLIP score as follows:

0 = 42.5 months
1 = 32.0 months
2 = 16.5 months
3 = 4.5 months
4 = 2.5 months
5 to 6 = 1 month

AFP, alpha-fetoprotein blood; CLIP, Cancer of the Liver Italian Program.

Source: U.S. Department of Veterans Affairs. (2018). *Viral hepatitis and liver disease.* https://www.hepatitis.va.gov/liver-cancer/clip-score.asp

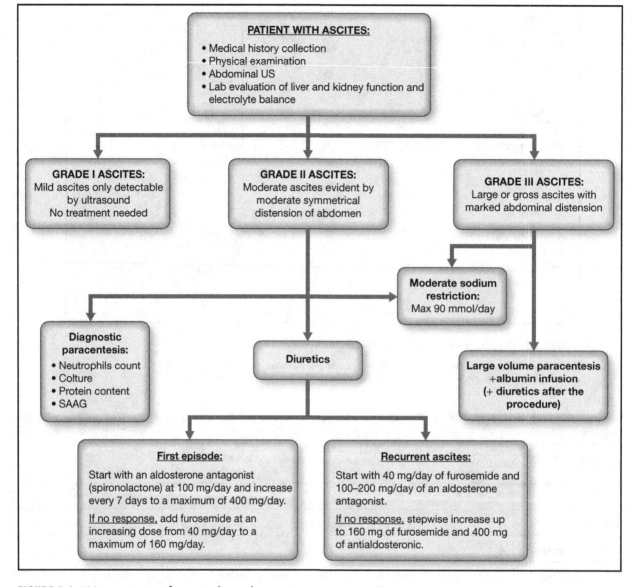

FIGURE 6.6   Management of uncomplicated ascites.

Note: No response to diuretic treatment defined by a weight loss of less than 1 kg in the first week or 2 kg every week thereafter.

US, ultrasound; SAAG, serum ascites albumin gradient.

Source: Piano, S., Tonon, M., & Angeli, P. (2018). Management of ascites and hepatorenal syndrome. *Hepatology International, 12*(1), 122–134. https://link.springer.com/article/10.1007/s12072-017-9815-0

SUBJECTIVE DATA

A. Fatigue.
B. Bloating.
C. Feeling of fullness.
D. Nausea.
E. Anorexia.
F. Weakness.
G. Pruritus (American Liver Foundation, 2017; Hubert & VanMeter, 2018).

OBJECTIVE DATA

A. Unintentional weight loss.

B. Fever.
C. Jaundice.
D. Vomiting.
E. Hepatomegaly.
F. Ascites (see Figure 6.6; American Liver Foundation, 2017; Hubert & VanMeter, 2018).

DIAGNOSTIC TESTS

A. See Appendix Table 6A.1 for listing of common diagnostic tests.
B. See Figure 6.5 and Tables 6.2 and 6.4 for liver cancer staging.

TABLE 6.3　PHARMACOLOGICAL INTERVENTIONS FOR HEPATIC ENCEPHALOPATHY

Drug	Dose	Undesirable effects
First-line therapy for acute episodic OHE in the United States		
Lactulose	20 g/30 mL–30 g/45 mL 3–4 per day titrated for 2–3 bowel movements a day orally. If unable to administer orally, use a similar dose via NG or 300 mL of enemas 3–4 per day until clinical improvement is noted.	Diarrhea, flatulence, and bloating. Unpleasant taste
Second-line therapy for acute episodic OHE in the United States (intolerant to lactulose)		
Rifaximin	400–550 mg PO twice daily indefinitely	No major side effects
Third-line (not approved by FDA) therapy for acute episodic OHE		
PEG	41 of PO or via NG tube × 1 single dose (in lieu of lactulose)	None clinically in short-term use
First-line therapy for prevention of recurrent OHE in the United States		
Lactulose	20 g/30 mL–30 g/45 mL 3–4 per day titrated for 2–3 bowel movements a day orally for low grades or use 300 mL of 3–4 per day enemas until clinical improvement is noted	Diarrhea, flatulence, and bloating. Unpleasant taste
Rifaximin	400–550 mg PO twice daily in conjunction with lactulose or as monotherapy for lactulose-intolerant patients	No major side effects
Experimental (not approved by FDA) therapy for secondary prophylaxis of OHE		
Probiotics	Dose dependent on the type of mixture used	No major side effects
FMT	One small open-label randomized clinical trial	Bloating and diarrhea

FDA, Food and Drug Administration; PEG, polyethylene glycol; FMT, fecal microbiota transplant; OHE, overt hepatic encephalopathy; NG, nasogastric.

Source: Acharya, C., & Bajaj, J. S. (2018). Current management of hepatic encephalopathy. *Official Journal of the American College of Gastroenterology, 113*(11), 1600–1612. https://www.proquest.com/publication/publications_2041977?accountid=28588.

DIFFERENTIAL DIAGNOSES
A. Cholangiocarcinoma.
B. Cirrhosis.
C. Hepatocellular adenoma (hepatic adenoma).
D. Appendicitis.
E. Cholecystitis.
F. Hepatomegaly.
G. Portal hypertension.
H. Viral infection.
I. Nonalcoholic fatty liver disease.
J. Pancreatitis.
K. Peptic ulcer disease (Small, 2021).

POTENTIAL COMPLICATIONS
A. Acute complications of advanced cancer (see Appendix C-7).
B. Ascites (see Figure 6.6).
C. Hepatic encephalopathy (see Table 6.3).
D. Portal hypertensive gastrointestinal bleeding.
E. Metastasis to the:

1. Lung.
2. Portal vein.
3. Portal lymph nodes (Small, 2021; Wright, 2019).

DISEASE-MODIFYING TREATMENTS
A. Hepatectomy.
B. Segmentectomy.
C. Radiofrequency ablation (RFA).
D. Chemotherapy (see Figure 5.2 in Chapter 5).
E. Radiation.
F. Immunotherapy.
G. Transplant (American Liver Foundation, 2017; Hubert & VanMeter, 2018).

PALLIATIVE INTERVENTIONS/SYMPTOM MANAGEMENT
A. See Appendix Table 6A.2 for listing of palliative interventions and symptom management.
B. See Appendix D-3 for overview of common symptoms.

PROGNOSIS
A. The 5-year survival rate is 20.3%.

TABLE 6.4 OKUDA STAGING SYSTEM FOR LIVER CANCER

Stage	Tumor size[a]	Ascites	Albumin	Bilirubin	Total score
I	>50% (+) <50% (−)	Present (+) Absent (−)	<3 g/dL (+) >3 g/dL (−)	>3 mg/dL (+) <3 mg/dL (−)	No +
II	>50% (+) <50% (−)	Present (+) Absent (−)	<3 g/dl (+) >3 g/dl (−)	>3 mg/dL (+) <3 mg/dL (−)	1 or 2+
III	>50% (+) <50% (−)	Present (+) Absent (−)	<3 g/dL (+) >3 g/dL (−)	>3 mg/dL (+) <3 mg/dL (−)	3 or 4+

[a]Largest cross-sectional area of tumor to largest cross-sectional area of liver.

Source: Modified from Okuda, K., Ohtsuki, T., Obata, H., Tomimatsu, M., Okazaki, N., Hasegawa, H., Nakajima, Y., & Ohnishi, K. (1985). Natural history of hepatocellular carcinoma and prognosis in relation to treatment study of 850 patients. *Cancer, 56*(4), 918–928. https://acsjournals.onlinelibrary.wiley.com/doi/pdfdirect/10.1002/1097-0142%2819850815%2956%3A4%3C918%3A%3AAID-CNCR2820560437%3E3.0.CO%3B2-E diseases/myasthenia-gravis#

B. In compensated liver disease, mortality is low (1%–3%).
C. Risk of mortality increases significantly in the presence of decompensated liver disease or portal hypertension (Mazzarelli et al., 2018; National Cancer Institute, 2023b).

NURSING INTERVENTIONS
A. Encourage hepatitis vaccination for patient and caregivers.
B. Encourage treatment for viral hepatitis.
C. Ensure proper symptom management.
D. Encourage smoking cessation (see Appendices B-10 and C-9).
E. Monitor effectiveness of interventions for ascites and modify plan of care as needed (see Figure 6.6 and Appendix B-1).
F. Monitor effectiveness of interventions for hepatic encephalopathy and modify plan of care as needed (see Table 6.3).
G. Teach patient to take all medications as prescribed.
H. Educate patient on disease trajectory.
I. Encourage patient to avoid alcohol use (see Appendix B-6).
J. Monitor caregiver stress (see Appendix B-5).
K. Encourage patient to complete advance directive.
L. Educate patient and family regarding availability of palliative care.
M. Educate patient and family regarding availability of hospice (when appropriate).

PANCREATIC CANCER

DEFINITION/CHARACTERISTICS
A. Malignancy that begins in the cells of pancreas.
B. Can occur in the head of the pancreas, the ampulla of Vater, the common bile duct, and/or the duodenum.
C. There are three types of pancreatic cancers:
   1. Exocrine (most common).
   2. Pancreatic neuroendocrine tumors or islet cell tumors (less than 20% of pancreatic cancers; American Cancer Society, 2021b; Sommers, 2019).

INCIDENCE AND PREVALENCE
A. There are more than 60,000 new cases of pancreatic cancer annually.
B. Pancreatic cancer represents 3.2% of all cancers.
C. The average risk of developing pancreatic cancer is 1% (National Cancer Institute, 2021).

ETIOLOGY
A. The exact cause of pancreatic cancer is not known.
B. Possible causes of pancreatic cancer include:
   1. Diabetes mellitus.
   2. Obesity.
   3. Chronic pancreatitis.
   4. Genetic mutations (Sommers, 2019).

PATHOPHYSIOLOGY
A. Adenocarcinoma is the most common exogenous pancreatic cancer.
B. Pancreatic adenocarcinoma spreads rapidly within the pancreas and to other organs.
C. Because symptoms are often vague, pancreatic cancer is not usually detected in early stages (Sommers, 2019).

PREDISPOSING FACTORS
A. Age (risk increases over age 45).
B. Sex (men are at higher risk).
C. Race and ethnicity (Black individuals and those of Ashkenazi Jewish heritage are at highest risk).
D. Smoking (increases risk by 2–3 times).
E. Diabetes.
F. Chronic pancreatitis.
G. Genetic mutations.
H. Diets high in fat, meat, dehydrated foods, fried foods, refined sugars, soybeans, and nitrosamines.
I. Occupational exposure to carcinogens.
J. High intake of coffee.
K. High alcohol intake.
L. Hepatitis B infection.
M. Cirrhosis.
N. Bacterial infection (such as Helicobacter pylori; American Society of Clinical Oncology, 2021; Sommers, 2019).

SUBJECTIVE DATA
A. Midepigastric pain (sign of advanced disease).
B. Bloating.
C. Gastrointestinal distress.
D. Flatulence.
E. Weakness.
F. Anorexia.
G. Nausea.
H. Malaise.
I. Pruritus.
J. Pain after eating.
K. Pain after activity that is alleviated by lying in supine position or sitting up (American Society for Clinical Oncology, 2021; Sommers, 2019).

OBJECTIVE DATA
A. Jaundice (follows a distinctive pattern beginning with mucus membranes, progressing to palms of hands, and finally becoming generalized).
B. Dark urine.
C. Clay-colored stools.
D. Foul-smelling, greasy stools that float.
E. Vomiting.
F. Unintentional weight loss.
G. Diarrhea or constipation.
H. Liver and/or spleen enlargement.
I. Ascites (see Figure 6.6).
J. Thromboembolism.
K. Dullness on percussion of upper abdomen (American Society for Clinical Oncology, 2021; Sommers, 2019).

DIAGNOSTIC TESTS
A. See Appendix Table 6A.1 for listing of common diagnostic tests.

DIFFERENTIAL DIAGNOSES
A. Abdominal aortic aneurysm.
B. Ampullary carcinoma.
C. Intestinal ischemia.
D. Gastric lymphoma.
E. Pancreatic lymphoma.
F. Hepatocellular carcinoma (hepatoma).
G. Bile duct strictures.
H. Bile duct tumors.
I. Neoplasms of the endocrine pancreas.
J. Acute pancreatitis.
K. Cholangitis.
L. Cholecystitis.
M. Choledochal cysts.
N. Chronic pancreatitis.
O. Gallstones (cholelithiasis).
P. Gastric cancer.
Q. Peptic ulcer disease (Dragovich, 2020).

POTENTIAL COMPLICATIONS
A. Acute complications of advanced cancer (see Appendix C-7).
B. Metastasis to the:
    1. Lung.
    2. Peritoneum.
    3. Spleen.
C. Bowel obstruction (Mayo Clinic, 2021b; Sommers, 2019).

DISEASE-MODIFYING TREATMENTS
A. Surgery:
    1. Laparoscopy.
    2. Whipple procedure.
    3. Distal pancreatectomy.
    4. Total pancreatectomy.
B. Radiation.
C. Chemotherapy (see Figure 5.2 in Chapter 5).
D. Immunotherapy.
E. Pancreatic enzyme supplements.
F. Targeted drug therapy:
    1. Erlotinib (Tarceva).
    2. Olaparib (Lynparza).
    3. Larotrectinib (Vitrakvi; American Cancer Society, 2021a).

PALLIATIVE INTERVENTIONS/SYMPTOM MANAGEMENT
A. See Appendix Table 6A.2 for listing of palliative interventions and symptom management.
B. See Appendix D-3 for overview of common symptoms.

PROGNOSIS
A. The 5-year survival rate is 10.8%.
B. Prognosis improves when disease is diagnosed at an earlier stage.
C. Because symptoms are vague, up to 80% of cases are diagnosed at a late stage.
D. Stage IV pancreatic cancer has a 5-year survival rate of 1% (Johns Hopkins Medicine, 2021; National Cancer Institute, 2021).

NURSING INTERVENTIONS
A. Ensure proper pain management.
B. Educate patient and family regarding expected symptoms.
C. Management of obstruction as indicated.
D. Teach patient to increase in fiber intake.
E. Encourage smoking cessation (see Appendices B-10 and C-9).
F. Teach patient to take all medications as prescribed.
G. Educate patient and family regarding disease trajectory (see Appendix B-1).
H. Encourage patient to verbalize fears.
I. Provide information regarding community support groups and evidence-based internet resources.
J. Ensure proper symptom management.
K. Monitor effectiveness of interventions for ascites and modify plan of care as needed (see Figure 6.6).
L. Encourage patient to avoid alcohol use (see Appendix B-6).
M. Monitor caregiver stress (see Appendix B-5).
N. Encourage completion of advance directives.

O. Educate patient and family regarding availability of palliative care.

P. Educate patient and family regarding availability of hospice (when appropriate; Center to Advance Palliative Care, 2021; Sommers, 2019).

COLORECTAL CANCER

DEFINITION/CHARACTERISTICS
A. Malignancy that originates in the colon or rectum.
B. About 65% of colorectal cancers occur in the rectum, sigmoid, and descending colon.
C. About 95% of colorectal tumors develop from an adenomatous polyp (Sommers, 2019).

INCIDENCE AND PREVALENCE
A. There are roughly 149,500 new cases annually in the United States.
B. Colorectal cancer is the third most commonly diagnosed cancer.
C. Colorectal cancer is the third leading cause of cancer deaths.
D. Colorectal cancer represents 7.9% of all new cancers diagnosed annually (National Cancer Institute, 2021a).

ETIOLOGY
A. Exact etiology is unknown.
B. Risk increases with age (Sommers, 2019).

PATHOPHYSIOLOGY
A. Colorectal cancer often begins as a polyp.
B. Once malignancy develops in the polyp, the tumor usually grows into the lumen of the colon, causing obstruction (Sommers, 2019).

PREDISPOSING FACTORS
A. Personal history of colorectal cancer or ovarian cancer.
B. History of:
    1. Ulcerative colitis.
    2. Crohn disease.
    3. Adenomatous colon polyps.
C. History of high-risk adenomas (polyps >1 cm or with abnormal microscopy).
D. Genetic predisposition.
E. Low-fiber, high-fat diet.
F. More than three alcoholic beverages daily.
G. Physical inactivity.
H. Tobacco use.
I. Diabetes mellitus.
J. Obesity (Sommers, 2019; Wright, 2019).

SUBJECTIVE DATA
A. Change in bowel habits.
B. Bowel fullness after defecation.
C. Gas pains.
D. Bloating.
E. Cramping.
F. Abdominal fullness.
G. Nausea (Sommers, 2019; Wright, 2019).

OBJECTIVE DATA
A. Thin stools.
B. Tarry stools.
C. Hematochezia.
D. Diarrhea.
E. Constipation.
F. Vomiting.
G. Unintentional weight loss (Sommers, 2019; Wright, 2019).

DIAGNOSTIC TESTS
A. See Appendix Table 6A.1 for listing of common diagnostic tests.
B. See Figure 6.7 for colon cancer staging.

DIFFERENTIAL DIAGNOSES
A. Arteriovenous malformation (AVM).
B. Carcinoid/neuroendocrine tumors and rare tumors of the gastrointestinal tract.
C. Ischemic bowel.
D. Small intestine carcinomas.
E. Gastrointestinal lymphoma.
F. Crohn disease.
G. Ileus.
H. Small intestinal diverticulosis.
I. Ulcerative colitis (Dragovich, 2021).

POTENTIAL COMPLICATIONS
A. Acute complications of advanced cancer (see Appendix C-7).
B. Metastasis to the:
    1. Lung.
    2. Liver.
    3. Peritoneum.
C. Bowel obstruction (Wright, 2019).

DISEASE-MODIFYING TREATMENTS
A. Surgery:
    1. Laparoscopic surgery.
    2. Colostomy for rectal cancer.
    3. Radiofrequency ablation (RFA) or cryoablation.
B. Radiation:
    1. External beam radiation therapy.
    2. Stereotactic radiation therapy.
    3. Intraoperative radiation therapy.
    4. Brachytherapy.
C. Chemotherapy (see Figure 5.2 in Chapter 5).
D. Targeted therapies.
E. Antiangiogenesis therapy.
F. Combined targeted therapies.
G. Tumor-agnostic treatment.
H. Immunotherapy (American Society of Clinical Oncology, 2021).

PALLIATIVE INTERVENTIONS/SYMPTOM MANAGEMENT
A. See Appendix Table 6A.2 for listing of palliative interventions and symptom management.
B. See Appendix D-3 for overview of common symptoms.

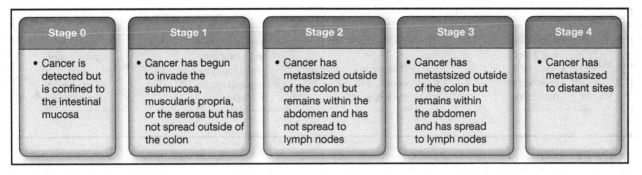

Stage 0	Stage 1	Stage 2	Stage 3	Stage 4
• Cancer is detected but is confined to the intestinal mucosa	• Cancer has begun to invade the submucosa, muscularis propria, or the serosa but has not spread outside of the colon	• Cancer has metastsized outside of the colon but remains within the abdomen and has not spread to lymph nodes	• Cancer has metastsized outside of the colon but remains within the abdomen and has spread to lymph nodes	• Cancer has metastasized to distant sites

FIGURE 6.7 Colon cancer staging.

Source: Adapted from Memorial Sloan Kettering Cancer Center. (2022). *Stages of colon cancer.* https://www.mskcc.org/cancer-care/types/colon/stages

PROGNOSIS
A. The 5-year survival rate is 64.7%.
B. Survival rates improve when detected early.
C. Survivorship has been increasing due to increased screening (National Cancer Institute, 2021a).

NURSING INTERVENTIONS
A. Ensure proper pain management.
B. Educate patient and family regarding expected symptoms (see Appendix B-1).
C. Management of bowel obstruction as indicated.
D. Teach patient to increase in fiber intake.
E. Encourage smoking cessation (see Appendices B-10 and C-9).
F. Teach patient to take all medications as prescribed.
G. Educate patient and family regarding disease trajectory.
H. Encourage patient to verbalize fears.
I. Provide information regarding community support groups and evidence-based internet resources.
J. Ensure proper symptom management.
K. Monitor effectiveness of interventions for ascites and modify plan of care as needed (see Figure 6.6).
L. Encourage patient to avoid alcohol use (see Appendix B-6).
M. Monitor caregiver stress (see Appendix B-5).
N. Encourage completion of advance directives.
O. Educate patient and family regarding availability of palliative care.
P. Educate patient and family regarding availability of hospice (when appropriate; Center to Advance Palliative Care, 2021; Sommers, 2019).

RENAL CANCER

DEFINITION/CHARACTERISTICS
A. Malignancy that originates in the cells of the kidney.
B. Most kidney cancers occur in only one kidney.
C. Masses tend to be large and nodular.
D. Types of kidney cancer:
   1. Renal cell cancer.
   2. Transitional cell cancer (urothelial carcinoma).
   3. Wilms tumor.
   4. Sarcoma.
   5. Lymphoma (American Society of Clinical Oncology, 2021; National Cancer Institute, 2023c; Sommers, 2019).

INCIDENCE AND PREVALENCE
A. There are about 76,000 new cases diagnosed annually.
B. Kidney cancer represents about 4% of all new cases of cancer.
C. Kidney cancer represents about 2.3% of all cancer deaths (National Cancer Institute, 2023c).

ETIOLOGY
A. The exact cause is not known (Sommers, 2019).

PATHOPHYSIOLOGY
A. Malignancy usually begins as a single mass in one kidney.
B. Because most kidney tumors are painless, kidney cancer is often not detected until the tumor is large and causing other symptoms.
C. If not detected or left untreated, metastasis usually begins in proximity to the affected kidney and then spreads to distant sites (Sommers, 2019).

PREDISPOSING FACTORS
A. Smoking.
B. Occupational exposure to carcinogens.
C. Chronic misuse of pain medications.
D. Obesity.
E. Hypertension.
F. Family history of renal cancer.
G. Genetic conditions such as von Hippel–Lindau disease.
H. Hereditary papillary renal cell carcinoma.
I. Sex (males are at higher risk).
J. Race and ethnicity (risk is heightened for those of African American and Alaskan/Native American heritage; Sommers 2019; Wright, 2019).

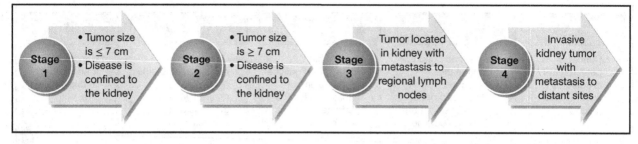

FIGURE 6.8 Staging of kidney cancer.

Source: Adapted from Rini, B. I., McKiernan, J. M., Chang, S. S., Choueiri, T. K., Kenney, P. A., Landman, J., Leibovich, B. C., Tickoo, S. T., Vikram., R., Zhou, M., & Stadler, W. M. (2018). *Kidney.* In M. B. Amin, S. Edge, F. Greene, D. R. Byrd, R. K Brookland, M. K., Washington, J. E. Gershenwald, C. C Compton, K. R. Hess, D. C. Sullivan, J. M. Jessup, J. D. Brierley, L. E. Gaspar, R. L. Schilsky, C. M. Balch, D. P. Winchester, E. A. Asare, M. Madera, D. M. Gress, & L. R. Meyer (Eds.), *AJCC cancer staging manual* (8th ed.). Springer International Publishing: American Joint Commission on Cancer. https://link.springer.com/book/9783319406176

SUBJECTIVE DATA
A. Flank pain.
B. Anorexia.
C. Fatigue.
D. Anxiety.
E. Mood swings.
F. Irritability.
G. Depression.
H. Insomnia.
I. Fever.
J. Night sweats.
K. Lethargy.
L. Weakness.
M. Edema (Sinabaldi et al., 2018; Sommers, 2019; Wright, 2019).

OBJECTIVE DATA
A. Hematuria.
B. Anemia.
C. Abdominal mass.
D. Cachexia.
E. Constipation.
F. Hypercalcemia.
G. Unintentional weight loss.
H. Change in mentation (Sinibaldi et al., 2018; Sommers, 2019; Wright, 2019).

DIAGNOSTIC TESTS
A. See Appendix Table 6A.1 for listing of common diagnostic tests.
B. See Figure 6.8 for kidney cancer staging.

DIFFERENTIAL DIAGNOSES
A. Abscess.
B. Benign mass.
C. Metastasis from a distant primary lesion.
D. Renal cyst.
E. Renal infarction.
F. Sarcoma.
G. Acute pyelonephritis.
H. Bladder cancer.

I. Chronic pyelonephritis.
J. Non-Hodgkin lymphoma (Sachdiva, 2021).

POTENTIAL COMPLICATIONS
A. Acute complications of advanced cancer (see Appendix C-7).
B. Metastasis to the:
　　1. Adrenal gland.
　　2. Bone.
　　3. Brain.
　　4. Liver.
　　5. Lung.
C. Toxicities related to treatments:
　　1. Hypertension.
　　2. Proteinuria.
　　3. Epistaxis.
　　4. Hemorrhage.
　　5. Thrombosis.
　　6. Gastrointestinal perforation (Sinibaldi et al., 2018; Wright, 2019).

DISEASE-MODIFYING TREATMENTS
A. Partial or total nephrectomy.
B. Immunotherapy.
C. Mechanistic target of rapamycin (mTOR) inhibitors.
D. Targeted therapies.
E. Chemotherapy (see Figure 5.2 in Chapter 5; Sinibaldi et al., 2018).

PALLIATIVE INTERVENTIONS/SYMPTOM MANAGEMENT
A. See Appendix Table 6A.2 for listing of palliative interventions and symptom management.
B. See Appendix D-3 for an overview of common symptoms.

PROGNOSIS
A. The overall 5-year survival rate is 75.6%.
B. Survival rates increase when detected in early stages.
C. If detected when only one kidney if affected, 5-year survival rate is 93%.
D. If detected when there is metastasis to nearby organs or surrounding tissues, 5-year survival rate is 70%. ▶

E. If detected when there is metastasis to distance sites, 5-year survival rate is 13% (American Society of Clinical Oncology, 2021; National Cancer Institute, 2023c).

NURSING INTERVENTIONS
A. Ensure proper pain management.
B. Implement interventions to reduce anxiety and depression.
C. Implement interventions for insomnia, if needed.
D. Provide incontinence care, if applicable.
E. Provide care of urinary catheter, if applicable.
F. Monitor amount, color, and clarity of urine.
G. Educate patient and family regarding possibility of hematuria.
H. Properly manage intractable hematuria.
I. Encourage smoking cessation (see Appendices B-10 and C-9).
J. Teach patient to avoid alcohol use (see Appendix B-6).
K. Educate patient and family regarding disease trajectory (see Appendix B-1).
L. Provide spiritual support.
M. Assess caregiver fatigue/burnout (see Appendix B-5).
N. Encourage completion of advance directives.
O. Educate patient and family regarding availability of palliative care.
P. Educate patient and family regarding availability of hospice services (when appropriate; Sinibaldi et al., 2018; Sommers, 2019).

BLADDER CANCER

DEFINITION/CHARACTERISTICS
A. Malignancy that originates in the bladder, renal pelvis, or ureters.
B. There are three types of bladder cancer:
   1. Urothelial carcinoma.
   2. Squamous cell carcinoma.
   3. Adenocarcinoma.
C. The most common type is urothelial cell carcinoma.
D. Benign bladder tumors are very rare.
E. The majority of cases occur in those >72 years old.
F. Bladder cancer is rare in those <40 years old (American Society of Clinical Oncology, 2021; National Cancer Institute, 2023d).

INCIDENCE AND PREVALENCE
A. There are over 83,700 new cases annually.
B. Bladder cancer represents 4.4% of all new cancer cases each year.
C. Bladder cancer represents 2.8% of all cancer deaths each year (National Cancer Institute, 2023d).

ETIOLOGY
A. The exact cause of bladder cancer is not known (Sommers, 2019).

PATHOPHYSIOLOGY
A. Cell mutations within the mucosa of the urinary tract lead to tumor growth.
B. Cancer cells can implant in multiple locations in the urinary tract as they are transported in urine (Sommers, 2019).

PREDISPOSING FACTORS
A. Cigarette smoking.
B. Occupational exposure to carcinogens.
C. History of radiation to the pelvis.
D. Treatment with cyclophosphamide or isophosphamide.
E. Use of *Aristolochia fangchi.*
F. Consumption of drinking water with high levels of arsenic or chlorine.
G. History of bladder cancer.
H. Chronic bladder infection.
I. Prolonged use of bladder catheter.
J. Vesical calculi.
K. Moderate to high caffeine intake.
L. Age >50 years.
M. Genetic predisposition.
N. European American heritage (Sommers, 2019; Wright, 2019).

SUBJECTIVE DATA
A. Dysuria.
B. Urinary frequency.
C. Diminished urine stream.
D. Flank pain.
E. Suprapubic pain after voiding.
F. Bladder irritability.
G. Lower back pain (Sommers, 2019; Wright, 2019).

OBJECTIVE DATA
A. Gross, painless hematuria.
B. Urinary dribbling.
C. Nocturia (Sommers, 2019).

DIAGNOSTIC TESTS
A. See Appendix Table 6A.1 for listing of common diagnostic tests.
B. See Figure 6.9 for staging of bladder cancer.

DIFFERENTIAL DIAGNOSES
A. Cystitis.
B. Hemorrhagic cystitis.
C. Nephrolithiasis.
D. Renal cell carcinoma.
E. Renal transitional cell carcinoma.
F. Ureteral trauma.
G. Urinary tract infection (Babaian, 2021).

POTENTIAL COMPLICATIONS
A. Acute complications of advanced cancer (see Appendix C-7).
B. Obstruction of the ureters, bladder neck, and prostatic urethra.

▶

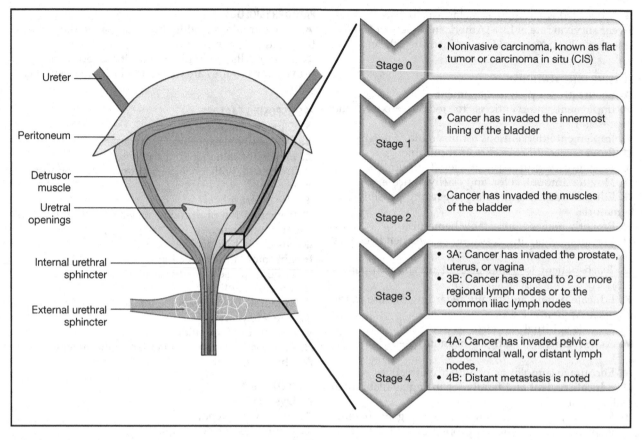

FIGURE 6.9   Stages of bladder cancer.

Source: Adapted from Bochner, B. H., Hansel, D. E., Efstathiou, J. A., Konety, B. K., Lee, C. T., McKiernan, J. M., Plimack, E. R., Reuter, V. E., Sridhar, S., Vikram, R., & Stader, W. M. Rini, B. I., McKiernan, J. M., Chang, S. S., Choueiri, T. K., Kenney, P. A., Landman, J., Leibovich (2018). *Urinary Bladder.* In M. B. Amin, S. Edge, F. Greene, D. R. Byrd, R. K Brookland, M. K., Washington, J. E. Gershenwald, C. C Compton, K. R. Hess, D. C. Sullivan, J. M. Jessup, J. D. Brierley, L. E. Gaspar, R. L. Schilsky, C. M. Balch, D. P. Winchester, E. A. Asare, M. Madera, D. M. Gress, & L. R. Meyer (Eds). *AJCC Cancer Staging Manual* (8th ed.). Springer International Publishing: American Joint Commission on Cancer. https://link.springer.com/book/9783319406176

C. Direct tumor extension into the sigmoid colon, rectum, prostate, uterus, and/or vagina.
D. Need for urinary diversion such as suprapubic catheter or Indiana pouch.
E. Impotence.
F. Female sexual dysfunction due to metastasis to vagina, ovaries, or uterus.
G. Metastasis to the:
    1. Bone.
    2. Liver.
    3. Lungs (Sommers, 2019).

DISEASE-MODIFYING TREATMENTS
A. Transurethral resection of the bladder (TURB).
B. Radical cystectomy.
C. Radiation.
D. Chemotherapy (see Figure 5.2 in Chapter 5).
E. Immunotherapy.
F. Ureteral stents.
G. Electrocautery fulguration.

H. Neodymium-doped yttrium-aluminum-garnet (Nd:YAG) laser (Sommers, 2019).

PALLIATIVE INTERVENTIONS/SYMPTOM MANAGEMENT
A. See Appendix Table 6A.2 for listing of palliative interventions and symptom management.
B. See Appendix D-3 for overview of common symptoms.

PROGNOSIS
A. Bladder cancer is often diagnosed at an early stage.
B. The 5-year survival rate is 77.1% (National Cancer Institute, 2023d; Sommers, 2019).

NURSING INTERVENTIONS
A. Ensure proper pain management.
B. Implement interventions to reduce anxiety and depression.
C. Implement interventions for insomnia, if needed.
D. Provide incontinence care, if applicable.
E. Provide care of urinary catheter, if applicable.

F. Monitor amount, color, and clarity of urine.

G. Educate patient and family regarding possibility of hematuria.

H. Properly manage intractable hematuria.

I. Educate patient and family regarding disease trajectory (see Appendix B-1).

J. Encourage smoking cessation (see Appendices B-10 and C-9).

K. Provide spiritual support.

L. Assess caregiver fatigue/burnout (see Appendix B-5).

M. Encourage completion of advance directives.

N. Educate patient and family regarding availability of palliative care.

O. Educate patient and family regarding availability of hospice services (when appropriate; Sinibaldi et al., 2018; Sommers, 2019).

STOMACH CANCER

DEFINITION/CHARACTERISTICS

A. Malignancy arising within the cells of the stomach.

B. Also called gastric cancer.

C. Most common sites are the antrum, pylorus, and in the area of the lesser curvature.

D. Most common type is adenocarcinoma (95%).

E. Other types include:

    1. Lymphoma.

    2. Gastric sarcoma.

    3. Neuroendocrine tumors (American Society of Clinical Oncology, 2021; Sommers, 2019).

INCIDENCE AND PREVALENCE

A. There are over 26,500 new cases diagnosed annually.

B. Stomach cancer represents 1.8% of all cancer deaths (National Cancer Institute, 2023e).

ETIOLOGY

A. The probable cause of most stomach cancers is H. pylori infection.

B. Other possible causes include:

    1. Dietary intake of carcinogens.

    2. Low-fiber diet.

    3. Occupational exposure to carcinogenic chemical.

    4. Personal history of gastric disease.

    5. Genetic predisposition (Sommers, 2019).

PATHOPHYSIOLOGY

A. Malignant cells within stomach cells lead to tumor growth.

B. Metastasis occurs via the lymphatic system and blood vessels to nearby structures such as the peritoneum.

C. Tumors can also directly metastasize into nearby tissues and organs (Sommers, 2019).

PREDISPOSING FACTORS

A. H. pylori infection in the stomach.

B. Chronic gastritis.

C. Pernicious anemia.

D. Intestinal metaplasia.

E. High dietary intake of salty or smoked foods.

F. Low-fiber diet.

G. Smoking.

H. Obesity.

I. Sex (males are at higher risk).

J. Gastric ulcers.

K. Gastric polyps.

L. Intestinal metaplasia.

M. Chronic peptic ulcers.

N. Genetic predisposition (first-degree relative with history of stomach cancer; Sommers, 2019; Wright, 2019).

SUBJECTIVE DATA

A. Indigestion.

B. Heartburn.

C. Bloating.

D. Stomach pain.

E. Nausea.

F. Anorexia.

G. Fatigue.

H. Persistent bad taste in the mouth (Sommers, 2019; Wright, 2019).

OBJECTIVE DATA

A. Vomiting.

B. Hematochezia.

C. Jaundice.

D. Ascites (see Figure 6.6).

E. Dysphagia.

F. Unintentional weight loss.

G. Hepatomegaly.

H. Palpable lymph nodes.

I. Pale skin and mucus membranes (later stages; Wright, 2019).

DIAGNOSTIC TESTS

A. See Appendix Table 6A.1 for listing of common diagnostic tests.

DIFFERENTIAL DIAGNOSES

A. Acute or chronic gastritis.

B. Atrophic gastritis.

C. Bacterial gastroenteritis.

D. Esophageal cancer.

E. Esophageal stricture.

F. Esophagitis.

G. Malignant neoplasms of the small intestine.

H. Non-Hodgkin lymphoma.

I. Peptic ulcer disease.

J. Viral gastroenteritis (Cabebe, 2021).

POTENTIAL COMPLICATIONS

A. Acute complications of advanced cancer (see Appendix C-7).

B. Metastasis to the:

    1. Liver.

    2. Lung.

    3. Peritoneum.

C. Malnutrition.

▶

D. Gastrointestinal obstruction.

E. Iron deficiency anemia.

F. Peritoneal effusions.

G. Jaundice (secondary to liver involvement).

H. Cachexia.

I. Gastrointestinal bleeding (Sommers, 2019; Wright, 2019).

DISEASE-MODIFYING TREATMENTS

A. Endoscopic mucosal resection (EMR).

B. Endoscopic submucosal dissection (ESD).

C. Partial (distal) gastrectomy.

D. Total gastrectomy.

E. Radiation.

F. Immunotherapy.

G. Chemotherapy (see Figure 5.2 in Chapter 5).

H. Targeted drug therapy (Johns Hopkins Medicine, 2021; Mayo Clinic, 2021b).

PALLIATIVE INTERVENTIONS/SYMPTOM MANAGEMENT

A. See Appendix Table 6A.2 for listing of palliative interventions and symptom management.

B. See Appendix D-3 for overview of common symptoms.

PROGNOSIS

A. The overall 5-year survival rate is 32.4%.

B. If stomach cancer is diagnosed in an early stage, the 5-year survival rate is 70%.

C. If stomach cancer is initially detected with distant metastasis, the 5-year survival rate is 6% (American Society of Clinical Oncology, 2021; National Cancer Institute, 2023e).

NURSING INTERVENTIONS

A. Teach patient to report symptoms promptly.

B. Symptom management.

C. Ensure management of nausea and vomiting.

D. Manage bleeding.

E. Review expected symptoms.

F. Management of bowel obstruction.

G. Teach patient to increase in fiber intake.

H. Encourage smoking cessation (see Appendices B-10 and C-9).

I. Gastrostomy tube care, if applicable.

J. Teach patient to take all medications as prescribed.

K. Review disease trajectory (see Appendix B-1).

L. Encourage patient to verbalize fears.

M. Provide information regarding community support groups and evidence-based internet resources.

N. Encourage completion of advance directives.

O. Educate patient and family regarding availability of palliative care.

P. Educate patient and family regarding availability of hospice care (when appropriate; Mahar et al., 2012; Sommers, 2019; Wright, 2019).

Q. Monitor caregiver stress (see Appendix B-5).

REFERENCES

Abt, D., Bywater, M., Engeler, D. S., & Schmid, H. P. (2013). Therapeutic options for intractable hematuria in advanced bladder cancer. *International Journal of Urology*, 20(7), 651–660. https://doi.org/10.1111/iju.12113

American Cancer Society. (2021a). *Cancer A to Z.* https://www.cancer.org/cancer.html

American Cancer Society. (2021b). *Melanoma skin cancer.* https://www.cancer.org/cancer/melanoma-skin-cancer.html

American Cancer Society. (2022). *Early detection, diagnosis, and staging.* https://www.cancer.org/cancer/liver-cancer/detection-diagnosis-staging/how-diagnosed.html

American Liver Foundation. (2017). *Liver cancer.* https://liverfoundation.org/for-patients/about-the-liver/diseases-of-the-liver/liver-cancer/#symptoms-of-liver-cancer

American Society of Clinical Oncology. (2021). *Types of cancer.* https://www.cancer.net/cancer-types

Babaian, K. N. (2021, February 23). *Bladder cancer differential diagnoses.* https://emedicine.medscape.com/article/438262-differential#

Cabebe, E. C. (2021, April 20). *Gastric cancer differential diagnoses.* https://emedicine.medscape.com/article/278744-differential

Center to Advance Palliative Care. (2021). *Disease types and palliative care.* https://getpalliativecare.org/whatis/disease-types/

Dragovich, T. (2020, October 2). *Pancreatic cancer differential diagnoses.* https://emedicine.medscape.com/article/280605-differential

Dragovich, T. (April 29, 2021). *Colorectal cancer differential diagnoses.* https://emedicine.medscape.com/article/277496-differential

Eldridge, L. (2020, December 20). *Lung cancer complications.* https://www.verywellhealth.com/lung-cancer-complications-and-emergencies-2248840

Hubert, R. J., & VanMeter, K. C. (2018). *Gould's pathophysiology for the health professions* (6th ed.). Elsevier Inc.

Johns Hopkins Medicine. (2021). *Conditions and diseases.* https://www.hopkinsmedicine.org/health/conditions-and-diseases

Kiziltas, S. (2016). Toll-like receptors in pathophysiology of liver diseases. *World Journal of Hepatology*, 8(32), 1354. https://doi.org/10.4254/wjh.v8.i32.1354

Kluger, B. M., Ney, D. E., Bagley, S. J., Mohile, N., Taylor, L. P., Walbert, T., & Jones, C. A. (2020). Top ten tips palliative care clinicians should know when caring for patients with brain cancer. *Journal of Palliative Medicine*, 23(3), 415–421. https://doi.org/10.1089/jpm.2019.0507

Mahar, A. L., Coburn, N. G., Karanicolas, P. J., Viola, R., & Helyer, L. K. (2012). Effective palliation and quality of life outcomes in studies of surgery for advanced, non-curative gastric cancer: A systematic review. *Gastric Cancer*, 15(1), 138–145. https://doi.org/10.1200/JCO.2014.55.1143

Mayo Clinic. (2021a). *Diseases and conditions.* https://www.mayoclinic.org/diseases-conditions

Mayo Clinic. (2021b). *Leukemia.* https://www.mayoclinic.org/diseases-conditions/leukemia/diagnosis-treatment/drc-20374378

Mayo Clinic. (2023). *Breast cancer.* https://www.mayoclinic.org/diseases-conditions/breast-cancer/symptoms-causes/syc-20352470

National Cancer Institute (2021a). *Cancer statistics.* https://seer.cancer.gov/statistics/

National Cancer Institute. (2023a). *Lung cancer: Health professional version.* https://www.cancer.gov/types/lung/hp

National Cancer Institute. (2023b). *Liver and bile duct cancer.* https://www.cancer.gov/types/liver

National Cancer Institute. (2023c). *Kidney (renal cell) cancer: Health professional version.* https://www.cancer.gov/types/kidney/hp

National Cancer Institute. (2023d). *What is bladder cancer?* https://www.cancer.gov/types/bladder

National Cancer Institute. (2023e). *Stomach (gastric) cancer: Health professional version.* https://www.cancer.gov/types/stomach/hp

National Organization for Rare Disorders. (2021). *Rare disease database.* https://rarediseases.org/rare-diseases/

Piano, S., Tonon, M., & Angeli, P. (2018). Management of ascites and hepatorenal syndrome. *Hepatology International, 12*(1), 122–134. https://link.springer.com/article/10.1007/s12072-017-9815-0

Robertson, D. (2021). Advanced health assessment of the respiratory system. In K.M. Myrick & L.M. Karosas (Eds.), *Advanced health assessment and differential diagnosis: Essentials for clinical practice* (pp. 207–237). Springer Publishing Company.

Sachdiva, K. (2021, February 19). *Renal cell carcinoma differential diagnoses.* https://emedicine.medscape.com/article/281340-differential

Seller, R. H., & Symons, A. B. (2018). *Differential diagnosis of common complaints.* Elsevier.

Siddiqui, F., & Siddiqui, A. H. (2020, November 20). *Lung cancer.* https://www.ncbi.nlm.nih.gov/books/NBK482357/

Sinibaldi, V. J., Pratz, C. F., & Yankulina, O. (2018). Kidney cancer: Toxicity management, symptom control, and palliative care. *Journal of Clinical Oncology, 36*(36), 3632–3638. https://doi.org/10.1200/JCO.2018.79.0188

Small, A. (2021). Advanced health assessment of the abdomen, rectum, and anus. In K.M. Myrick & L. M. Karosas (Eds.), *Advanced health assessment and differential diagnosis: Essentials for clinical practice* (pp. 207–237). Springer Publishing Company.

Sommers, M. S. (2019). *Davis's diseases and disorders: A nursing therapeutics manual* (6th ed.). F.A. Davis Co.

Watson, M., Campbell, R., Vallath, N., Ward, S., & Wells, J. (2019). *Oxford handbook of palliative care.* Oxford University Press.

Wright, P. M. (2019). *Certified hospice and palliative nurse (CHPN®) exam review.* Springer Publishing Company.

TABLE 6A.1   DIAGNOSTIC TESTS FOR CANCERS OF THE CHEST AND ABDOMEN

TYPE	NOTES
Physical examination	• Thorough physical examination with focused system assessment
Imaging	• Mammogram, ultrasound (with or without elastography), breast MRI, breast tomosynthesis (3D mammography), MBI, also called scintimammography or BSGI, PEM, CEM, also known as CESM, EIT (breast) • CT or CAT scan with contrast (lung, liver, pancreatic, renal, stomach) • PET scan (bladder, lung, pancreatic, stomach) • Invasive staging bronchoscopic ultrasound-TBNA, endoscopic TBNA, mediastinoscopy thoracoscopy VATS (lung) • Ultrasound (liver, renal, pancreatic) • MRI (liver, pancreatic, renal, bladder, stomach) • ERCP, PTC (pancreatic) • Endoscopy of the colon (colorectal) • X-ray (bladder, renal, stomach) • Cystoscopy and nephro-ureteroscopy (renal) • Cystoscopy, CT urogram, or retrograde pyelogram (bladder) • Bone scan (bladder) • Upper endoscopy, upper gastrointestinal series, endoscopic ultrasound, esophagogastroduodenoscopy (stomach)
Laboratory tests	• Biomarkers (lung cancer) • AFP test, LFTs, hepatitis B and C antibody testing, coagulation testing (e.g., CBC, fibrinogen level, factor-V assay, prothrombin time, platelet count)—liver • Tumor marker antigen; CA 19-9, bilirubin level (pancreatic) • Fecal occult blood test (colorectal, stomach) • Serum CEA (lung, breast, liver, pancreas, stomach, colorectal, bladder) • Urinalysis (renal cancer) • CBC • CMP • Urine cytology (bladder)
Pathology	• Biopsy (fine needle, open, or core biopsy) • Bronchoscopy biopsy, thoracentesis, sputum cytology (lung) • Liver biopsy (liver) • Molecular testing of the tumor (pancreatic) • Biopsy (HER2 testing)—stomach

(continued)

TABLE 6A.1   DIAGNOSTIC TESTS FOR CANCERS OF THE CHEST AND ABDOMEN (*CONTINUED*)

TYPE	NOTES
Disease staging	<ul><li>TNM tumor staging (see Appendix C-7)</li><li>The BCLC system (liver; see Figure 6.5)</li><li>The CLIP system (liver; see Table 6.2)</li><li>The Okuda system (liver; see Table 6.4)</li><li>Stages 1–4 (colon; see Figure 6.7)</li><li>Stages 1–4 (renal; see Figure 6.8)</li><li>Stages 1–4 (bladder; see Figure 6.9)</li></ul>

AFP, alpha-fetoprotein blood; BCLC, Barcelona Clinic Liver Cancer; BSGI, breast-specific gamma imaging; CA, cancer; CBC, complete blood count; CEA, carcinoembryonic antigen; CEM, contrast-enhanced mammography; CESM, contrast-enhanced spectral mammography; CLIP, Cancer of the Liver Italian Program; CMP, complete metabolic profile; EIT, electrical impedance imaging; ERCP, endoscopic retrograde cholangiopancreatography; LFTs, liver function tests; MBI, molecular breast imaging; PEM, positron emission mammography; PTC, percutaneous transhepatic cholangiography; TBNA, transbronchial needle aspiration; VATS, video-assisted thoracoscopy; TNM, tumor, node, metastasis.

Sources: American Cancer Society. (2021a). *Cancer A to Z.* https://www.cancer.org/cancer.html; American Cancer Society. (2021b). *Melanoma skin cancer.* https://www.cancer.org/cancer/melanoma-skin-cancer.html; American Cancer Society. (2022). *Early detection, diagnosis, and staging.* https://www.cancer.org/cancer/liver-cancer/detection-diagnosis-staging/how-diagnosed.html; American Liver Foundation. (2017). *Liver cancer.* https://liverfoundation.org/for-patients/about-the-liver/diseases-of-the-liver/liver-cancer/#symptoms-of-liver-cancer; American Society of Clinical Oncology. (2021). *Types of cancer.* https://www.cancer.net/cancer-types; Hubert, R. J., & VanMeter, K. C. (2018). *Gould's pathophysiology for the health professions* (6th ed). Elsevier Inc.; Mayo Clinic. (2021a). *Diseases and conditions.* https://www.mayoclinic.org/diseases-conditions; Mayo Clinic. (2021b). *Leukemia.* https://www.mayoclinic.org/diseases-conditions/leukemia/diagnosis-treatment/drc-20374378; Siddiqui, F., & Siddiqui, A. H. (2020, November 20). *Lung cancer.* https://www.ncbi.nlm.nih.gov/books/NBK482357/; Sommers, M. S. (2019). *Davis's diseases and disorders: A nursing therapeutics manual* (6th ed). F.A. Davis Co.

TABLE 6A.2   PALLIATIVE INTERVENTIONS/SYMPTOM MANAGEMENT FOR CANCERS OF THE CHEST AND ABDOMEN

SYMPTOM	INTERVENTION
Anorexia	<ul><li>Use of appetite stimulants (see Appendix D-1)</li><li>Offer small, frequent meals and snacks</li><li>Offer nutritional supplements</li></ul>
Anxiety and depression	<ul><li>Antidepressants, anxiolytics, or benzodiazepines as indicated by patient's condition, age, and life expectancy (see Appendix D)</li><li>Non-pharmacological interventions</li></ul>
Ascites (see Figure 6.6)	<ul><li>Abdominal ultrasound (liver, pancreatic, stomach)</li><li>Paracentesis with peritoneal fluid analysis (liver, pancreatic, stomach)</li><li>PleurX drain for ascites if patient is homebound (liver, pancreatic, stomach)</li><li>Albumin infusion if indicated (liver, pancreatic, stomach)</li><li>Diuretics (liver, pancreatic, stomach; see Appendix D-1)</li></ul>
Bile duct obstruction	<ul><li>Endoscopic retrograde cholangiopancreatography (liver, pancreatic, stomach)</li><li>Chemotherapy (liver, pancreatic, stomach; see Figure 5.2)</li><li>Radiation therapy (liver, pancreatic, stomach)</li><li>Stent placement, if possible (liver, pancreatic, stomach)</li></ul>
Bleeding (hematemesis, melena, anemia)	<ul><li>Stent placement (liver, stomach)</li><li>Cauterization (liver, stomach)</li></ul>
Bone-modifying interventions (see Appendix D-1)	<ul><li>Bisphosphonates to strengthen bones and reduce bone loss (breast)</li></ul>

(continued)

TABLE 6A.2   PALLIATIVE INTERVENTIONS/SYMPTOM MANAGEMENT FOR CANCERS OF THE CHEST AND ABDOMEN (*CONTINUED*)

SYMPTOM	INTERVENTION
Bowel dysfunction	• Management of constipation and/or diarrhea (colon) • Management of proctitis (colon) • Anti-inflammatory medications (colon; see Appendix D-1)
Bowel obstruction	• Surgery to remove or debulk tumor (colon, stomach) • Bowel rest (colon, stomach) • Bowel decompression (colon, stomach) • Placement of nasogastric tube to reduce gastric pressure (colon, stomach)
Dyspnea (see Appendix D)	• Corticosteroids for reducing inflammation (breast, lung) • Opioids to reduce inspiratory effort and tachypnea (breast, lung) • Bronchodilators for opening airways (mechanism of action of relaxation of muscular bands that surround bronchi, thus widening the airway)—breast, lung • Diuretics to reduce systemic congestion (breast, lung) • Anticholinergics to reduce secretions, especially at the end of life (breast, lung) • Use of fans (breast, lung) • Lower temperature in the room (breast, lung)
Fatigue and somnolence	• Alternate periods of rest with periods of activity • Utilize energy conversation techniques • Psychostimulants (see Appendix D)
Hepatic encephalopathy (see Table 6.3)	• Lactulose (liver; see Appendix D, diuretics) • Antibiotic therapy (liver) • Polyethylene glycol (liver)
Insomnia (see Appendix D)	• Use of benzodiazepines, antidepressants, or antihistaminic agents, as indicated by patient's condition, age, and life expectancy • Provide proper sleep hygiene • Use non-pharmacological interventions for relaxation • Address underlying anxiety and depression
Intractable hematuria	• Orally administered epsilon-aminocaproic acid (bladder, renal) • Intravesical formalin (bladder, renal) • Alum or prostaglandin irrigation (bladder, renal) • Urinary diversion (bladder, renal) • Radiation therapy (bladder, renal) • Embolization (bladder, renal) • Intra-arterial mitoxantrone perfusion (bladder, renal)
Lymphedema	• Topical application of emollients containing lactic acid, urea, ceramides, glycerin, dimethicone, olive oil, or salicylic acid • Frequently assess for and promptly treat secondary infection • Use of topical steroids if skin becomes inflamed • Silver-containing polymer dressing for ulcers associated with primary lymphedema • Frequent dressing changes if lymphorrhea (drainage of lymphatic fluid directly through the skin) occurs to prevent skin breakdown • Application of low-pressure (40–60 mmHg) compression therapy • Physical and/or occupational therapy to increase muscle mass and stimulate lymphatic flow • Assess and treat pain associated with limb heaviness, fluid retention, and immobility • Address body image issues related to lymphedema

(continued)

TABLE 6A.2   PALLIATIVE INTERVENTIONS/SYMPTOM MANAGEMENT FOR CANCERS OF THE CHEST AND ABDOMEN (*CONTINUED*)

SYMPTOM	INTERVENTION
Nausea	• Antiemetics (see Appendix D-1) • Non-pharmacological interventions (see Appendix D-2)
Pain management	• See Appendix E
Psychosocial distress/body image changes	• Antidepressants • Non-pharmacological interventions (see Appendix D-2)
Renal/cancer-induced anemia	• Iron supplementation (bladder, renal) • ESA (bladder, renal) • Red blood cell transfusions (in refractory cases when patient is symptomatic; bladder, renal)
Tumor reduction	• Palliative chemotherapy (stomach; see Figure 5.3 in Chapter 5) • Palliative radiation (stomach) • Surgical interventions (if indicated; stomach)
Urinary fistulas	• Urinary drainage (bladder) • Pain management (bladder) • Incontinence care (bladder) • Bowel rest with intravenous hyperalimentation (bladder) • Use of a somatostatin analog, such as octreotide (bladder; see Appendix D-1) • Surgical interventions such as reconstruction, ileostomy, colostomy, urostomy, or stenting, depending on the patient's prognosis and ability to tolerate anesthesia (bladder)
Ureteral obstruction	• Review medications and reduce dose or discontinue those that cause urinary retention, if possible (anticholinergics, antidepressants, antihistamines, antipsychotics, muscle relaxants)—bladder • Insert urinary catheter, if possible. If not possible, placement of a suprapubic catheter may be necessary (bladder) • If obstruction is due to prostate enlargement, consider use of tamsulosin or finasteride (bladder) • Consider palliative TURP, if appropriate (bladder) • Monitor for post-obstructive diuresis and replace fluids orally or intravenously (bladder)

ESA, erythropoiesis-stimulating agents; TURP, transurethral prostatectomy.

Source: Abt, D., Bywater, M., Engeler, D. S., & Schmid, H. P. (2013). Therapeutic options for intractable hematuria in advanced bladder cancer. *International Journal of Urology, 20*(7), 651–660. https://doi.org/10.1111/iju.12113; Center to Advance Palliative Care. (2021). *Disease types and palliative care.* https://getpalliativecare.org/whatis/disease-types/; Guyer, D. L., Almhanna, K., & McKee, K. Y. (2020). Palliative care for patients with esophageal cancer: A narrative review. *Annals of Translational Medicine, 8*(17). https://doi.org.10.21037/atm-20-3676; Kluger, B. M., Ney, D. E., Bagley, S. J., Mohile, N., Taylor, L. P., Walbert, T., & Jones, C. A. (2020). Top ten tips palliative care clinicians should know when caring for patients with brain cancer. *Journal of Palliative Medicine, 23*(3), 415–421. https://doi.org/10.1089/jpm.2019.0507; Mahar, A. L., Coburn, N. G., Karanicolas, P. J., Viola, R., & Helyer, L. K. (2012). Effective palliation and quality of life outcomes in studies of surgery for advanced, non-curative gastric cancer: a systematic review. *Gastric Cancer, 15*(1), 138–145. https://doi.org/10.1200/JCO.2014.55.1143; Mazzarelli, C., Prentice, W. M., Heneghan, M. A., Belli, L. S., Agarwal, K., & Cannon, M. D. (2018). Palliative care in end-stage liver disease: Time to do better? *Liver Transplantation, 24*(7), 961–968.; Piano, S., Tonon, M., & Angeli, P. (2018). Management of ascites and hepatorenal syndrome. *Hepatology International, 12*(1), 122–134. https://link.springer.com/article/10.1007/s12072-017-9815-0; Sinibaldi, V. J., Pratz, C. F., & Yankulina, O. (2018). Kidney cancer: Toxicity management, symptom control, and palliative care. *Journal of Clinical Oncology, 36*(36), 3632–3638. https://doi.org/10.1200/JCO.2018.79.0188; Sommers, M. S. (2019). *Davis's diseases and disorders: A nursing therapeutics manual* (6th ed.). F.A. Davis Co.

CHAPTER 7

CANCERS OF THE REPRODUCTIVE SYSTEM

CERVICAL CANCER

DEFINITION/CHARACTERISTICS
A. Malignancy that originates in the cells that line the cervix.
B. The two most common types are:
   1. Squamous cell carcinoma.
   2. Adenocarcinoma (American Cancer Society, 2021).

INCIDENCE AND PREVALENCE
A. There are approximately 14,000 new cases annually.
B. Cervical cancer represents about 0.8% of all new cancer cases each year.
C. Most common in women 35 to 55 years of age (Johnson et al., 2019; National Cancer Institute, 2023; Sommers, 2019).

ETIOLOGY
A. Human papillomavirus (HPV) is associated with most cases of cervical cancer.
B. Subtypes HPV 16 and 18 together account for over 60% of all cases.
C. Up to 80% of women will become infected with HPV at some point in their lives (Johnson et al., 2019; Mayo Clinic, 2021b).

PATHOPHYSIOLOGY
A. HPV is often contracted in adolescence or early adulthood.
B. Because cervical cancer is often asymptomatic, it may take a decade or more before cervical changes and symptoms emerge.
C. Cervical changes are typically detected on Pap test.
D. If left untreated, cervical cancer can metastasize into adjacent tissue or to distant sites.
E. Metastasis to distant sites occurs through the lymphatic system (Johnson et al., 2019; Sommers, 2019).

PREDISPOSING FACTORS
A. Multiple sexual partners.
B. History of sexually transmitted infections such as gonorrhea and chlamydia.
C. Immunodeficiency.
D. Tobacco use.
E. History of cervicitis.
F. Prenatal exposure to diethylstilbestrol (DES).
G. Long-term use of oral contraceptives (>5 years).
H. Family or personal history of cervical cancer.
I. First pregnancy before age 17 years.
J. Personal history of more than four pregnancies.
K. Latina and Black women are at highest risk.
L. Women of lower socioeconomic status are at heightened risk (Johnson et al., 2019; Mayo Clinic, 2021b; Sommers, 2019).

SUBJECTIVE DATA
A. Often asymptomatic.
B. In advanced disease, pelvic or lower pain that radiates to the back of the legs.
C. Fatigue (Johnson et al., 2019).

OBJECTIVE DATA
A. Abnormal menstrual bleeding.
B. Increased vaginal discharge.
C. Painful intercourse.
D. Hematuria.
E. Hematochezia.
F. Unintentional weight loss.
G. Lymphedema.
H. Vaginal passage of urine or stool (Johnson et al., 2019; Mayo Clinic, 2021b).

DIAGNOSTIC TESTS
A. See Appendix Table 7A.1 for listing of common diagnostic tests.
B. See Figure 7.1 for the FIGO staging system.

DIFFERENTIAL DIAGNOSES
A. Cervicitis/infection.
B. Primary melanoma and Paget disease.
C. Vaginal cancer.
D. Endometrial carcinoma.
E. Pelvic inflammatory disease.
F. Vaginitis (Boardman, 2021).

POTENTIAL COMPLICATIONS
A. Acute complications of advanced cancer (see Appendix C-7).
B. Bowel obstruction.

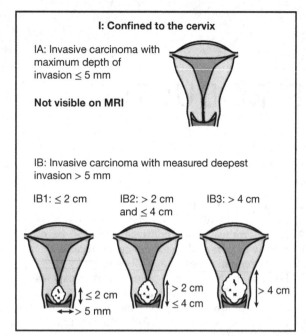

I: Confined to the cervix

IA: Invasive carcinoma with maximum depth of invasion ≤ 5 mm

Not visible on MRI

IB: Invasive carcinoma with measured deepest invasion > 5 mm

IB1: ≤ 2 cm   IB2: > 2 cm and ≤ 4 cm   IB3: > 4 cm

≤ 2 cm   > 2 cm ≤ 4 cm   > 4 cm

> 5 mm

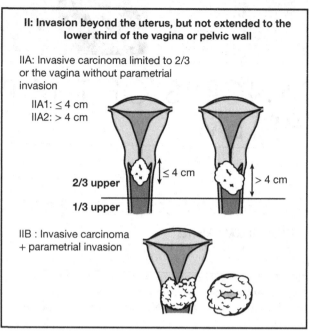

II: Invasion beyond the uterus, but not extended to the lower third of the vagina or pelvic wall

IIA: Invasive carcinoma limited to 2/3 or the vagina without parametrial invasion

IIA1: ≤ 4 cm
IIA2: > 4 cm

2/3 upper   ≤ 4 cm   > 4 cm

1/3 upper

IIB : Invasive carcinoma + parametrial invasion

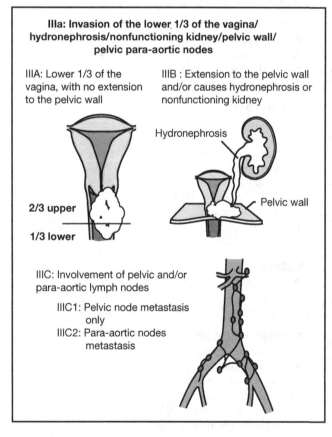

IIIa: Invasion of the lower 1/3 of the vagina/ hydronephrosis/nonfunctioning kidney/pelvic wall/ pelvic para-aortic nodes

IIIA: Lower 1/3 of the vagina, with no extension to the pelvic wall

IIIB : Extension to the pelvic wall and/or causes hydronephrosis or nonfunctioning kidney

Hydronephrosis

Pelvic wall

2/3 upper

1/3 lower

IIIC: Involvement of pelvic and/or para-aortic lymph nodes

IIIC1: Pelvic node metastasis only
IIIC2: Para-aortic nodes metastasis

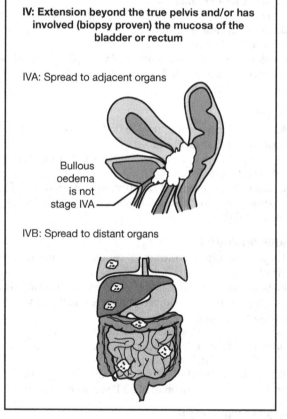

IV: Extension beyond the true pelvis and/or has involved (biopsy proven) the mucosa of the bladder or rectum

IVA: Spread to adjacent organs

Bullous oedema is not stage IVA

IVB: Spread to distant organs

FIGURE 7.1 FIGO staging system.

Source: Adapted from Manganaro, L., Lakhman, Y., Bharwani, N., Gui, B., Gigli, S., Vinci, V., Rizzo, S., Kido, A., Cunha, T. M., Sala, E., Rockall, A., Forstner, R., & Nougaret, S. (2021). Staging, recurrence and follow-up of uterine cervical cancer using MRI: Updated Guidelines of the European Society of Urogenital Radiology after revised FIGO staging 2018. *European Radiology*, 1–15. https://link.springer.com/article/10.1007/s00330-020-07632-9

C. Urinary obstruction.
D. Sexual dysfunction.
E. Fecal urgency and incontinence.
F. Incomplete bowel emptying.
G. Metastasis to the:
  1. Liver.
  2. Lung.
  3. Peritoneum (Johnson et al., 2019; Sommers, 2019; Wright, 2019).

DISEASE-MODIFYING TREATMENTS
A. Loop electrosurgical excision procedure (LEEP).
B. Partial or total hysterectomy.
C. Pelvic lymph node dissection.
D. Para-aortic lymphadenectomy.
E. Sentinel lymph node mapping.
F. Pelvic exenteration.
G. Radiation.
H. Chemotherapy (see Figure 5.2 in Chapter 5).
I. Immunotherapy (Johns Hopkins Medicine, 2021; Johnson et al., 2019).

PALLIATIVE INTERVENTIONS/SYMPTOM MANAGEMENT
A. See Appendix Table 7A.2 for listing of palliative interventions and symptom management.
B. See Appendix D-3 for overview of common symptoms.

PROGNOSIS
A. The 5-year survival rate is 66.3%.
B. Prognosis is improved when detected early.
C. Routine Pap tests improve chance of early detection.
D. Vaccination reduces risk of cervical cancer (98% effective; Centers for Disease Control and Prevention, 2020; Johnson et al., 2019; National Cancer Institute, 2023).

NURSING INTERVENTIONS
A. Teach patient to report pain and other symptoms promptly.
B. Educate patient to take all medications as prescribed.
C. Implement interventions for lymphedema.
D. Implement interventions for incontinence and for protection of skin.
E. Teach smoking cessation interventions (see Appendices B-10 and C-9).
F. Educate patient and family regarding disease trajectory (see Appendix B-1).
G. Provide spiritual support.
H. Assess caregiver fatigue/burnout (see Appendix B-5).
I. Encourage completion of advance directives.
J. Educate patient and family regarding availability of palliative care.
K. Educate patient and family regarding availability of hospice services (when appropriate).

OVARIAN CANCER

DEFINITION/CHARACTERISTICS
A. Malignancy that originates in the epithelium of the ovaries.
B. Types of ovarian cancer:
  1. Epithelial tumors: begin in the tissue that covers the ovaries (most common type).
  2. Stromal tumors: begin in hormone-producing cells.
  3. Germ cell tumors: begin in egg-producing cells.
C. About 20% of ovarian cancers are diagnosed at an early stage.
D. Extra-ovarian primary peritoneal carcinoma is closely related to ovarian cancer. It occurs in the peritoneum; women with a history of oophorectomy are still at risk for this type of cancer (American Cancer Society, 2021; Johns Hopkins Medicine, 2021; Mayo Clinic, 2021b; Sommers, 2019).

INCIDENCE AND PREVALENCE
A. There are approximately 21,000 new cases annually.
B. Most originate in the fallopian tube.
C. White women are at higher risk.
D. Ovarian cancer is the primary cause of death from reproductive cancers in women (American Society of Clinical Oncology, 2021; Sommers, 2019).

ETIOLOGY
A. The exact etiology is unknown (American Cancer Society, 2021; Mayo Clinic, 2021a).

PATHOPHYSIOLOGY
A. Cell mutations cause proliferation of abnormal cells and rapid cell growth.
B. Once malignant cells begin to multiply, metastasis can occur to nearby tissues and organs as well as distant sites (Mayo Clinic, 2021b).

PREDISPOSING FACTORS
A. Advanced age.
B. Obesity.
C. Nulliparity.
D. Infertility.
E. Hormonal therapy after menopause.
F. Personal or family history of breast, ovarian, or colorectal cancer.
G. Genetic predisposition.
H. Estrogen hormone replacement therapy.
I. Early menarche.
J. Late menopause.
K. Celibacy.
L. Exposure to asbestos and talc (American Cancer Society, 2021; Mayo Clinic, 2021a; Sommers, 2019).

SUBJECTIVE DATA

A. Nausea.
B. Frequent gas.
C. Indigestion.
D. Dyspnea.
E. Early satiety
F. Abdominal pain that resembles appendicitis.
G. Back pain.
H. Fatigue.
I. Pelvic pressure.
J. Urinary frequency and urgency.
K. Painful intercourse.
L. Pelvic discomfort and/or cramping (American Cancer Society, 2021; Johns Hopkins Medicine, 2021; Mayo Clinic, 2021a; Sommers, 2019).

OBJECTIVE DATA

A. Abdominal bloating.
B. Constipation.
C. Diarrhea.
D. Vaginal bleeding.
E. Unintentional weight loss.
F. Wasting of extremities.
G. Palpable enlarged of nodular ovaries.
H. Late stage: malignant pleural effusion (American Cancer Society, 2021; Johns Hopkins Medicine, 2021; Mayo Clinic, 2021b; Sommers, 2019).

DIAGNOSTIC TESTS

A. See Appendix Table 7A.1 for listing of common diagnostic tests.

DIFFERENTIAL DIAGNOSES

A. Appendiceal tumors.
B. Benign lesions of the uterine corpus.
C. Bladder distention/urinary retention.
D. Bowel/omental adhesions.
E. Colon cancer.
F. Fecal impaction.
G. Metastatic gastrointestinal carcinoma.
H. Ovarian torsion.
I. Pelvic abscess.
J. Peritoneal cyst.
K. Uterine anomalies.
L. Uterine fibroids.
M. Adnexal tumors.
N. Anovulation.
O. Appendicitis.
P. Cervicitis.
Q. Colon cancer.
R. Bowel obstruction.
S. Ectopic pregnancy.
T. Endometriosis.
U. Gastric cancer.
V. Irritable bowel syndrome (IBS).
W. Ovarian cysts.
X. Pelvic inflammatory disease.
Y. Peritoneal cancer.
Z. Urinary tract obstruction.
AA. Uterine cancer (Green, 2022; Shetty, 2019).

POTENTIAL COMPLICATIONS

A. Acute complications of advanced cancer (see Appendix C-7).
B. Metastasis to the:
   1. Liver.
   2. Lung(s).
   3. Peritoneum.
C. Malignant ascites.
D. Malignant pleural effusion.
E. Infection or sepsis.
F. Bowel obstruction.
G. Ileus.
H. Peripheral edema.
I. Ascites.
J. Pneumonia (Miller & Nevadunsky, 2018; Sommers, 2019).

DISEASE-MODIFYING TREATMENTS

A. Chemotherapy (see Figure 5.2 in Chapter 5).
B. Radiation.
C. Targeted therapies.
D. Immunotherapies.
E. Clinical trials (Sommers, 2019).

PALLIATIVE INTERVENTIONS/SYMPTOM MANAGEMENT

A. See Appendix Table 7A.2 for listing of palliative interventions and symptom management.
B. See Appendix D-3 for overview of common symptoms.

PROGNOSIS

A. The overall 5-year survival rate is 49%.
B. For women over the age of 65 years, the 5-year survival rate is 32%.
C. For women younger than 65 years, the 5-year survival rate is 61%.
D. If diagnosed and treated before the cancer metastasizes, the 5-year survival rate is 93%. Only 16% of cases are identified at this stage.
E. If ovarian cancer is diagnosed after metastasis to nearby organs or tissues, the 5-year survival rate is 75%.
F. If diagnosed after metastasis to a distant body part, the 5-year survival rate is 30%. Approximately 58% of cases are diagnosed at this stage.
G. If brain metastasis has occurred, the prognosis is between 2 weeks to 9 months.
H. If multiple areas of metastasis are present, the prognosis is very poor.
I. If bowel obstruction has occurred, the prognosis is weeks to months (American Society of Clinical Oncology, 2021; Miller & Nevadunsky, 2018).

NURSING INTERVENTIONS

A. Teach patient to report pain and other symptoms promptly.
B. Educate patient to take all medications as prescribed. ▶

C. Implement interventions for lymphedema.
D. Implement interventions for incontinence and for protection of skin.
E. Teach smoking cessation interventions (see Appendices B-10 and C-9).
F. Educate patient and family regarding disease trajectory (see Appendix B-1).
G. Provide spiritual support.
H. Assess caregiver fatigue/burnout (see Appendix B-5).
I. Encourage completion of advance directives.
J. Educate patient and family regarding availability of palliative care.
K. Educate patient and family regarding availability of hospice services (when appropriate).
L. Provide referral to community support groups, as needed.

UTERINE CANCER

DEFINITION/CHARACTERISTICS
A. Malignancy that arises within the cells of the uterus.
B. There are two types:
    1. Endometrial cancer (common).
    2. Uterine sarcoma (rare).
C. Uterine cancer is the most common reproductive cancer in women (National Cancer Institute, 2021a).

INCIDENCE AND PREVALENCE
A. There are over 66,000 new cases each year.
B. Uterine cancers make up about 3.5% of all new cancer cases annually (National Cancer Institute, 2021a).

ETIOLOGY
A. The etiology is unknown.
B. May be associated with endogenous or exogenous hormone levels (Sommers, 2019).

PATHOPHYSIOLOGY
A. Disease begins with mutations in the uterine cells.
B. Malignant cells coalesce into a tumor that can then metastasize to other areas (American Society of Clinical Oncology, 2021).

PREDISPOSING FACTORS
A. Genetic predisposition.
B. Risk factors include:
    1. Age over 50 years; peak age of diagnosis is 58 to 60.
    2. Race (White women are at increased risk).
    3. Diabetes.
    4. Obesity.
    5. Metabolic syndrome.
    6. Hypothyroidism.
    7. History of retinoblastoma.
    8. Personal or family history of breast, colon, or ovarian cancers.
    9. Endometrial hyperplasia.
    10. Polycystic ovary syndrome (PCOS).
    11. Ovarian tumors.
    12. Tamoxifen use.
    13. Personal history of radiation to abdomen or pelvis.
    14. Use of estrogen.
    15. Early menarche (before age 12).
    16. Late menopause (after age 52).
    17. Nulliparity (American Society of Clinical Oncology, 2021; Cancer Treatment Centers of America, 2021; Sommers, 2019).

SUBJECTIVE DATA
A. Pelvic pain.
B. Abnormal, painless, vaginal bleeding (American Society for Clinical Oncology, 2021; Sommers, 2019).

OBJECTIVE DATA
A. Fever.
B. Abnormal Pap test.
C. Abnormal vaginal bleeding or discharge.
D. Mucosanguineous, odorous vaginal discharge (late stage).
E. Weight loss (late stage).
F. Bowel or bladder dysfunction (late stage).
G. Dyspareunia (American Society of Clinical Oncology, 2021; Sommers, 2019).

DIAGNOSTIC TESTS
A. See Appendix Table 7A.1 for listing of common diagnostic tests.

DIFFERENTIAL DIAGNOSES
A. Endometriosis.
B. Fibroids.
C. Adenomyosis.
D. Ovulatory dysfunction.
E. Endometrial polyp.
F. Endometrial hyperplasia.
G. Hematometra.
H. Incomplete abortion.
I. Uterine lymphoma (Brenner, 1996; Faizan & Muppidi, 2020).

POTENTIAL COMPLICATIONS
A. Acute complication of advanced cancer (see Appendix C-7).
B. Metastasis to the:
    1. Pelvic organs or bony structures.
    2. Para-aortic nodes.
    3. Peritoneum.
    4. Lungs.
C. Bowel obstruction.
D. Severe radiation enterocolitis (treatment-related).
E. Refractory and severe lower extremity edema (Gupta et al., 2014; Wright, 2019).

DISEASE-MODIFYING TREATMENTS
A. Partial or total hysterectomy.
B. Salpingo-oophorectomy.
C. Radiation.

▶

D. Chemotherapy (see Figure 5.2 in Chapter 5).
E. Hormone therapy.
F. Targeted drug therapy.
G. Immunotherapy (Mayo Clinic, 2021b).

PALLIATIVE INTERVENTIONS/SYMPTOM MANAGEMENT

A. See Appendix Table 7A.2 for listing of palliative interventions and symptom management.
B. See Appendix D-3 for overview of common symptoms.

PROGNOSIS

A. The 5-year survival rate is 81.1%.
B. Uterine sarcoma is often aggressive with a poor prognosis.
C. Endometrial cancer is often curable.
D. Prognosis increases with early detection. When uterine cancer is detected prior to metastasis, the survival rate is 95%.
E. If uterine cancer has metastasized regionally, the survival rate is 69%.
F. If uterine cancer has spread to distant sites, the survival rate is 17% (National Cancer Institute, 2021a).

NURSING INTERVENTIONS

A. Teach patient to report pain and other symptoms promptly.
B. Implement pain and symptom management interventions.
C. Educate patient to take all medications as prescribed.
D. Teach deep breathing and relaxation techniques.
E. Encourage smoking cessation (see Appendices B-10 and C-9).
F. Implement interventions for incontinence and for protection of skin.
G. Monitor for fistulas and urinary obstruction and implement corrective measures as appropriate.
H. Educate patient and family regarding disease trajectory (see Appendix B-1).
I. Provide spiritual support.
J. Assess caregiver fatigue/burnout (see Appendix B-5).
K. Encourage completion of advance directives.
L. Educate patient and family regarding availability of palliative care.
M. Educate patient and family regarding availability of hospice services (when appropriate).
N. Provide referral to community support groups, as needed.

PENILE CANCER

DEFINITION/CHARACTERISTICS

A. Malignancy that arises in the cells of the penis.
B. Often begins as squamous cell carcinoma, and this type accounts for nearly 95% of all penile cancers.
C. Other types include:
  1. Sarcoma.
  2. Melanoma.
  3. Basal cell carcinoma (Ratini, 2022).

INCIDENCE AND PREVALENCE

A. Rare in the United States and Europe; accounts for only 0.2% of cancers in these areas (1 in 100,00 men are affected).
B. Most common in Africa and South Africa where it accounts for up to 10% of cancers (Rodway & McCance, 2019).

ETIOLOGY

A. Exact etiology is unknown (Ratini, 2022).

PATHOPHYSIOLOGY

A. Penile cancer often begins as squamous cell carcinoma involving small, fat, ulcerative, or papillary lesions on the glans or foreskin.
B. If left untreated, it can metastasize to the penile shaft (Rodway & McCance, 2019).

PREDISPOSING FACTORS

A. Age over 55.
B. History of human papillomavirus (HPV) infection.
C. Exposure to ultraviolet light (most commonly related to treatment for psoriasis).
D. HIV infection or AIDS.
E. Uncircumcised penis (circumcision at birth reduces risk of penile cancer by up to 50%).
F. Phimosis (Rodway & McCance, 2019).

SUBJECTIVE DATA

A. Pain is a late sign and is associated with poorer outcomes (Rodway & McCance, 2019).

OBJECTIVE DATA

A. Leukoplakia (thick, white plaque generally noticed at the meatus).
B. Red, inflamed areas of the penis or glans.
C. Ulcerative lesions noted on the glans or penis.
D. Red encrustations of Bowen disease.
E. In situ carcinoma that affects the penile shaft (Rodway & McCance, 2019).

DIAGNOSTIC TESTS

A. See Appendix Table 7A.1 for listing of common diagnostic tests.

DIFFERENTIAL DIAGNOSES

A. Sexually transmitted infections.
B. Benign mass.
C. Erythroplasia of Queyrat.
D. Leukoplakia.
E. Bowen disease.
F. Psoriasis (Chipollini et al., 2019; Rodway & McCance, 2019).

POTENTIAL COMPLICATIONS

A. Acute complications of advanced cancer (see Appendix C-7).

B. Metastasis to the:

1. Bladder.
2. Prostate.
3. Rectum.
4. Kidneys (Rodway & McCance, 2019).

DISEASE-MODIFYING TREATMENTS

A. Circumcision in low-risk neoplasms.

B. Mohs micrographic surgery for small, superficial shaft lesions.

C. For more extensive lesions, a wide, local excision is necessary with a margin of a few millimeters, up to 2 cm.

D. In advanced disease, a glansectomy or partial or total penectomy may be required (Chipollini et al., 2019; Rodway & McCance, 2019).

PALLIATIVE INTERVENTIONS/SYMPTOM MANAGEMENT

A. See Appendix Table 7A.2 for listing of palliative interventions and symptom management.

B. See Appendix D-3 for overview of common symptoms.

PROGNOSIS

A. Extensive metastasis is associated with poorer prognosis.

B. Early squamous cell lesions are easily treated, but often ignored, leading to more advanced disease at the time of diagnosis.

C. About 30% of penile cancers have spread to nearby lymph nodes by the time of diagnosis.

D. When the cancer is confined to the penis, the 5-year survival rate is approximately 85%.

E. When the cancer has metastasized to nearby tissues or lymph nodes, the 5-year survival rate is approximately 59% (Rodway & McCance, 2019).

NURSING INTERVENTIONS

A. Individualize plan of care to patient's lifestyle needs.

B. Implement interventions for pain and symptoms management.

C. Educate patient to take all medications as prescribed.

D. Teach deep breathing and relaxation techniques.

E. Encourage smoking cessation (see Appendices B-10 and C-9).

F. Educate patient and family regarding disease trajectory (see Appendix B-1).

G. Provide spiritual support.

H. Assess caregiver fatigue/burnout (see Appendix B-5).

I. Encourage completion of advance directives.

J. Educate patient and family regarding availability of palliative care.

K. Educate patient and family regarding availability of hospice services (when appropriate).

L. Provide referral to community support groups, as needed.

PROSTATE CANCER

DEFINITION/CHARACTERISTICS

A. Malignancy that arises in the cells of the prostate.

B. Nearly all prostate cancers are adenocarcinomas.

C. Other types include:

1. Small cell carcinomas.
2. Neuroendocrine tumors.
3. Transitional cell carcinomas.
4. Sarcomas.

D. Median age of diagnosis is 66 years.

E. Prostate cancer is the second most common type of cancer in men (National Cancer Institute, 2021b).

INCIDENCE AND PREVALENCE

A. There are over 248,000 new cases diagnosed annually.

B. Prostate cancer represents 13% of all cancers.

C. Adenocarcinomas account for >95% of all prostate cancers.

D. Deaths from prostate cancer represent about 5% of all cancer deaths annually (National Cancer Institute, 2021b; Sommers, 2019).

ETIOLOGY

A. Exact etiology is unknown (National Cancer Institute, 2021b; Sommers, 2019).

PATHOPHYSIOLOGY

A. May begin with a condition called prostatic intraepithelial neoplasia (PIN).

B. Typically, prostate cancer is initially identified in the outer portion of the posterior lobe in the glandular cells of the prostate gland.

C. Local metastasis first occurs in the seminal vesicles, bladder, and/or peritoneum.

D. Metastasis occurs to distant sites via the hematologic and lymphatic systems.

E. The pelvic and perivesicular lymph nodes and bones of the pelvis, sacrum, and lumbar spine are the first sites affected by distant metastasis followed by metastasis to the lungs, liver, and kidneys (National Cancer Institute, 2021b; Sommers, 2019).

PREDISPOSING FACTORS

A. Age over 50

B. Race (African Americans have higher risk).

C. Family history.

D. Cigarette smoking.

E. High-fat diet.

F. Overuse of alcohol.

G. Exposure to Agent Orange.

H. Environmental exposure to cadmium.
I. Prostatitis.
J. High-grade PIN.
K. First-degree relative diagnosed with prostate cancer before the age of 65 (National Cancer Institute, 2021b; Sommers, 2019).

SUBJECTIVE DATA

A. Often asymptomatic but when symptoms occur, they may include:
    1. Urinary frequency.
    2. Urinary urgency.
    3. Urinary hesitancy.
    4. Nocturia.
    5. Dysuria.
    6. Back pain (National Cancer Institute, 2021b; Sommers, 2019).

OBJECTIVE DATA

A. Hematuria.
B. Urinary retention.
C. Diminished urinary stream.
D. Erectile dysfunction.
E. Prostate irregularity on digital rectal exam (National Cancer Institute, 2021b; Sommers, 2019).

DIAGNOSTIC TESTS

A. See Table 7.1 for prostate cancer grading.
B. See Appendix Table 7A.1 for listing of common diagnostic tests.

DIFFERENTIAL DIAGNOSES

A. Acute bacterial prostatitis and prostatic abscess.
B. Bacterial prostatitis.
C. Benign prostatic hyperplasia (BPH).

D. Nonbacterial prostatitis.
E. Tuberculosis of the genitourinary system (Tracy, 2021).

POTENTIAL COMPLICATIONS

A. Acute complications of advanced cancer (see Appendix C-7).
B. Metastasis.
C. Bone pain.
D. Pathological fractures.
E. Myelosuppression.
F. Urinary retention (National Cancer Institute, 2021b).

DISEASE-MODIFYING TREATMENTS

A. Active surveillance.
B. Cryotherapy.
C. Transurethral resection of the prostate (TURP).
D. Radical prostatectomy.
E. Radiation therapy.
F. Chemotherapy (see Figure 5.2 in Chapter 5).
G. Hormone therapy (National Cancer Institute, 2021b; Sommers, 2019).

PALLIATIVE INTERVENTIONS/SYMPTOM MANAGEMENT

A. See Appendix Table 7A.2 for listing of palliative interventions and symptom management.
B. See Appendix D-3 for overview of common symptoms.

PROGNOSIS

A. The Gleason score/grade group is the best predictor of life expectancy (see Table 7.1).
B. Prostate cancer responds well to treatment when detected in its early stages.
C. The 5-year survival rate is 99% for local and regional disease.

TABLE 7.1   GRADING OF PROSTATE CANCER

GLEASON SCALE	GRADE	TNM	PSA
≤ 6 → low risk, low potential for metastasis	1	T1a-c, T2a, N0, M0	<10
7 → moderate risk, likely to metastasize	2 or 3	T1a-c, T2a, T2b, N0, M0	≥10 or <20
8 to 10 → high risk, aggressive with high potential for metastasis	Gleason score 8 = Grade 4 Gleason score 9–10 = Grade 5	T3a-b, T4 with N0, M0 or Any T with N1, M0 or Any T with any N and M1	≥ 20 or any PSA if Gleason score ≥ 8

TNM, tumor, node, metastasis; PSA, prostate-specific antigen.

Source: Adapted from Buyyounouski, M. K., Choyke, P. L., Kattan, M. W., McKenney, J. K., Srigley, J. R., Barocas, D. A., Brimi, F., Brookland, R. K., Epstein, J. I., Fine, S. W. Halabi, S., Hamstra, D. A., Mason, M. D., Oh, W. K., Pettaway, C. A., Sartor, O., Schymura, M. J., Touijer, K. M., Zelefsky, M. J., . . . Cooper, K. (2018). Prostate. In M. B. Amin, S. Edge, F. Greene, D. R. Byrd, R. K. Brookland, M. K. Washington, J. E. Gershenwald, C. C Compton, K. R. Hess, D. C. Sullivan, J. M. Jessup, J. D. Brierley, L. E. Gaspar, R. L. Schilsky, C. M. Balch, D. P. Winchester, E. A. Asare, M. Madera, & D. M. Gress (Eds.), *AJCC cancer staging manual* (8th ed.). Springer International Publishing: American Joint Commission on Cancer. https://link.springer.com/book/97833194 06176. Used with permission.

D. The 5-year survival rate when widespread metastasis is present is 30%.

E. The overall 5-year survival rate is 98%.

F. Overall prognosis is dependent on:

   1. Extent of disease.

   2. Tumor grade.

   3. Patient's overall health.

   4. Patient's age.

   5. Prostate-specific antigen (PSA) level.

   6. Serum acid phosphate levels.

   7. Postoperative nomograms (National Cancer Institute, 2021b).

NURSING INTERVENTIONS

A. Individualize plan of care to patient's lifestyle needs.

B. Provide teaching regarding blood in urine or semen.

C. Teach Kegel exercises.

D. Implement interventions for pain and symptom management.

E. Educate patient to take all medications as prescribed.

F. Teach deep breathing and relaxation techniques.

G. Encourage smoking cessation (see Appendices B-10 and C-9).

H. Implement interventions for incontinence and for protection of skin.

I. Monitor for urinary obstruction and implement corrective measures as appropriate.

J. Educate patient and family regarding disease trajectory (see Appendix B-1).

K. Provide spiritual support.

L. Assess caregiver fatigue/burnout (see Appendix B-5).

M. Encourage completion of advance directives.

N. Educate patient and family regarding availability of palliative care.

O. Educate patient and family regarding availability of hospice services (when appropriate).

P. Provide referral to community support groups, as needed.

TESTICULAR CANCER

DEFINITION/CHARACTERISTICS

A. Malignancy that arises in the cells of one or both testicles.

B. Classified as either seminomas or nonseminomas.

C. Seminomas are the most common (30%) and the least aggressive.

D. Nonseminomas make up about 1% of all testicular cancers and are highly aggressive (National Cancer Institute, 2022; Rodway & McCance, 2019).

INCIDENCE AND PREVALENCE

A. Testicular cancer is rare.

B. It is most common in men between the ages of 15 and 35 years.

C. Approximately 8,900 new cases are diagnosed annually in the United States.

D. There are about 410 deaths each year in the United States resulting from testicular cancer.

E. White men have about a 0.2% chance of developing testicular cancer within their lifetimes.

F. The lifetime risk for Black men is about 4 times higher than in White men (Rodway & McCance, 2019).

ETIOLOGY

A. Exact etiology is unknown (Rodway & McCance, 2019).

PATHOPHYSIOLOGY

A. Testicular cancer most often begins in germ cells (spermatozoa or sperm cells).

B. Although highly treatable, if left untreated, the malignancy can metastasize to proximal and distant sites.

C. Testicular tumors are slightly more common in the right testicle.

D. About 1% to 2% of testicular tumors are bilateral (Rodway & McCance, 2019).

PREDISPOSING FACTORS

A. Genetic predisposition.

B. History of cryptorchidism.

C. Abnormal testicular development.

D. HIV infection.

E. AIDS.

F. Klinefelter syndrome.

G. Personal history of testicular cancer (Rodway & McCance, 2019).

SUBJECTIVE DATA

A. Testicular heaviness.

B. Dull ache in lower abdomen.

C. Acute pain secondary to rapid tumor growth.

D. Lumbar pain (Rodway & McCance, 2019).

OBJECTIVE DATA

A. Painless enlargement of testicle(s); this is the first sign.

B. Hydrocele.

C. Gynecomastia.

D. Firm, nontender testicular mass (Rodway & McCance, 2019).

DIAGNOSTIC TESTS

A. See Appendix Table 7A.1 for listing of common diagnostic tests.

DIFFERENTIAL DIAGNOSES

A. Hydrocele.

B. Epididymo-orchitis.

C. Spermatocele.

D. Epididymitis (Rodway & McCance, 2019).

POTENTIAL COMPLICATIONS

A. Acute complications of advanced cancer (see Appendix C-7).

B. Paresthesias.

▶

C. Raynaud phenomenon.
D. Infertility (Rodway & McCance, 2019).

DISEASE-MODIFYING TREATMENTS

A. Orchiectomy.
B. Radiation therapy.
C. Chemotherapy (see Figure 5.3 in Chapter 5; Rodway & McCance, 2019).

PALLIATIVE INTERVENTIONS/SYMPTOM MANAGEMENT

A. See Appendix Table 7A.2 for listing of palliative interventions and symptom management.
B. See Appendix D-3 for overview of common symptoms.

PROGNOSIS

A. Dependent on histology of tumor and stage at time of diagnosis.
B. The 5-year survival rate is 95.4% if confined to testes at the time of diagnosis.
C. The 5-year survival rate is 73.9% if distant metastasis is present at the time of diagnosis (Rodway & McCance, 2019).

NURSING INTERVENTIONS

A. Individualize plan of care to patient's lifestyle needs.
B. Provide teaching regarding blood in urine or semen.
C. Teach Kegel exercises.
D. Implement interventions for pain and symptom management.
E. Educate patient to take all medications as prescribed.
F. Teach deep breathing and relaxation techniques.
G. Encourage smoking cessation (see Appendices B-10 and C-9.
H. Implement interventions for incontinence and for protection of skin.
I. Educate patient and family regarding disease trajectory (see Appendix B-1).
J. Provide spiritual support.
K. Assess caregiver fatigue/burnout (see Appendix B-5).
L. Encourage completion of advance directives.
M. Educate patient and family regarding availability of palliative care.
N. Educate patient and family regarding availability of hospice services (when appropriate).
O. Provide referral to community support groups, as needed.

REFERENCES

American Cancer Society. (2021). *Melanoma skin cancer.* https://www.cancer.org/cancer/melanoma-skin-cancer.html

American Society of Clinical Oncology. (2021). *Types of cancer.* https://www.cancer.net/cancer-types

Boardman, C. H. (2021, March 4). *Cervical cancer differential diagnoses.* https://emedicine.medscape.com/article/253513-differential

Brenner, P. F. (1996). Differential diagnosis of abnormal uterine bleeding. *American Journal of Obstetrics and Gynecology, 175*(3), 766–769. https://doi.org/10.1016/S0002-9378(96)80082-2

Cancer Treatment Centers of America. (2021). *Risk factors for uterine cancer.* https://www.cancercenter.com/cancer-types/uterine-cancer/risk-factors

Center to Advance Palliative Care. (2021). *Disease types and palliative care.* https://getpalliativecare.org/whatis/disease-types/

Centers for Disease Control and Prevention. (2020). *Vaccines and preventable disease.* https://www.cdc.gov/vaccines/vpd/hpv/hcp/vaccines.html

Chipollini, J., De la Rosa, A, H., Azizi, M., Shayegan, B., Zorn, K. C., & Spiess, P. E. (2019). Patient presentation, differential diagnosis, and management of penile lesions. *Canadian Urological Association Journal, 13*(2 Suppl 1), S2. https://doi.org/10.5489/cuaj.5712

Cornish, L. (2019). Holistic management of malignant wounds in palliative patients. *British Journal of Community Nursing, 24*(Suppl 9), S19–S23. https://www.magonlinelibrary.com/toc/bjcn/current

Eleje, G. U., Eke, A. G., Igberase, G. O., Igwegbe, A. O., & Eleje, L., I. (2019). Palliative interventions for controlling vaginal bleeding in advanced cervical cancer. *Cochrane Database of Systematic Reviews, 3.* https://doi.org/10.1002/14651858.CD011000.pub3

Enclara Pharmacia. (2019). *Palliative management of sweating at end of life.* https://enclarapharmacia.com/wp-content/uploads/2020/06/PALLIATIVE_MANAGEMENT_OF_SWEATING_AT_END_OF_LIFE_MAY-2019_.pdf

Faizan, U., & Muppidi, V. (2020). *Uterine cancer.* https://www.ncbi.nlm.nih.gov/books/NBK562313/

Fife, C. E., Farrow, W., Hebert, A. A., Armer, N. C., Stewart, B. R., Cormier, J. N., & Armer, J. M. (2017). Skin and wound care in lymphedema patients: A taxonomy, primer, and literature review. *Advances in Skin & Wound Care, 30*(7), 305–318. https://journals.lww.com/aswcjournal/pages/default.aspx

Green, A. E. (2022). *Ovarian cancer: Differential diagnoses.* https://emedicine.medscape.com/article/255771-differential

Gupta, P., Aich, R. K., & Deb, A. R. (2014). Acute complications following intracavitary high-dose-rate brachytherapy in uterine cancer. *Journal of Contemporary Brachytherapy, 6*(3), 276. https://www.ncbi.nlm.nih.gov/pmc/articles/PMC4200184/

Habib, M. H., & Arnold, R. (2021). Urinary incontinence in palliative care settings: Part 2 Management #426. *Journal of Palliative Medicine, 24*(11), 1734–1735. https://doi.org/10.1089/jpm.2021.0373

Hoppenot, C., Littell, R. D., DeEulis, T., & Hartenbach, E. M. (2021). Top ten tips palliative care clinicians should know about caring for patients with cervical cancer. *Journal of Palliative Medicine, 24*(3), 438–442. https://www.liebertpub.com/doi/abs/10.1089/jpm.2021.0006

Johns Hopkins Medicine. (2021). *Conditions and diseases.* https://www.hopkinsmedicine.org/health/conditions-and-diseases

Johnson, C. A., James, D., Marzan, A., & Armaos, M. (2019). Cervical cancer: An overview of pathophysiology and management. *Seminars in Oncology Nursing, 35*(2), 166–174. WB Saunders. https://doi.org/10.1016/j.soncn.2019.02.003

Kim, M. J., & Tanco, K. (2021). Genitourinary issues in palliative care. In N. Dimitrov & K. Kemle (Eds.), *Palliative and serious illness patient management for physician assistants* (pp. 198–213). Oxford University Press. https://oxfordmedicine.com/view/10.1093/med/9780190059996.001.0001/med-9780190059996

Kluger, B. M., Ney, D. E., Bagley, S. J., Mohile, N., Taylor, L. P., Walbert, T., & Jones, C. A. (2020). Top ten tips palliative care clinicians should know when caring for patients with brain cancer. *Journal of Palliative Medicine, 23*(3), 415–421. https://doi.org/10.1089/jpm.2019.0507

Krakauer, E. L., Kane, K., Kwete, X., Afshan, G., Bazzett-Matabele, L., Bien-Aimé, D. D. R., Borges, L. F., Byrne-Martelli, S., Connor, S., Correa, R., Devi, C. R. B., Diop, M., Elmore, S. N., Gafer, N., Goodman, A., Grover, S., Hasenburg, A., Irwin, K., Kamdar, M., . . . Fidarova, E. (2021a). Augmented package of palliative care for women with cervical cancer: Responding to refractory suffering. *JCO Global Oncology, 7,* 886–895. https://doi.org/10.1200/GO.21.00027

Lambert, L. A., & Wiseman, J. (2018). Palliative management of peritoneal metastases. *Annals of Surgical Oncology, 25*(8), 2165–2171. https://link.springer.com/content/pdf/10.1245/s10434-018-6335-7.pdf

Mayo Clinic. (2021a). *Diseases and conditions.* https://www.mayoclinic.org/diseases-conditions

Mayo Clinic. (2021b). *Leukemia.* https://www.mayoclinic.org/diseases-conditions/leukemia/diagnosis-treatment/drc-20374378

Miller, D., & Nevadunsky, N. (2018). Palliative care and symptom management for women with advanced ovarian cancer. *Hematology/Oncology Clinics, 32*(6), 1087–1102. https://doi.org/10.1016/j.hoc.2018.07.012

Mosti, G., & Cavezzi, A. (2019). Compression therapy in lymphedema: Between past and recent scientific data. *Phlebology, 34*(8), 515–522. https://journals.sagepub.com/home/phl

National Cancer Institute. (2021a). *Uterine cancer—Health professional version.* https://www.cancer.gov/types/uterine/hp

National Cancer Institute. (2021b). *Prostate cancer—Health professional version.* https://www.cancer.gov/types/prostate/hp

National Cancer Institute. (2022). *Testicular cancer.* https://www.cancer.gov/types/testicular

National Cancer Institute. (2023). *Cancer stat facts: Cervical cancer.* https://seer.cancer.gov/statfacts/html/cervix.html

Palmer, S. J. (2019). Faecal incontinence in palliative and end of life care. *British Journal of Community Nursing, 24*(11), 528–532. https://pubmed.ncbi.nlm.nih.gov/31674223/

Ratini, M. (2022). *Penile cancer.* https://www.webmd.com/cancer/penile-cancer-overview

Rodway, G. W., & McCance, K. L. (2019). Alternations of the make reproductive system. In K. L. McCance & S. E. Huether (Eds.), *Pathophysiology: The biologic basis for disease in adults and children* (8th ed.). Elsevier-Mosby.

Rubinsak, L. (2021). *Palliative care of the patient with advanced gynecologic cancer.* https://emedicine.medscape.com/article/270646-overview

Shetty, M. (2019). Imaging and differential diagnosis of ovarian cancer. *Seminars in Ultrasound, CT and MRI, 40*(4), 302–318. https://www.sciencedirect.com/science/article/abs/pii/S0887217119300023X

Sommers, M. S. (2019). *Davis's diseases and disorders: A nursing therapeutics manual* (6th ed.). F.A. Davis Co.

Tracy, C. R. (2021, October 4). *Prostate cancer differential diagnosis.* https://emedicine.medscape.com/article/1967731-differential

Wright, P. M. (2019). *Certified hospice and palliative nurse (CHPN) exam review.* Springer Publishing Company.

TABLE 7A.1 DIAGNOSTIC TESTS FOR CANCERS OF THE REPRODUCTIVE SYSTEM

TYPE	NOTES
Physical examination	• Thorough physical exam with focused pelvic and abdominal examination. Attention to sexual history, urinary symptoms, or sexual dysfunction
Imaging	• Colposcopy, cystoscopy, proctoscopy (cervical) • Positron emission testing (cervical) • CT scan (cervical cancer, penile cancer, testicular cancer) • MRI (cervical, penile) • Exploratory laparoscopy (ovarian) • Ultrasound (ovarian, uterine, penile, prostate, testicular) • Hysteroscopy (uterine) • Endometrial biopsy (uterine) • MRI-directed biopsy (prostate) • Intravenous pyelogram (testicular) • Lymphangiogram (uterine, testicular)
Laboratory tests	• Pap test (cervical) • HPV DNA test (cervical) • CA-125 blood test (ovarian, uterine) • Complete blood count • CEA (penile) • Screening for sexually transmitted infections (penile) • PSA test (prostate) • Tumor markers (testicular) • AFP (testicular)
Pathology	• LEEP (cervical) • Endocervical curettage (cervical) • Cone biopsy (conization; cervical) • Cold knife cone biopsy (cervical) • Punch biopsy (cervical) • Fine-needle aspiration (penile) • Needle biopsy (prostate) • Biopsy (ovarian cancer, uterine cancer, penile) • Inguinal biopsy (testicular) • Orchiectomy with biopsy (testicular) • FIGO staging (cervical, ovarian, uterine; see Figure 7.1) • TNM criteria (ovarian, uterine, penile, prostate, testicular; see Appendix C-8)

AFP, alpha-fetoprotein; CEA, carcinoembryonic antigen; HPV, herpes papillomavirus; LEEP, loop electrosurgical excision procedure; PSA, prostate-specific antigen; TNM, tumor, node, metastasis.

Sources: American Cancer Society. (2021). *Melanoma skin cancer.* https://www.cancer.org/cancer/melanoma-skin-cancer.html; Center to Advance Palliative Care. (2021). *Disease types and palliative care.* https://getpalliativecare.org/whatis/disease-types/; Johns Hopkins Medicine. (2021). *Conditions and diseases.* https://www.hopkinsmedicine.org/health/conditions-and-diseases; Johnson, C. A., James, D., Marzan, A., & Armaos, M. (2019). Cervical cancer: An overview of pathophysiology and management. *Seminars in Oncology Nursing, 35*(2), 166–174. WB Saunders. https://doi.org/10.1016/j.soncn.2019.02.003; Mayo Clinic. (2021b). *Leukemia.* https://www.mayoclinic.org/diseases-conditions/leukemia/diagnosis-treatment/drc-20374378; National Cancer Institute. (2021b). *Prostate cancer- Health professional version.* https://www.cancer.gov/types/prostate/hp; Rodway, G. W., & McCance, K. L. (2019). Alternations of the make reproductive system. In K. L. McCance & S. E. Huether, (Eds.), *Pathophysiology: The biologic basis for disease in adults and children* (8th ed.). Elsevier-Mosby; Sommers, M. S. (2019). *Davis's diseases and disorders: A nursing therapeutics manual* (6th ed). F.A. Davis Co.

TABLE 7A.2 PALLIATIVE INTERVENTIONS/SYMPTOM MANAGEMENT FOR CANCERS OF THE REPRODUCTIVE SYSTEM

SYMPTOM	INTERVENTION
Anorexia	• Use of appetite stimulants (see Appendix D-1) • Offer small, frequent meals and snacks • Offer nutritional supplements
Anxiety and depression (see Appendix D)	• Antidepressants, anxiolytics, or benzodiazepines as indicated by patient's condition, age, and life expectancy • Non-pharmacological interventions
Ascites (see Figure 6.6)	• Abdominal ultrasound (ovarian, uterine) • Paracentesis with peritoneal fluid analysis (ovarian, uterine) • PleurX drain for ascites if patient is homebound (ovarian, uterine) • Albumin infusion if indicated (ovarian, uterine) • Diuretics (ovarian, uterine; see Appendix D-1)
Bowel obstruction	• Surgery to remove or debulk tumor (ovarian, uterine) • Bowel rest (ovarian, uterine) • Bowel decompression (ovarian, uterine) • Placement of nasogastric tube to reduce gastric pressure (ovarian, uterine)
Constipation	• Promotility agents (see Appendix D-1) • Laxatives (see Appendix D-1) • Ambulation • Increased dietary fiber • Increased fluids (as tolerated)
Fatigue and somnolence	• Alternate periods of rest with periods of activity • Utilize energy conversation techniques • Psychostimulants (see Appendix D)
Gas	• Antacids (ovarian, uterine; see Appendix D-1) • Ambulation (ovarian, uterine) • Small, frequent meals (ovarian, uterine) • Limit intake of fatty foods (ovarian, uterine)
Gastrointestinal symptoms (see Appendix D-1)	• Antacids • Antiemetics • Promotility agents • Laxatives • Antidiarrheals
Incontinence	• Identify and correct causes of incontinence, if possible (i.e., urinary tract infection, Clostridium difficile, etc.) • Use protective pads/undergarments • Utilize urinary diversion devices (indwelling catheter, condom catheter, etc.), as appropriate • Provide meticulous skin care and reposition patient at least every 2 hours • Utilize fecal collection devices as indicated (i.e., external pouch, rectal tubes)

(continued)

TABLE 7A.2 PALLIATIVE INTERVENTIONS/SYMPTOM MANAGEMENT FOR CANCERS OF THE REPRODUCTIVE SYSTEM (*CONTINUED*)

SYMPTOM	INTERVENTION
Insomnia (see Appendix D)	• Use of benzodiazepines, antidepressants, or antihistaminic agents, as indicated by patient's condition, age, and life expectancy • Provide proper sleep hygiene • Use non-pharmacological interventions for relaxation • Address underlying anxiety and depression
Intractable hematuria	• Orally administer epsilon-aminocaproic acid (prostrate) • Intravesical formalin (prostrate) • Alum or prostaglandin irrigation (prostrate) • Hydrostatic pressure (prostrate) • Urinary diversion (prostrate) • Radiation therapy (prostrate) • Embolization (prostrate) • Intra-arterial mitoxantrone perfusion (prostrate)
Lymphedema	• Topical application of emollients containing lactic acid, urea, ceramides, glycerin, dimethicone, olive oil, or salicylic acid (cervical, penile) • Frequently assess for and promptly treat secondary infection (cervical, penile) • Use of topical steroids if skin becomes inflamed (cervical, penile) • Silver-containing polymer dressing for ulcers associated with primary lymphedema (cervical, penile) • Frequent dressing changes if lymphorrhea (drainage of lymphatic fluid directly through the skin) occurs to prevent skin breakdown (cervical, penile) • Application of low-pressure (40–60 mmHg) compression therapy (cervical, penile) • Physical and/or occupational therapy to increase muscle mass and stimulate lymphatic flow (cervical, penile) • Assess and treat pain associated with limb heaviness, fluid retention, and immobility (cervical, penile) • Address body image issues related to lymphedema (cervical, penile)
Malodorous vaginal discharge	• Sitz bath (cervical, ovarian, uterine) • Systemic antibiotics and metronidazole (cervical, ovarian, uterine) • Application of skim emollients to prevent vulvar skin excoriation (cervical, ovarian, uterine) • Dressings containing charcoal (cervical, ovarian, uterine) • Use of diffused essential oils (cervical, ovarian, uterine) • Placement of odor-absorbing cat litter or shaving cream under the patient's bed or in another unobtrusive area in the room (cervical, ovarian, uterine)

(*continued*)

TABLE 7A.2 PALLIATIVE INTERVENTIONS/SYMPTOM MANAGEMENT FOR CANCERS OF THE REPRODUCTIVE SYSTEM (*CONTINUED*)

SYMPTOM	INTERVENTION
Nausea	• Antiemetics (see Appendix D-1) • Non-pharmacological interventions (see Appendix D-2)
Neuropathy	• Antidepressants (see Appendix D-1) • Anticonvulsants (i.e., gabapentin) • Anesthetics (i.e., ketamine) • Opioids
Pain management	• See Appendix E
Pleural effusion	• Medical/chemical pleurodesis (if prognosis is > 12 weeks; uterine) • Small bore or tunneled pleural catheter (uterine) • Thoracentesis (uterine) • Chest tube (uterine) • Opioids for pain management and dyspnea (uterine) • Supplemental oxygen (uterine) • Moving air and pursed-lip breathing to combat feelings of breathlessness (uterine)
Psychosocial distress/body image changes	• Antidepressants • Non-pharmacological interventions (see Appendix D-2)
Tumor reduction	• Palliative chemotherapy (prostate; see Figure 5.3 in Chapter 5) • Palliative radiation (prostate) • Surgical interventions (if indicated; prostate)
Urinary fistulas	• Urinary drainage (ovarian, prostate, uterine) • Pain management (ovarian, prostate, uterine) • Incontinence care (ovarian, prostate, uterine) • Bowel rest with intravenous hyperalimentation (ovarian, prostate, uterine) • Use of a somatostatin analog, such as octreotide (ovarian, prostate, uterine; see Appendix D-1) • Surgical interventions such as reconstruction, ileostomy, colostomy, urostomy, or stenting, depending on the patient's prognosis and ability to tolerate anesthesia (ovarian, prostate, uterine)
Ureteral obstruction (uterine, penile, prostate)	• Review medications and reduce dose or discontinue those that cause urinary retention, if possible (anticholinergics, antidepressants, antihistamines, antipsychotics, muscle relaxants)—penile, prostate, uterine • Insert urinary catheter, if possible. If not possible, placement of a suprapubic catheter may be necessary (penile, prostate, uterine) • If obstruction is due to prostate enlargement, consider use of tamsulosin or finasteride (penile, prostate, uterine) • Consider palliative TURP, if appropriate (penile, prostate, uterine) • Monitor for post-obstructive diuresis and replace fluids orally or intravenously (penile, prostate, uterine)

(continued)

TABLE 7A.2   PALLIATIVE INTERVENTIONS/SYMPTOM MANAGEMENT FOR CANCERS OF THE REPRODUCTIVE SYSTEM (CONTINUED)

SYMPTOM	INTERVENTION
Vaginal bleeding	• Vaginal bleeding (cervical, ovarian, uterine) • Palliative radiation therapy (cervical, ovarian, uterine) • Vaginal packing (cervical, ovarian, uterine) • Use of formalin-soaked vaginal packs (cervical, ovarian, uterine) • QuikClot combat gauze (cervical, ovarian, uterine) • Cautery (cervical, ovarian, uterine) • Endoscopic hemostatic forceps (cervical, ovarian, uterine) • Tranexamic acid (cervical, ovarian, uterine) • Interventional radiology techniques, such as uterine artery embolization; uterine artery resection; uterine artery ligation adonizing radiation/radiation therapy (cervical, ovarian, uterine)

TURP, transurethral resection of the prostate.

Sources: Center to Advance Palliative Care. (2021). *Disease types and palliative care.* https://getpalliativecare.org/whatis/disease-types/; Cornish, L. (2019). Holistic management of malignant wounds in palliative patients. *British Journal of Community Nursing, 24*(Suppl. 9), S19–S23. https://www.magonlinelibrary.com/toc/bjcn/current; Eleje, G. U., Eke, A. G., Igberase, G. O, Igwegbe A. O., & Eleje L. I. (2019). Palliative interventions for controlling vaginal bleeding in advanced cervical cancer. *Cochrane Database of Systematic Reviews, 3.* https://doi.org/10.1002/14651858.CD011000.pub3; Enclara Pharmacia. (2019). *Palliative management of sweating at end of life.* https://enclarapharmacia.com/wp-content/uploads/2020/06/PALLIATIVE_MANAGEMENT_OF_SWEATING_AT_END _OF_LIFE_MAY-2019_.pdf; Fife, C. E., Farrow, W., Hebert, A. A., Armer, N. C., Stewart, B. R., Cormier, J. N., & Armer, J. M. (2017). Skin and wound care in lymphedema patients: A taxonomy, primer, and literature review. *Advances in Skin & Wound Care, 30*(7), 305–318. https://journals.lww.com/aswcjournal/pages/default.aspx; Guyer, D. L., Almhanna, K., & McKee, K. Y. (2020). Palliative care for patients with esophageal cancer: A narrative review. *Annals of Translational Medicine, 8*(17). https://doi.org.10.21037/atm-20-3676; Habib, M. H., & Arnold, R. (2021). Urinary incontinence in palliative care settings: Part 2 Management #426. *Journal of Palliative Medicine, 24*(11), 1734–1735. https://doi.org/10.1089/jpm.2021.0373; Hoppenot, C., Littell, R. D., DeEulis, T., & Hartenbach, E. M. (2021). Top ten tips palliative care clinicians should know about caring for patients with cervical cancer. *Journal of Palliative Medicine, 24*(3), 438–442. https://www.liebertpub.com/doi/abs/10.1089/jpm.2021.0006; Kim, M. J., & Tanco, K. (2021). Genitourinary issues in palliative care. In N. Dimitrov & K. Kemle, (Eds.), *Palliative and serious illness patient management for physician assistants* (pp. 198–213). Oxford University Press. https://oxfordmedicine.com/view/10.1093/med/9780190059996.001.0001/med-9780190059996; Krakauer, E. L., Kane, K., Kwete, X., Afshan, G., Bazzett-Matabele, L., Ruthnie Bien-Aimé, D. D., Borges, L. F., Byrne-Martelli, S., Connor, S., Correa, R., Devi, C. R. B., Diop, M., Elmore, S. N., Gafer, N., Goodman, A., Grover, S., Hasenburg, A., Irwin, K., Kamdar, M., . . . Fidarova, E. (2021a). Augmented package of palliative care for women with cervical cancer: Responding to refractory suffering. *JCO Global Oncology, 7,* 886–895. https://doi.org/10. 1200/GO.21.00027; Krakauer, E. L., Kwete, X., Kane, K., Afshan, G., Bazzett-Matabele, L., Bien-Aimé, D. D. R., ... & Fidarova, E. (2021b). Cervical cancer-associated suffering: Estimating the palliative care needs of a highly vulnerable population. *JCO Global Oncology, 7,* 862–872. https://doi.org.10.1200/GO.21.00025; Lambert, L. A., & Wiseman, J. (2018). Palliative management of peritoneal metastases. *Annals of Surgical Oncology, 25*(8), 2165–2171. https://link.springer.com/content/pdf/10.1245/s10434-018-6335-7.pdf; Miller, D., & Nevadunsky, N. (2018). Palliative care and symptom management for women with advanced ovarian cancer. *Hematology/Oncology Clinics, 32*(6), 1087–1102. https://doi.org/10.1016/j.hoc.2018.07.012; Mosti, G., & Cavezzi, A. (2019). Compression therapy in lymphedema: Between past and recent scientific data. *Phlebology, 34*(8), 515–522. https://journals.sagepub.com/home/phl; Palmer, S. J. (2019). Faecal incontinence in palliative and end of life care. *British Journal of Community Nursing, 24* (11), 528–532. https://pubmed.ncbi.nlm.nih.gov/31674223/; Rodway, G. W., & McCance, K. L. (2019). Alternations of the make reproductive system. In K. L. McCance & S. E. Huether, (Eds.), *Pathophysiology: The biologic basis for disease in adults and children* (8th ed.). Elsevier-Mosby; Rubinsak, L. (2021). Palliative care of the patient with advanced gynecologic cancer. https://emedicine.medscape.com/article/270646-overview; Sommers, M. S. (2019). *Davis's diseases and disorders: A nursing therapeutics manual* (6th ed.). F.A. Davis Co; Wright, P. M. (2020). *Certified hospice and palliative nurse (CHPN®) exam review.* Springer Publishing Company.

CHAPTER 8

CANCERS OF THE BLOOD, SKIN, AND BONE

BONE CANCER

DEFINITION/CHARACTERISTICS
A. Malignancy that arises from bone cells.
B. The most common forms are:
   1. Osteosarcoma.
   2. Chondrosarcoma.
   3. Ewing sarcoma (Kneisl et al., 2018).

INCIDENCE AND PREVALENCE
A. Relatively rare, representing only 0.2% of all cancers.
B. Osteosarcoma and Ewing sarcoma develop mainly in children and young adults.
C. Chondrosarcoma generally develops in middle-aged adults.
D. Nearly 4,000 new cases of bone cancer are diagnosed annually in the United States.
E. Approximately 200 deaths are attributable to bone cancer each year in the United States (American Society of Clinical Oncology, 2022; Ferguson & Turner, 2018).

ETIOLOGY
A. The etiology is unknown (Johns Hopkins Medicine, 2022).

PATHOPHYSIOLOGY
A. Osteosarcoma arises from the primitive mesenchymal cells that become osteoblasts.
B. The origin of Ewing sarcoma is unknown but may arise from primitive neuroectodermal or neural crest cells.
C. Chondrosarcoma originates in cartilage cells but may also arise from a bone or cartilage tumor (Ferguson & Turner, 2018; Johns Hopkins Medicine, 2022).

PREDISPOSING FACTORS
A. Risk factors for chondrosarcoma include:
   1. Enchondromas.
   2. Multiple exostoses.
   3. Ollier disease.
   4. Maffucci syndrome.
B. Risk factors for osteosarcoma include:
   1. Metal implants within bone tissue.
   2. Paget disease.
   3. History of radiation therapy.

C. There are no known risk factors for Ewing sarcoma, but incidence rates are higher in Blacks than in Whites (Ferguson & Turner, 2018; Johns Hopkins Medicine, 2022).

SUBJECTIVE DATA
A. Pain that wakes the person from sleep (Ferguson & Turner, 2018; Kneisl et al., 2018).

OBJECTIVE DATA
A. Palpable mass (may not be palpable in bones with fatty tissue over malignancy).
B. Swelling at tumor site.
C. Decreased range of motion (Ferguson & Turner, 2018; Kneisl et al., 2018).

DIAGNOSTIC TESTS
A. See Appendix Table 8A.1 for listing of common diagnostic tests.

DIFFERENTIAL DIAGNOSES
A. Musculoskeletal injuries (Ferguson & Turner, 2018).

POTENTIAL COMPLICATIONS
A. Acute complications of advanced cancer (see Appendix C-7).
B. Metastasis to lungs, lymph nodes, or other bones (Ferguson & Turner, 2018).

DISEASE-MODIFYING TREATMENTS
A. Surgical excision.
B. Chemotherapy (see Figure 5.2 in Chapter 5).
C. Radiation (Johns Hopkins Medicine, 2022).

PALLIATIVE INTERVENTIONS/SYMPTOM MANAGEMENT
A. See Appendix Table 8A.2 for listing of palliative interventions and symptom management.
B. See Appendix D-3 for overview of common symptoms.

PROGNOSIS
A. The 5-year survival rate for those with chondrosarcoma is 78% if metastasis is present. If localized, the 5-year survival rate is 75%. If distant metastasis is present, the 5-year survival rate is 22%.
B. The 5-year survival rate for those with Ewing sarcoma is 61%. If metastasis is present but localized, the ▶

5-year survival rate is 81%. If distant metastasis is present, the 5-year survival rate is 38%.

C. The 5-year survival rate for those with osteosarcoma is 60%. If metastasis is present but localized, the 5-year survival rate is 74%. If distant metastasis is present, the 5-year survival rate is 27% (American Society of Clinical Oncology, 2022).

NURSING INTERVENTIONS

A. Effectively manage symptoms.

B. Educate patient and family on disease trajectory (see Appendix B-1).

C. Use and teach patient and family infection control measures.

D. Teach patient to take all medications as prescribed.

E. Maintain nutritional status.

F. Provide spiritual support.

G. Assess caregiver fatigue/burnout (see Appendix B-5).

H. Encourage completion of advance directives.

I. Educate patient and family regarding availability of palliative care.

J. Educate patient and family regarding availability of hospice services (when appropriate).

K. Provide referral to community support groups, as needed.

MELANOMA SKIN CANCER

DEFINITION/CHARACTERISTICS

A. Melanoma skin cancer arises from the melanocytes, typically nevus or moles.

B. There are three types of melanoma:

1. Basal cell.
2. Squamous cell.
3. Melanoma.

C. Of the three types of skin cancer, melanoma is most likely to metastasize (National Cancer Institute, 2021c; Sommers, 2019).

INCIDENCE AND PREVALENCE

A. Melanoma is the most common type of cancer in the United States.

B. There are over 100,000 new cases of melanoma diagnosed annually.

C. Melanoma accounts for 5.6% of all new cancer cases each year.

D. Melanoma accounts for 1% of all cancers.

E. The lifetime risk for melanoma is 1 in 54 (National Cancer Institute, 2021c; Sommers, 2019).

ETIOLOGY

A. Melanoma is associated with prolonged exposure to ultraviolet radiation either through direct sun exposure or the use of tanning beds (Sommers, 2019).

PATHOPHYSIOLOGY

A. Prolonged exposure to UV radiation damages the DNA of melanocytes, causing malignant changes.

B. Melanomas may develop in precursor skin lesions or in otherwise healthy skin.

C. Melanomas metastasize radially first and then vertically.

D. Vertical growth of melanomas indicates that malignant cells have developed the ability to metastasize (Heistein & Acharya, 2021; Sommers, 2019).

PREDISPOSING FACTORS

A. Genetic predisposition: first-degree relative diagnosed with melanoma before age 50.

B. Fair skin.

C. Blonde or red hair.

D. Tendency to develop freckles.

E. Presence of a large number of nevi.

F. Chronic skin inflammation.

G. Sex (higher incidence among males).

H. Race (higher incidence among Whites).

I. Exposure to environmental carcinogens.

J. Sunburns during childhood.

K. Use of tanning beds.

L. Prolonged exposure to direct sunlight.

M. Immunosuppression (National Cancer Institute, 2021c; Sommers, 2019).

SUBJECTIVE DATA

A. A sore or open area that seems to be slow healing.

B. Changes in sensation such as tenderness or itchiness (American Cancer Society, 2021b).

OBJECTIVE DATA

A. A mole or skin lesion that is asymmetric, has irregular borders, and/or has changed in color, diameter, size, shape, and elevation, or if new symptoms appear (see Figure 8.1).

B. New-onset scaliness or bleeding of a mole.

C. Ugly duckling sign (a mole that appears different from all other moles on the body).

D. Erythema around the border of a mole (American Cancer Society, 2021b).

DIAGNOSTIC TESTS

A. See Appendix Table 8A.1 for listing of common diagnostic tests.

DIFFERENTIAL DIAGNOSES

A. Benign melanocytic lesions.

B. Dysplastic nevus.

C. Squamous cell carcinoma.

D. Metastatic tumors to the skin.

E. Blue nevus.

F. Epithelioid (Spitz) tumor.

G. Pigmented spindle cell tumor.

H. Halo nevus.

I. Atypical fibroxanthoma.

J. Pigmented actinic keratosis.

K. Sebaceous carcinoma.

L. Histiocytoid hemangioma (Tan, 2020).

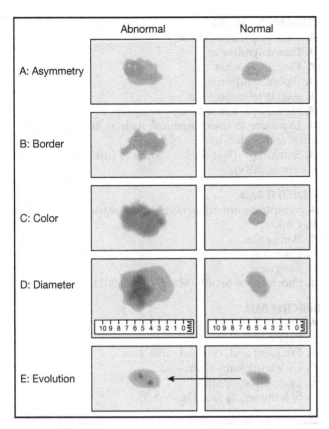

	Abnormal	Normal
A: Asymmetry		
B: Border		
C: Color		
D: Diameter		
E: Evolution		

FIGURE 8.1 ABCDE of melanoma.

POTENTIAL COMPLICATIONS

A. Acute complications of advanced cancer (see Appendix C-7).
B. Secondary infection.
C. Scarring.
D. Lymphedema.
E. Metastasis to the:
  1. Bone.
  2. Brain.
  3. Liver.
  4. Lung(s).
  5. Muscle.
F. Recurrence.
G. Altered body image (Heistein & Acharya, 2021; Sommers, 2019).

DISEASE-MODIFYING TREATMENTS

A. Surgical resection.
B. Chemotherapy (see Figure 5.2 in Chapter 5).
C. Immunotherapy.
D. Targeted drug therapy.
E. Excision of lesion.
F. Partial amputation of finger or toe if this is the site of the lesion (American Cancer Society, 2021b; Sommers, 2019).

PALLIATIVE INTERVENTIONS/SYMPTOM MANAGEMENT

A. See Appendix Table 8A.2 for listing of palliative interventions and symptom management.
B. See Appendix D-3 for overview of common symptoms.
C. See also the video "Palliative Care for the Melanoma Patient" available at www.aimatmelanoma.org/support-resources/palliative-care/ (Martin, 2018).

PROGNOSIS

A. The 5-year survival rate for melanoma is 93.3%.
B. Prognosis for metastatic melanoma is poor.
C. Melanoma is highly resistant to chemotherapy.
D. Factors associated with poor prognosis:
  1. Distant metastasis.
  2. Neural involvement.
  3. Immunosuppression.
  4. Tobacco use.
  5. Poor overall health of patient.
  6. Multiple comorbidities (National Cancer Institute, 2021c; Sommers, 2019).

NURSING INTERVENTIONS

A. Implement interventions to maintain skin integrity to the greatest extent possible.
B. Educate patient and family on disease trajectory (see Appendix B-1).
C. Use and teach patient and family infection control measures.
D. Teach patient to take all medications as prescribed.
E. Maintain nutritional status.
F. Encourage smoking cessation (see Appendices B-10 and C-9).
G. Implement interventions to effectively manage pain and other symptoms.
H. Provide wound care as needed.
I. Provide spiritual support.
J. Assess caregiver fatigue/burnout (see Appendix B-5).
K. Encourage completion of advance directives.
L. Educate patient and family regarding availability of palliative care.
M. Educate patient and family regarding availability of hospice services (when appropriate).
N. Provide referral to community support groups, as needed.

LEUKEMIA

DEFINITION/CHARACTERISTICS

A. Malignancy that affects the production of blood cells.
B. Results in the overproduction of abnormal leukocytes.
C. Leukemia can be categorized as acute or chronic.
  1. Acute leukemias include:
    a. Acute lymphocytic leukemia (ALL).
    b. Acute myeloid leukemia (AML).
  2. Chronic leukemias include:
    a. Chronic lymphocytic leukemia (CLL).
    b. Chronic myeloid leukemia (CML).
    c. Chronic myelomonocytic leukemia (CMML). ▶

D. Leukemia can also be classified as:

  1. Lymphocytic, meaning that lymphocytes, and thus the lymphatic system, are primarily affected.

  2. Myelogenous, meaning that myeloid cells are primarily affected. Erythrocytes, leukocytes, and plasma cells develop from myeloid cells (Mayo Clinic, 2021a; National Cancer Institute, 2021d).

INCIDENCE AND PREVALENCE

A. Leukemia occurs most often in those over the age of 55, but it is also the most common cancer among those younger than 15 years of age.

B. There are more than 61,000 new cases diagnosed annually.

C. Leukemia represents 3.2% of all new cancer cases each year (National Cancer Institute, 2021d).

ETIOLOGY

A. The exact cause of leukemia is not known.

B. Genetic link is often present (see Figure 8.2; National Cancer Institute, 2021d; Sommers, 2019).

PATHOPHYSIOLOGY

A. Malignant transformation of cells leads to unregulated production of abnormal blood cells (Mayo Clinic, 2021a).

PREDISPOSING FACTORS

A. Genetic predisposition.

B. Down syndrome.

C. Fanconi anemia.

D. Bloom syndrome.

E. Ataxia telangiectasia.

F. History of chemotherapy or radiation treatments.

G. Exposure to toxic chemical such as benzene, herbicides, and pesticides.

H. Smoking (National Cancer Institute, 2021d; Sommers, 2019).

SUBJECTIVE DATA

A. Symptoms are often vague and nonspecific.

B. Chills.

C. Bone pain.

D. Dizziness.

E. Fatigue.

F. Shortness of breath (Mayo Clinic, 2021a).

OBJECTIVE DATA

A. Fever.

B. Pallor.

C. Frequent and/or severe infection.

D. Unintentional weight loss.

E. Lymphadenopathy.

F. Splenomegaly (see Figure 8.3).

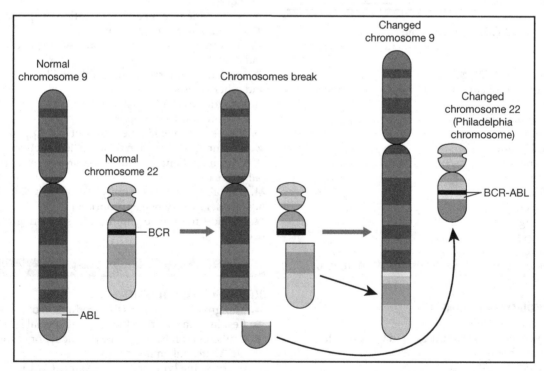

FIGURE 8.2 Chromosomal changes in leukemia.

Note: A chromosomal translocation activates an oncogene. Chromosomal translocation between chromosomes 9 and 22 produces a mutant Philadelphia chromosome that positions a breakpoint cluster region (BCR) gene next to the ABL (Abelson murine leukemia) proto-oncogene. The protein encoded by the fusion gene BCR-ABL is a continually activated protein tyrosine kinase that stimulates cells to continually divide, bypassing normal controls of the cell cycle. Presence of this gene is common in leukemias, particularly in chronic myeloid leukemia.

G. Hepatomegaly.
H. Recurrent epistaxis.
I. Petechiae.
J. Retinal hemorrhage.
K. Night sweats.
L. Anemia.
M. Pallor.
N. Ascites.
O. Sternal or rib tenderness (indication of infiltration of the periosteum; Mayo Clinic, 2021a; Sommers, 2019).

DIAGNOSTIC TESTS

A. See Appendix Table 8A.1 for listing of common diagnostic tests.

DIFFERENTIAL DIAGNOSES

A. Anemia.
B. B-cell lymphoma.
C. Bone marrow failure.
D. Lymphoblastic lymphoma.
E. Myelodysplastic syndrome (MDS).
F. Chronic myeloid leukemia (CML).
G. Hematolymphoid disorders with neutrophilia and/or monocytosis.
H. Common myeloproliferative neoplasms (Seiter, 2021; Stanford Medicine, 2021).

POTENTIAL COMPLICATIONS

A. Acute complications of advanced cancer (see Appendix C-7).
B. Myelosuppression.
C. Neutropenia.
D. Thrombocytopenia.
E. Peripheral neuropathy.
F. Osteonecrosis of the jaw.
G. Renal impairment.
H. Thrombosis and embolism.
I. AML.

J. Hyperviscosity syndrome.
K. Cryoglobulinemia (Leukemia & Lymphoma Society, 2015).

DISEASE-MODIFYING TREATMENTS

A. Chemotherapy (see Figure 5.2 in Chapter 5).
B. Clinical trials.
C. Central nervous system prophylaxis.
D. Dasatinib.
E. Autologous or allogeneic bone marrow transplantation.
F. Immunomodulation.
   1. Chimeric antigen receptor (CAR) T-cell therapy (National Cancer Institute, 2021d).

PALLIATIVE INTERVENTIONS/SYMPTOM MANAGEMENT

A. See Appendix Table 8A.2 for listing of palliative interventions and symptom management.
B. See Appendix D-3 for overview of common symptoms.

PROGNOSIS

A. The overall 5-year survival rate for all leukemias is 66.4%.
B. ALL: The 5-year relative survival rate is 40%.
C. AML: The 5-year relative survival rate is 27%.
D. CLL: The 5-year relative survival rate is 87%.
E. CML: The 5-year relative survival rate is 70% (American Cancer Society, 2022a; Leukemia & Lymphoma Society, 2023).

NURSING INTERVENTIONS

A. Use and teach patient and family infection control measures.
B. Teach patient to take all medications as prescribed.
C. Maintain nutritional status.
D. Implement interventions for pain and symptom management.

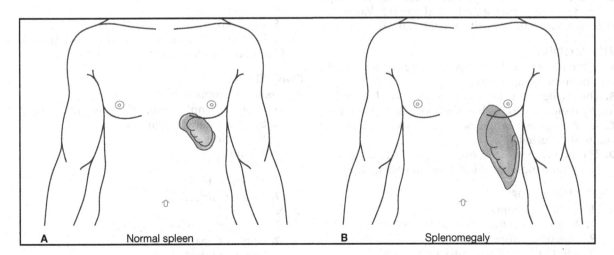

| A | Normal spleen | B | Splenomegaly |

FIGURE 8.3 Splenomegaly.

E. Encourage smoking cessation (see Appendices B-10 and C-9).
F. Provide wound care as needed.
G. Prepare for and manage bleeding.
H. Provide spiritual support.
I. Assess caregiver fatigue/burnout (see Appendix B-5).
J. Encourage completion of advance directives.
K. Educate patient and family regarding availability of palliative care.
L. Educate patient and family regarding availability of hospice services (when appropriate).
M. Provide referral to community support groups, as needed.

LYMPHOMA

DEFINITION/CHARACTERISTICS
A. A term for all types of cancers that begin within the lymphatic system.
B. There are two main types:
   1. Hodgkin.
   2. Non-Hodgkin (National Cancer Institute, 2021f).

INCIDENCE AND PREVALENCE
A. Hodgkin lymphoma:
   1. Accounts for 0.5% of all new cancer cases in the United States each year.
   2. There are an estimated 8,800 new cases each year.
B. Non-Hodgkin lymphoma (NHL):
   1. Accounts for about 4% of all new cancer cases each year.
   2. It is one of the most common cancers in the United States.
   3. Approximately 81,000 new cases are diagnosed annually (National Cancer Institutes, 2021g, 2021h).

ETIOLOGY
A. Malignancy that originates in the lymphatic cells.
B. Hodgkin lymphoma typically originates in lymph nodes in the upper part of the body (Hubert & VanMeter, 2018; National Cancer Institute, 2021e, 2021f).

PATHOPHYSIOLOGY
A. Lymphoma usually begins in a single lymph node, most often in the upper body.
B. The malignancy then begins to spread to other, nearby lymph nodes, such as the nodes in the neck area.
C. As the disease progresses, T-cell and lymphocyte counts are affected.
D. The presence of Reed–Sternberg cells is diagnostic for Hodgkin lymphoma (Hubert & VanMeter, 2018).

PREDISPOSING FACTORS
A. Hodgkin lymphoma:
   1. Age: younger than 20 or over 55 years.
   2. Genetic predisposition.
   3. Infection with Epstein–Barr virus (EBV).
   4. Male sex.
   5. Immunosuppression.
B. NHL:
   1. HIV infection.
   2. Genetic predisposition.
   3. Age over 60 years.
   4. Male sex.
   5. Overweight or obesity.
   6. White race.
   7. History of breast implants.
   8. Exposure to certain chemicals such as benzene as well as those in certain herbicides and insecticides.
   9. Previous exposure to chemotherapeutic agents.
   10. Previous exposure to radiation.
   11. Immunosuppression.
   12. Autoimmune diseases such as rheumatoid arthritis, systemic lupus erythematosus, Sjogren disease, or celiac disease.
   13. History of infections such as human T-cell lymphotropic virus (HTLV-1), EBV, or human herpesvirus 8 (HHV-8).
   14. Chronic immune stimulation from infections such as *Helicobacter pylori*, *Chlamydophila psittaci*, *Campylobacter jejuni*, or hepatitis C (American Cancer Society, 2021a; Hubert & VanMeter, 2018).

SUBJECTIVE DATA
A. Hodgkin lymphoma:
   1. Fatigue.
   2. Pruritus.
   3. Weakness.
B. NHL:
   1. Chills.
   2. Night sweats.
   3. Weakness.
   4. Fatigue.
   5. Ascites.
   6. Early satiety.
   7. Dyspnea.
   8. Nausea.
   9. Headache.
   10. Diplopia (American Cancer Society, 2021a; Hubert & VanMeter, 2018).

OBJECTIVE DATA
A. Hodgkin lymphoma:
   1. Painless lymphadenopathy (usually cervical).
   2. Splenomegaly (see Figure 8.2).
   3. Weight loss.
   4. Anemia.
   5. Fever.
   6. Bleeding/bruising.
   7. Frequent infections.
B. NHL:
   1. Enlarged, painless lymph node.
   2. Unintentional weight loss.
   3. Frequent infections.

4. Shortness of breath.

5. Vomiting.

6. Initial presentation may include diffuse, non-organized lymph node involvement consistent with widespread metastasis.

7. Intestinal nodes and organs are often involved in early stages (American Cancer Society, 2021a; Hubert & VanMeter, 2018).

DIAGNOSTIC TESTS

A. See Appendix Table 8A.1 for listing of common diagnostic tests.

DIFFERENTIAL DIAGNOSES

A. Hodgkin lymphoma:

    1. Cytomegalovirus (CMV).

    2. EBV infectious mononucleosis (mono).

    3. NHL.

    4. Sarcoidosis.

    5. Serum sickness.

    6. Small cell lung cancer (SCLC).

    7. Syphilis.

    8. Toxoplasmosis.

    9. Tuberculosis (TB).

B. NHL:

    1. Hodgkin lymphoma.

    2. EBV infectious mono (Lash, 2020; Vinjamaram, 2021).

PALLIATIVE INTERVENTIONS/SYMPTOM MANAGEMENT

A. See Appendix Table 8A.2 for listing of palliative interventions and symptom management.

B. See Appendix D-3 for overview of common symptoms.

POTENTIAL COMPLICATIONS

A. Immunosuppression.

B. Increased risk for other types of cancers.

C. Increased risk for heart and lung disease.

D. Rectal bleeding (if the gastrointestinal system is affected).

E. Bone marrow suppression.

F. Infertility.

G. Hormonal disorders (Myhre & Sifris, 2021; National Health Service, 2021).

DISEASE-MODIFYING TREATMENTS

A. Radiation.

B. Chemotherapy (see Figure 5.2 in Chapter 5).

C. Surgical interventions.

D. Immunotherapy.

E. Targeted drug therapy (American Cancer Society, 2021a; Hubert & VanMeter, 2018).

PROGNOSIS

A. The 5-year survival rate for Hodgkin lymphoma is about 88%.

B. The 5-year survival rate for NHL is about 73%.

C. The stage of disease at the time of diagnosis impacts survival rate; treatment is more challenging in the presence of widespread disease (see Table 8.1; Hubert & VanMeter, 2018; National Cancer Institute, 2021e, 2021f).

NURSING INTERVENTIONS

A. Individualize plan of care to patient's age and lifestyle needs.

B. Provide teaching regarding treatments and treatment side effects (see Appendix B-1).

C. Teach patient to monitor for signs of infection.

D. Teach patient to decrease risk for infection through handwashing, avoiding crowded areas, and wearing a mask.

E. Teach patient how to manage bruising and bleeding.

F. Encourage smoking cessation (see Appendices B-10 and C-9).

G. Encourage small, frequent meals and high-calorie snacks.

H. Teach patient to take medications as prescribed.

I. Implement interventions for pain and symptom management.

J. Offer reputable online resources.

K. Provide spiritual support.

L. Assess caregiver fatigue/burnout (see Appendix B-5).

M. Encourage completion of advance directives.

N. Educate patient and family regarding availability of palliative care.

O. Educate patient and family regarding availability of hospice services (when appropriate).

P. Provide referral to community support groups, as needed.

TABLE 8.1	LUGANO CLASSIFICATION
STAGE	**AREA OF INVOLVEMENT**
I	One lymph node region
IE	One extra-nodal site
II	Two or more lymph node regions
IIE	Localized extra-nodal sites on the same side of the diaphragm
III	Lymph node regions or lymphoid structures (e.g., thymus and Waldeyer ring) on both sides of the diaphragm
IV	Diffuse or disseminated extra-lymphatic organ involvement

Source: Yoon, D. H., Cao, J., Chen, T. Y., Izutsu, K., Kim, S. J., Kwong, Y. L., Lin, T. Y., Thye, L. S., Xu, B., Yang, D. H., & Kim, W. S. (2020). Treatment of mantle cell lymphoma in Asia: A consensus paper from the Asian Lymphoma Study Group. *Journal of Hematology & Oncology, 13*(1), 1–11.

MULTIPLE MYELOMA

DEFINITION/CHARACTERISTICS
A. A type of cancer that affects the plasma cells.
B. When plasma cells accumulate in multiple bony areas, the disease is called multiple myeloma.
C. When only a single lesion is found, it is called plasmacytoma rather than multiple myeloma (Hubert & VanMeter, 2018; National Cancer Institute, 2021b).

INCIDENCE AND PREVALENCE
A. There are nearly 35,000 new cases diagnosed annually.
B. Multiple myeloma represents about 1.8% of all new cancer cases.
C. About 2% of all deaths attributed to cancer each year are from multiple myeloma (National Cancer Institute, 2021a).

ETIOLOGY
A. Etiology is unknown (Hubert & VanMeter, 2018).

PATHOPHYSIOLOGY
A. Bone marrow is gradually replaced with malignant plasma cells.
B. With bone marrow function impaired, production of blood cells and antibodies is affected.
C. The malignant plasma cells in the bone marrow erode bone tissue.
D. Metastatic tumors often affect the vertebrae, ribs, pelvis, and skull (Hubert & VanMeter, 2018).

PREDISPOSING FACTORS
A. Increased age.
B. Black race.
C. Male sex.

D. Personal history of monoclonal gammopathy of undetermined significance (MGUS) or plasmacytoma.
E. Exposure to radiation or carcinogenic materials (National Cancer Institute, 2021b).

SUBJECTIVE DATA
A. Pain, especially bone pain at rest.
B. Fatigue.
C. Dyspnea.
D. Weakness.
E. Poor endurance.
F. Restlessness.
G. Anorexia.
H. Nausea.
I. Increased thirst (as a result of hypercalcemia; Hubert & VanMeter, 2018; National Cancer Institute, 2021b).

OBJECTIVE DATA
A. Frequent infections.
B. Pathological fractures.
C. Bone fragility.
D. Anemia.
E. Bleeding.
F. Proteinuria.
G. Impaired kidney function.
H. Vomiting.
I. Confusion.
J. Constipation.
K. Urinary frequency (Hubert & VanMeter, 2018; National Cancer Institute, 2021b).

DIAGNOSTIC TESTS
A. See Appendix Table 8A.1 for listing of common diagnostic tests.
B. See Table 8.2 CRAB criteria.

TABLE 8.2   CRAB CRITERIA FOR DIAGNOSING MULTIPLE MYELOMA

FEATURE	SYMPTOM	DIAGNOSTIC CRITERIA	MANAGEMENT
C	Calcium	Corrected serum calcium >11 mg/dL	Hydration and IV bisphosphonates; additional agents include corticosteroids and calcitonin
R	Renal insufficiency	SCr >2 mg/dL	Correct hypercalcemia and possible dehydration. Avoid nephrotoxic agents such as NSAIDs
A	Anemia	Hemoglobin <10 g/dL or >2 g/dL below LLN	Correct iron, folate, and vitamin B$_{12}$, deficiency. If patient is symptomatic, consider use of an erythropoietic agent; however, recognize that myeloma therapy may increase risk of thrombosis
B	Bone disease	One or more osteolytic lesions, pathological fractures, severe osteopenia, and/or pain	Bisphosphonates or denosumab for lytic bone disease; pain control may be necessary

LLN, lower limit of normal; NSAIDs, nonsteroidal anti-inflammatory drugs; SCr, serum creatinine.

Source: American Cancer Society (2022a). *Cancer facts and figures.* https://www.cancer.org/content/dam/cancer-org/research/cancer-facts-and-statistics/annual-cancer-facts-and-figures/2022/2022-cancer-facts-and-figures.pdf; Cornish, L. (2019). Holistic management of malignant wounds in palliative patients. *British Journal of Community nursing, 24*(Supp. 9), S19–S23. https://www.magonlinelibrary.com/toc/bjcn/current; Düll, M. M., & Kremer, A. E. (2019). Treatment of pruritus secondary to liver disease. *Current Gastroenterology Reports, 21*(9), 1–9. https://link.springer.com/article/10.1007/s11894-019-0713-6#Sec9; https://www.uspharmacist.com/article/multiple-myeloma-updates-in-management

DIFFERENTIAL DIAGNOSES

A. Primary (malignant) lymphoma of bone.
B. Metastatic bone disease.
C. MGUS.
D. Waldenstrom macroglobulinemia (Shah, 2021).

POTENTIAL COMPLICATIONS

A. Acute complications of advanced cancer (see Appendix C-7).
B. Pathological fractures.
C. Hypercalcemia results from breakdown of bone tissue.
D. Metastasis to lymph nodes and organs.
E. Amyloidosis (Hubert & VanMeter, 2018).

DISEASE-MODIFYING TREATMENTS

A. Chemotherapy (see Figure 5.2 in Chapter 5).
B. Radiation.
C. Immunomodulating agents.
D. Proteasome inhibitors.
E. Histone deacetylase (HDAC) inhibitors.
F. Monoclonal antibodies.
G. Antibody-drug conjugates.
H. Nuclear export inhibitor.
I. Surgical interventions:
   1. Typically used in the case of plasmacytomas.
   2. Used in cases in multiple myeloma when spinal cord compression occurs to stabilize the spinal column (if patient's condition permits surgical intervention; American Cancer Society, 2021a; Hubert & VanMeter, 2018).

PALLIATIVE INTERVENTIONS/SYMPTOM MANAGEMENT

A. See Appendix Table A8.2 for listing of palliative interventions and symptom management.
B. See Appendix D-3 for overview of common symptoms.

PROGNOSIS

A. Multiple myeloma is staged using the Revised International Staging System (RISS; see Table 8.3), which takes four factors into account:
   1. The amount of albumin in the blood.
   2. The amount of beta-2-microglobulin in the blood.
   3. The amount of lactate dehydrogenase (LDH) in the blood.
   4. The specific gene abnormalities (cytogenetics) of the cancer.
B. Mean survival rate is 3 years.
C. The 5-year year survival rate is 55.6%.
D. Age-adjusted death rates have been falling by about 1% each year.
E. Prognosis is affected by:
   1. The type of plasma cell cancer.
   2. The stage of the disease at the time of diagnosis.
   3. Pre-existing medical conditions.
   4. Responsiveness of the malignancy to treatments (American Cancer Society, 2021a; Hubert & VanMeter, 2018; National Cancer Institute, 2021a).

TABLE 8.3 REVISED INTERNATIONAL STAGING SYSTEM

STAGE	CRITERIA	SURVIVAL (MONTHS)
I	• β_2-microglobulin <3.5 mg/L • Albumin ≥3.5 g/dL • Standard-risk chromosomal abnormalities • Normal LDH (defined as less than ULN)	82
II	• Not RISS stage I or III	62
III	• β_2-microglobulin ≥5.5 mg/L regardless of albumin levels • High-risk chromosomal abnormalities: del 17p, t(4;14), or t(14;16) • High LDH (defined as higher than ULN)	40

del, deletion; LDH, lactate dehydrogenase; RISS, Revised International Staging System; t, translocation; ULN, upper limit of normal.

Sources: American Cancer Society. (2022a). *Cancer facts and figures.* https://www.cancer.org/content/dam/cancer-org/research/cancer-facts-and-statistics/annual-cancer-facts-and-figures/2022/2022-cancer-facts-and-figures.pdf; Ferguson, J. L., & Turner, S. P. (2018). Bone cancer: diagnosis and treatment principles. *American Family Physician, 98*(4), 205–213. https://www.aafp.org/pubs/afp/issues/2018/0815/p205.html; https://www.uspharmacist.com/article/multiple-myeloma-updates-in-management

NURSING INTERVENTIONS

A. Individualize plan of care to patient's age and lifestyle needs.
B. Provide teaching regarding treatments and treatment side effects.
C. Teach patient to monitor for signs of infection.
D. Teach patient to decrease risk for infection through handwashing, avoiding crowded areas, and wearing a mask.
E. Teach patient how to manage bruising and bleeding.
F. Encourage small, frequent meals and high-calorie snacks.
G. Encourage smoking cessation (see Appendices B-10 and C-9).
H. Teach patient to take medications as prescribed.
I. Implement interventions for pain and symptom management.
J. Offer reputable online resources.
K. Provide spiritual support.
L. Assess caregiver fatigue/burnout (see Appendix B-5).
M. Encourage completion of advance directives.
N. Educate patient and family regarding availability of palliative care.
O. Educate patient and family regarding availability of hospice services (when appropriate).
P. Provide referral to community support groups, as needed.

SQUAMOUS CELL CARCINOMA

DEFINITION/CHARACTERISTICS
A. Malignancy of the epidermis with uncontrolled growth of keratinocytes (see Figure 8.4).
B. There are two types of squamous cell carcinomas:
    1. In situ (Bowen disease).
    2. Invasive (McCance & Huether, 2019).

INCIDENCE AND PREVALENCE
A. Squamous cell carcinoma is the second most common type of cancer in humans.
B. There are approximately 1.8 million new cases of squamous cell carcinoma diagnosed annually.
C. The incidence of squamous cell carcinoma has increased by 200% in the past 30 years (McCance & Huether, 2019; Skin Cancer Foundation, 2022).

ETIOLOGY
A. Etiology is unknown (McCance & Huether, 2019; Rice et al., 2018).

PATHOPHYSIOLOGY
A. Development of actinic keratosis is a precursor to squamous cell carcinoma.
B. Malignancy arises from the epithelium and penetrates the basement membrane.
C. Characterized by keratinization (McCance & Huether, 2019; Rice et al., 2018).

PREDISPOSING FACTORS
A. Age over 50 years.
B. Light-colored skin.
C. Male sex.
D. Personal history of skin cancer, xeroderma pigmentosum, or human papillomavirus (HPV).
E. Unprotected exposure to ultraviolet light.
F. Genetic predisposition.
G. Chronic arsenic exposure.
H. Chronic, nonhealing wound.
I. Radiation exposure
J. Immunosuppression (McCance & Huether, 2019; Skin Cancer Foundation, 2022).

SUBJECTIVE DATA
A. Pain at site of lesion (McCance & Huether, 2019).

OBJECTIVE DATA
A. Firm lesion with elevation and increasing diameter (see Figure 8.1).
B. Surface of the lesion may be granular and bleed easily (McCance & Huether, 2019).

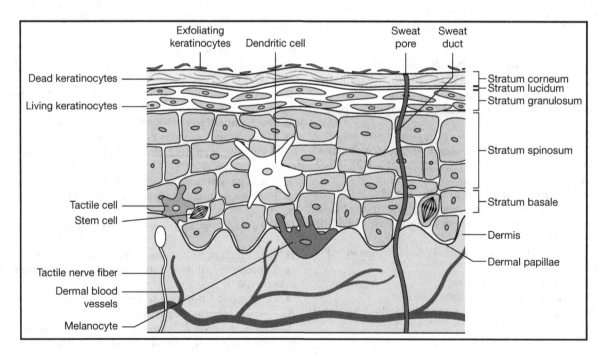

FIGURE 8.4 Layers of the epidermis.

Note: Cell types and layers of the epidermis. The epidermis is divided into four layers: basal cell, stratum spinosum, stratum granulosum, and stratum corneum. Basal layer is responsible for cell division and the process of cell differentiation. Stratum spinosum is abundant in keratinocytes. Stratum granulosum involves the process of differentiation that gives rise to cells that provide the granular layer with further structural support. Stratum corneum is the superficial layer composed of dead cells that protect the skin from microbes.

DIAGNOSTIC TESTS

A. See Appendix Table 8A.1 for listing of common diagnostic tests.

DIFFERENTIAL DIAGNOSES

A. Congenital tumors.
B. Actinic keratosis.
C. Papillomas.
D. Vascular lesions.
E. Xanthomatous lesions.
F. Allergic contact dermatitis.
G. Benign skin lesions.
H. Chemical burns.
I. Bowenoid papulosis (Wells, 2021).

POTENTIAL COMPLICATIONS

A. Acute complications of advanced cancer (see Appendix C-7).
B. Metastasis to the:
   1. Lymph nodes.
   2. Lung(s).
   3. Skin.
   4. Liver.
   5. Bone (Goto et al., 2019; McCance & Huether, 2019).

DISEASE-MODIFYING TREATMENTS

A. Chemotherapy (see Figure 5.2 in Chapter 5).
B. Radiation.
C. Cryotherapy.
D. Photodynamic therapy.
E. Microsurgical excision.
F. Topical medications.
G. Laser surgery.
H. Mohs chemosurgery (McCance & Huether, 2019; Skin Cancer Foundation, 2022).

PALLIATIVE INTERVENTIONS/SYMPTOM MANAGEMENT

A. See Appendix Table 8A.2 for listing of palliative interventions and symptom management.
B. See Appendix D-3 for overview of common symptoms.

PROGNOSIS

A. Highly treatable when diagnosed early.
B. Over 15,000 deaths in the United States are attributable to squamous cell carcinoma each year (Skin Cancer Foundation, 2022).

NURSING INTERVENTIONS

A. Individualize plan of care to patient's age and lifestyle needs (see Appendix B-1).
B. Provide teaching regarding treatments and treatment side effects.
C. Teach patient to monitor for signs of infection.
D. Teach patient to decrease risk for infection through handwashing, avoiding crowded areas, and wearing a mask.
E. Encourage smoking cessation (see Appendices B-10 and C-9).
F. Encourage small, frequent meals and high-calorie snacks.
G. Teach patient to take medications as prescribed.
H. Implement interventions for pain and symptom management.
   I. Offer reputable online resources.
J. Provide spiritual support.
K. Assess caregiver fatigue/burnout (see Appendix B-5).
L. Encourage completion of advance directives.
M. Educate patient and family regarding availability of palliative care.
N. Educate patient and family regarding availability of hospice services (when appropriate).
O. Provide referral to community support groups, as needed.

REFERENCES

AIM at Melanoma Foundation. (2018). *Palliative care for the melanoma patient.* https://www.youtube.com/watch?v=4JooncxfRD4&t=3s

AIM at Melanoma Foundation. (2021). *What is palliative care?* https://www.aimatmelanoma.org/support-resources/palliative-care/

American Cancer Society. (2021a). *Cancer A to Z.* https://www.cancer.org/cancer.html

American Cancer Society. (2021b). *Melanoma skin cancer.* https://www.cancer.org/cancer/melanoma-skin-cancer.html

American Cancer Society. (2022a). *Cancer facts and figures.* https://www.cancer.org/content/dam/cancer-org/research/cancer-facts-and-statistics/annual-cancer-facts-and-figures/2022/2022-cancer-facts-and-figures.pdf

American Cancer Society. (2022b). *Supportive treatments for patients with multiple myeloma.* https://www.cancer.org/cancer/multiple-myeloma/treating/supportive.html

American Society of Clinical Oncology. (2022). *Bone cancer (sarcoma of the bone): Statistics.* https://www.cancer.net/cancer-types/bone-cancer-sarcoma-bone/statistics#:~:text=This%20year%2C%20an%20estimated%203%2C910,people%20age%2015%20to%2019

Center to Advance Palliative Care. (2021). *Disease types and palliative care.* https://getpalliativecare.org/whatis/disease-types/

Cornish, L. (2019). Holistic management of malignant wounds in palliative patients. *British Journal of Community Nursing, 24*(Supp. 9), S19–S23. https://www.magonlinelibrary.com/toc/bjcn/current

Düll, M. M., & Kremer, A. E. (2019). Treatment of pruritus secondary to liver disease. *Current Gastroenterology Reports, 21*(9), 1–9. https://link.springer.com/article/10.1007/s11894-019-0713-6#Sec9

Ferguson, J. L., & Turner, S. P. (2018). Bone cancer: Diagnosis and treatment principles. *American Family Physician, 98*(4), 205–213. https://www.aafp.org/pubs/afp/issues/2018/0815/p205.html

Goto, H., Kiyohara, Y., Shindo, M., & Yamamoto, O. (2019). Symptoms of and palliative treatment for unresectable skin cancer. *Current Treatment Options in Oncology, 20*(4), 1–10. https://link.springer.com/content/pdf/10.1007/s11864-019-0626-5.pdf

Guyer, D. L., Almhanna, K., & McKee, K. Y. (2020). Palliative care for patients with esophageal cancer: A narrative review. *Annals of Translational Medicine, 8*(17). https://doi.org/10.21037/atm-20-3676

Heistein, J. B., & Acharya, U. (2021). *Malignant melanomas.* https://www.ncbi.nlm.nih.gov/books/NBK470409/

Hubert, R. J., & VanMeter, K. C. (2018). *Gould's pathophysiology for the health professions* (6th ed.). Elsevier Inc.

Johns Hopkins Medicine. (2022). *Chondrosarcoma.* https://www.hopkinsmedicine.org/health/conditions-and-diseases/sarcoma/chondrosarcoma#:~:text=Most%20often%2C%20chondrosarcoma%20happens%20from,noncancerous)%20bone%20or%20cartilage%20tumor

Kneisl, J. S., Rosenberg, A. E., Anderson, P. M., Antonescu, C. R., Bruland, O. S., Cooper, K., Horvai, A. E., Holt, G. E., O'Sullivan, B., Patel, S. R., & Rose, P. S. (2018). Bone. In M. B. Amin, S. B. Edge, F. L. Greene, D. R. Byrd, R. K. Brookland, M. K. Washington, J. E. Gershenwald, C. C. Compton, K. R. Hess, D. C. Sullivan, J. M. Jessup, J. D. Brierley, L. E. Gaspar, R. L. Schilsky, C. M. Balch, D. P. Winchester, E. A. Asare, M. Madera, D. M. Gress, & L. R. Meyer (Eds.), *AJCC cancer staging manual* (8th ed.). Springer International Publishing: American Joint Commission on Cancer. https://link.springer.com/book/9783319406176

Lash, B. W. (2020, August 3). *Hodgkin lymphoma differential diagnoses.* https://emedicine.medscape.com/article/201886-differential

Leukemia & Lymphoma Society. (2015). *Disease complications.* https://lls.org/myeloma/disease-complications

Leukemia & Lymphoma Society (2023). *Facts and statistics overview.* https://www.lls.org/facts-and-statistics/facts-and-statistics-overview

Martin, S. (2018). *Palliative care for the melanoma patient* [YouTube video]. https://www.youtube.com/watch?v=4JooncxfRD4&t=3s.

Mayo Clinic. (2021a). *Leukemia.* https://www.mayoclinic.org/diseases-conditions/leukemia/diagnosis-treatment/drc-20374378

McCance, K. L., & Huether, S. E. (2019). Structure, function, and disorders of the integument. In K. L. McCance & S. E. Huether (Eds.), *Pathophysiology: The biologic basis for disease in adults and children* (8th ed.). Elsevier-Mosby.

Moffitt Cancer Center. (2018). *Stages of leukemia.* https://moffitt.org/cancers/leukemia/diagnosis/stages/

Myhre, J., & Sifris, D. (2021). *Symptoms of lymphoma.* https://www.verywellhealth.com/warning-signs-of-lymphoma-2252446#complications

National Cancer Institute. (2021a). *Cancer statistics.* https://seer.cancer.gov/statistics/

National Cancer Institute. (2021b). *NCI dictionary of cancer terms.* https://www.cancer.gov/publications/dictionaries/cancer-terms

National Cancer Institute. (2021c). *Skin cancers (including melanoma—Health professional version.* https://www.cancer.gov/types/skin/hp

National Cancer Institute. (2021d). *Leukemia.* https://www.cancer.org/cancer/leukemia.html

National Cancer Institute. (2021e). *Cancer stat facts: Hodgkin lymphoma.* https://seer.cancer.gov/statfacts/html/hodg.html

National Cancer Institute. (2021f). *Non-Hodgkin lymphoma.* https://seer.cancer.gov/statfacts/html/nhl.html

National Health Service. (2021). *Complications: Hodgkin lymphoma.* https://www.nhs.uk/conditions/hodgkin-lymphoma/complications/

Rice, T. W., Kelsen, D., Blackstone, E. H., Ishwaran, H., Patil, D. T., Bass, A. J., Erasmus, J. J., Gerdes, H., & Hofstetter, W. L. (2018). *Urinary Bladder.* In M. B. Amin, S. B. Edge, F. L. Greene, D. R. Byrd, R. K. Brookland, M. K. Washington, J. E. Gershenwald, C. C. Compton, K. R. Hess, D. C. Sullivan, J. M. Jessup, J. D. Brierley, L. E. Gaspar, R. L. Schilsky, C. M. Balch, D. P. Winchester, E. A. Asare, M. Madera, D. M. Gress, & L. R. Meyer (Eds.), *AJCC cancer staging manual* (8th ed.). Springer International Publishing: American Joint Commission on Cancer. https://link.springer.com/book/9783319406176

Seiter, K. (2021, March 16). *Acute myeloid leukemia (AML) differential diagnoses.* https://emedicine.medscape.com/article/197802-differential

Shah, D. (2021, May 11). *Multiple myeloma differential diagnoses.* https://emedicine.medscape.com/article/204369-differential

Skin Cancer Foundation. (2022). *Squamous cell carcinoma.* https://www.skincancer.org/skin-cancer-information/squamous-cell-carcinoma/scc-treatment-options/

Sommers, M. S. (2019). *Davis's diseases and disorders: A nursing therapeutics manual* (6th ed.). F.A. Davis Co.

Stanford Medicine. (2021). *Chronic myelogenous leukemia (CML).* http://surgpathcriteria.stanford.edu/mdsmps/chronic-myeloid-myelogenous-leukemia/differential-diagnosis.html

Tan, W. W. (2020, September 1). *Malignant melanoma differential diagnosis.* https://emedicine.medscape.com/article/280245-differential

Vinjamaram, S. (2021, August 3). *Non-Hodgkin lymphoma (NHL) differential diagnoses.* https://emedicine.medscape.com/article/203399-differential

Wells, J. W. (2021). *Cutaneous squamous cell carcinoma: Differential diagnoses.* https://emedicine.medscape.com/article/1965430-differential

Yoon, D. H., Cao, J., Chen, T. Y., Izutsu, K., Kim, S. J., Kwong, Y. L., Lin, T. Y., Thye, L. S., Xu, B., Yang, D. H., & Kim, W. S. (2020). Treatment of mantle cell lymphoma in Asia: A consensus paper from the Asian Lymphoma Study Group. *Journal of Hematology & Oncology, 13*(1), 1–11.

APPENDIX

TABLE 8A.1   DIAGNOSTIC TESTS FOR CANCERS OF THE SKIN AND BLOOD

TYPE	NOTES
Physical examination	• Thorough physical examination • Attention to history of pain or tumor growth (bone cancer) • Focused dermatological assessment (melanoma skin cancer, squamous cell carcinoma) • Laboratory studies and abdominal assessment (Hodgkin lymphoma, non-Hodgkin lymphoma, multiple myeloma leukemia)
Imaging	• Chest x-ray (bone cancer, melanoma skin cancer, leukemia, non-Hodgkin lymphoma) • CT scan (bone cancer, melanoma skin cancer, leukemia, Hodgkin lymphoma, non-Hodgkin lymphoma, multiple myeloma) • PET (bone cancer, melanoma skin cancer, leukemia, Hodgkin lymphoma, non-Hodgkin lymphoma, multiple myeloma) • MRI (bone cancer, leukemia, Hodgkin lymphoma, non-Hodgkin lymphoma, multiple myeloma) • Ultrasound, including regional lymph nodes (melanoma skin cancer leukemia, non-Hodgkin lymphoma) • Bone scan (bone cancer, non-Hodgkin lymphoma, multiple myeloma)
Laboratory tests	• Complete blood count • IHC (bone cancer, melanoma skin cancer, Hodgkin lymphoma) • FISH (melanoma skin cancer, multiple myeloma) • CGH (melanoma skin cancer) • GEP (melanoma skin cancer) • Flow cytometry and IHC (non-Hodgkin lymphoma, multiple myeloma) • Chromosome tests (to determine type of lymphoma; non-Hodgkin lymphoma) • Blood and urine immunoglobulin studies (multiple myeloma) • 24-hour urine test (multiple myeloma) • Cryogenic analysis (multiple myeloma)

(continued)

TABLE 8A.1   DIAGNOSTIC TESTS FOR CANCERS OF THE SKIN AND BLOOD (*CONTINUED*)

TYPE	NOTES
Pathology	<ul><li>Biopsy (bone cancer, Hodgkin lymphoma, non-Hodgkin lymphoma)</li><li>Biopsy for melanoma skin cancer may include shave, punch, incisional, excisional, fine-needle aspiration, and/or lymph node biopsy</li><li>Bone marrow aspiration and biopsy (bone cancer, leukemia, Hodgkin lymphoma, multiple myeloma)</li><li>Lymphadenectomy (Hodgkin lymphoma, non-Hodgkin lymphoma)</li><li>Lumbar puncture (non-Hodgkin lymphoma)</li><li>Pleural fluid testing (non-Hodgkin lymphoma)</li><li>Peritoneal fluid testing (non-Hodgkin lymphoma)</li><li>Multiple myeloma is diagnosed using the CRAB criteria (see Table 8.1)</li><li>Squamous cell carcinoma is staged using the TNM method (see Appendix C-8)</li><li>Bone cancer is staged according to general staging criteria (see Appendix C-8)</li><li>Hodgkin and non-Hodgkin lymphoma are staged using the Lugano classification system</li><li>Leukemia staging<ul><li>Acute lymphocytic leukemia is staged according to the type of lymphocyte and the maturity of the cells</li><li>Acute myeloid leukemia is staged using the FAB system</li><li>Chronic lymphocytic leukemia is staged using the Rai system</li><li>Chronic myeloid leukemia is staged according to the number of diseased cells identified in blood and bone marrow</li></ul></li></ul>

CGH, comparative genomic hybridization; FAB, French American-British; FISH, fluorescence in situ hybridization; GEP, gene expression profiling; IHC, immunohistochemistry; TNM, tumor, node, metastasis.

Sources: American Cancer Society. (2021b). *Melanoma skin cancer.* https://www.cancer.org/cancer/melanoma-skin-cancer.html; American Cancer Society. (2021a). *Cancer A to Z.* https://www.cancer.org/cancer.html; Ferguson, J. L., & Turner, S. P. (2018). Bone cancer: Diagnosis and treatment principles. *American Family Physician, 98*(4), 205–213. https://www.aafp.org/pubs/afp/issues/2018/0815/p205.html; Kneisl, J. S., Rosenberg, A. E., Anderson, P. M., Antonescu, C. R., Bruland, O. S., Cooper, K., Horvai, A. E., Holt, G. E., O'Sullivan, B., Patel, S. R., & Rose, P. S. (2018). Bone. In M. B. Amin, S. B. Edge, F. L. Greene, D. R. Byrd, R. K Brookland, M. K., Washington, J. E. Gershenwald, C. C Compton, K. R. Hess, D. C. Sullivan, J. M. Jessup, J. D. Brierley, L. E. Gaspar, R. L. Schilsky, C. M. Balch, D. P. Winchester, E. A. Asare, M. Madera, D. M. Gress, & L. R. Meyer (Eds.), *AJCC cancer staging manual* (8th ed.). Springer International Publishing: American Joint Commission on Cancer. https://link.springer.com/book/9783319406176; Mayo Clinic (2021a). *Leukemia.* https://www.mayoclinic.org/diseases-conditions/leukemia/diagnosis-treatment/drc-20374378; McCance, K. L., & Huether, S. E. (2019). Structure, function, and disorders of the integument. In K. L. McCance & S. E. Huether (Eds.), *Pathophysiology: The biologic basis for disease in adults and children* (8th ed.). Elsevier-Mosby; Moffitt Cancer Center. (2018). *Stages of leukemia.* https://moffitt.org/cancers/leukemia/diagnosis/stages/; National Cancer Institute. (2021b). *NCI dictionary of cancer terms.* https://www.cancer.gov/publications/dictionaries/cancer-terms; National Cancer Institute. (2021c). *Skin cancers (including melanoma—health professional version.* https://www.cancer.gov/types/skin/hp; Skin Cancer Foundation. (2022). *Squamous cell carcinoma.* https://www.skincancer.org/skin-cancer-information/squamous-cell-carcinoma/scc-treatment-options/; Sommers, M. S. (2019). *Davis's diseases and disorders: A nursing therapeutics manual* (6th ed.). F.A. Davis Co.

TABLE 8A.2   PALLIATIVE INTERVENTIONS/SYMPTOM MANAGEMENT FOR CANCERS OF THE SKIN AND BLOOD

SYMPTOM	INTERVENTION
Abnormal blood cell counts	<ul><li>Blood transfusions</li><li>IVIG</li><li>Plasmapheresis</li><li>Pharmacological interventions (see Appendix D-1)<ul><li>Epoetin (Procrit)</li><li>Darbepoetin (Aranesp)</li><li>Iron supplementation</li></ul></li></ul>
Anorexia	<ul><li>Use of appetite stimulants (see Appendix D-1)</li><li>Offer small, frequent meals and snacks</li><li>Offer nutritional supplements</li></ul>

(continued)

TABLE 8A.2   PALLIATIVE INTERVENTIONS/SYMPTOM MANAGEMENT FOR CANCERS OF THE SKIN AND BLOOD (*CONTINUED*)

SYMPTOM	INTERVENTION
Anxiety and depression	• Antidepressants, anxiolytics, or benzodiazepines as indicated by patient's condition, age, and life expectancy (see Appendix D-1) • Non-pharmacological interventions (see Appendix D-2)
Ascites (see Figure 6.7)	• Abdominal ultrasound (leukemia, lymphoma) • Paracentesis with peritoneal fluid analysis (leukemia, lymphoma) • PleurX drain for ascites if patient is homebound (leukemia, lymphoma) • Albumin infusion if indicated (leukemia, lymphoma) • Diuretics (leukemia, lymphoma; see Appendix D-1)
Bleeding	• Cauterization • QuikClot combat gauze
Bone-modifying interventions	• Bisphosphonates to strengthen bones and reduce bone loss (see Appendix D-1)
Constipation	• Promotility agents (see Appendix D-1) • Laxatives (see Appendix D-1) • Ambulation • Increased dietary fiber • Increased fluids (as tolerated)
Dyspnea (see Appendix D)	• Corticosteroids for reducing inflammation (see Appendix D) • Bronchodilators for opening airways (mechanism of action of relaxation of muscular bands that surround bronchi, thus widening the airway; see Appendix D) • Diuretics to reduce systemic congestion (see Appendix D) • Anticholinergics to reduce secretions, especially at the end of life (see Appendix D) • Use of fans • Lower temperature in the room
Fatigue and somnolence	• Alternate periods of rest with periods of activity • Utilize energy conversation techniques • Psychostimulants (see Appendix D)
Fever	• Address underlying cause, when possible • Use of antipyretics • Application of cool compresses • Increase fluids to address dehydration, if applicable
Frequent infection	• Avoid crowds or large gatherings • Wear mask when in the company of others • Wash hands frequently • Use of antibiotics or anti-infectives as indicated • Avoid animals and live plants • Avoid dental work • Avoid vaccines unless otherwise directed • Avoid raw foods
Inflammation	• NSAIDS • Corticosteroids (see Appendix D)

(*continued*)

TABLE 8A.2 PALLIATIVE INTERVENTIONS/SYMPTOM MANAGEMENT FOR CANCERS OF THE SKIN AND BLOOD (*CONTINUED*)

SYMPTOM	INTERVENTION
Insomnia	• Use of benzodiazepines, antidepressants, or antihistaminic agents, as indicated by patient's condition, age, and life expectancy • Provide proper sleep hygiene • Use non-pharmacological interventions for relaxation (see Appendix D-2) • Address underlying anxiety and depression
Lymphedema	• Topical application of emollients containing lactic acid, urea, ceramides, glycerin, dimethicone, olive oil, or salicylic acid • Frequently assess for and promptly treat secondary infection • Use of topical steroids if skin becomes inflamed • Silver-containing polymer dressing for ulcers associated with primary lymphedema • Frequent dressing changes if lymphorrhea (drainage of lymphatic fluid directly through the skin) occurs to prevent skin breakdown • Application of low-pressure (40–60 mmHg) compression therapy • Physical and/or occupational therapy to increase muscle mass and stimulate lymphatic flow • Assess and treat pain associated with limb heaviness, fluid retention, and immobility • Address body image issues related to lymphedema
Malodorous wound	• Systemic antibiotics and metronidazole (SCC) • Application of skin emollients to prevent skin excoriation (SCC) • Dressings containing charcoal (SCC) • Use of diffused essential oils (SCC) • Placement of odor-absorbing cat litter or shaving cream under the patient's bed or in another unobtrusive area in the room (SCC)
Nausea	• Antiemetics (see Appendix D-1) • Non-pharmacological interventions (see Appendix D-2)
Night sweats	• Review medications and lower dosages on or discontinue medications that can cause hyperhidrosis (i.e., hormones, antidepressants, aromatase inhibitors, etc.)—lymphoma • Use cotton bed linens and light pajamas (lymphoma) • Offer cool washcloths to forehead and underarms (lymphoma) • Open window and/or use fan (lymphoma) • Increase fluid intake as appropriate (lymphoma) • Avoid alcohol use (lymphoma) • Consider use of NSAIDs and/or corticosteroids (lymphoma)
Pain management	• See Appendix E
Palliative radiation	• If melanoma has metastasized to the brain (melanoma skin cancer)
Pathological fractures	• Treatment of localized pain (bone cancer, multiple myeloma) • Joint stabilization (bone cancer, multiple myeloma) • For lower extremity compression fractures, surgical stabilization with or without joint replacement, if patient's condition and prognosis are favorable (bone cancer, multiple myeloma) • For vertebral compression fractures, VP or BKP may be considered, depending on patient's condition and prognosis (bone cancer, multiple myeloma)

(continued)

TABLE 8A.2 PALLIATIVE INTERVENTIONS/SYMPTOM MANAGEMENT FOR CANCERS OF THE SKIN AND BLOOD (*CONTINUED*)

SYMPTOM	INTERVENTION
Pruritus	• Thorough dermatological exam to establish cause • Depending on cause, topical agents such as ointments, barrier creams, or soaks can be trialed (e.g., calamine, menthol, oatmeal bath, antihistamine cream) • Systemic antihistamines may be used but are not recommended for older adults (see Appendix D) • Maintain short fingernails
Psychosocial distress/body image changes	• Antidepressants • Non-pharmacological interventions (see Appendix D-2)
Wound care	• See Appendix F

Note: See also the video "Palliative Care for the Melanoma Patient" by S. Martin (2018) at: https://www.youtube.com/watch?v=4JooncxfRD4&t=3s

BKP, balloon kyphoplasty; IVIG, intravenous immunoglobulin; NSAIDS, nonsteroidal anti-inflammatory drugs; VP, vertebroplasty.

NONCANCER DIAGNOSES

CHAPTER 9

CARDIAC DISEASE

ADVANCED AND END-STAGE HEART FAILURE

DEFINITION/CHARACTERISTICS
A. Progressive deterioration of heart function in which the heart cannot produce adequate cardiac output.
B. This underperformance of the heart muscle leads to inadequate perfusion of all tissues and organs and an inability to meet the body's metabolic needs.
C. Heart failure may be described as left-sided or right-sided (Brashers, 2019; Sommers, 2019; Wright, 2019).

INCIDENCE AND PREVALENCE
A. Heart failure affects about 6.2 million adults in the United States.
B. Roughly 600,000 Americans ≥ age 20 have advanced heart failure.
C. Heart failure affects approximately 10% of American seniors (American Heart Association, 2022; Centers for Disease Control and Prevention, 2022a).

ETIOLOGY
A. About 70% of cardiovascular disease-related events are attributable to poor cardiovascular health.
B. Heart failure usually occurs secondary to:
   1. Altered preload (poor venous return) related to:
     a. Incompetent valves.
     b. Renal failure.
     c. Fluid volume overload.
     d. Congenital left-to-right shunt.
   2. Altered afterload related to:
     a. Hypertension.
     b. Valvular stenosis.
     c. Hypertrophic cardiomyopathy.
   3. Diminished heart contractility secondary to:
     a. Cardiomyopathy.
     b. Coronary artery disease (CAD).
     c. Acute myocardial infarction.
     d. Amyloidosis.
     e. Sarcoidosis.
     f. Hypocalcemia.
     g. Hypomagnesemia.
     h. Iatrogenic cardiomyopathy (commonly caused by drugs or radiation; Sommers, 2019; Tsao et al., 2022).

PATHOPHYSIOLOGY
A. Low production of angiotensin II leads to increased cardiac workload, progressive loss of cardiac function, and cardiac hypertrophy.
B. The diseased cardiac muscle produces inadequate cardiac output, which leads to poor tissue perfusion and increased pulmonary capillary pressure (Brashers, 2019; Sommers, 2019).

PREDISPOSING FACTORS
A. Ischemic heart disease.
B. Hypertension.
C. Advanced age.
D. Smoking.
E. Obesity.
F. Diabetes.
G. Renal failure.
H. Valvular heart disease (VHD).
I. Cardiomyopathies.
J. Congenital heart disease.
K. Alcohol abuse.
L. Genetic predisposition (American Heart Association, 2022; Brashers, 2019; Tsao et al., 2022).

SUBJECTIVE DATA
A. Symptoms vary by cause and severity but may include:
   1. Anxiety.
   2. Irritability.
   3. Fatigue.
   4. Lethargy.
   5. Dyspnea.
   6. Anorexia.
   7. Nausea.
   8. Syncope (Sommers, 2019).

OBJECTIVE DATA
A. Signs vary by cause and severity but may include:
   1. Shortness of breath at rest or with activity (most common).
   2. Muscle weakness.
   3. Orthopnea.
   4. Cough with frothy sputum.
   5. Vomiting.
   6. Unintentional weight loss or weight gain.
   7. Hepatojugular reflux (see Table 9.1).

▶

TABLE 9.1   ASSESSMENT OF HEPATOJUGULAR REFLUX

STEP		WATCH FOR	TEACH PATIENT
Wash hands and obtain patient's verbal consent for the procedure.		Patient's openness to the procedure and understanding of the technique	Purpose of the procedure and what they will experience
Position patient in supine position with head turned to their left.		Distention of jugular veins	Breathe normally
Raise head of bed 30°–45° and measure jugular vein distention, if present. If patient cannot tolerate this position, raise head of bed to 90° for procedure.		Changes in jugular vein distention	Relax abdomen
Apply steady and firm pressure to the pre-umbilical area for approximately 10–15 seconds. If abdominal guarding is noted, stop procedure.		Sustained elevation (>3 cm) of jugular vein pressure if head is at 30–45 degree angle is considered positive for hepatojugular reflux. Any elevation of jugular vein pressure that is sustained for >10 seconds if head is at a 90 degree angle is considered positive for hepatojugular reflux.	Results of the procedure and meaning of those results

Sources: Thibodeau, J. T., & Drazner, M. H. (2018). The role of the clinical examination in patients with heart failure. *JACC: Heart Failure, 6*(7), 543–551, https://www.jacc.org/doi/abs/10.1016/j.jchf.2018.04.005; Vaidya, Y., Bhatti, H., & Dhamoon, A. S. (2018). *Hepatojugular reflux.* https://www.ncbi.nlm.nih.gov/books/NBK526097/

8. Inspiratory crackles or wheezes.
9. Tachypnea.
10. Tachycardia.
11. S3 or S4 on heart auscultation (see Figure 9.1).
12. presence of murmurs (see Figures 9.2 and 9.3).
13. Pale, cyanotic, cool, clammy skin (Sommers, 2019).

DIAGNOSTIC TESTS
A. See Appendix Table 9A.1 for listing of common diagnostic tests.

DIFFERENTIAL DIAGNOSES
A. Acute renal failure.
B. Acute respiratory distress syndrome (ARDS).

C. Cirrhosis.
D. Pulmonary fibrosis.
E. Nephrotic syndrome.
F. Respiratory failure.
G. Venous insufficiency.
H. Pulmonary embolism (PE).
I. Bacterial pneumonia.
J. Cardiogenic pulmonary edema.
K. Chronic obstructive pulmonary disease (COPD).
L. Cirrhosis.
M. Emphysema (Dumitru, 2022; Malik et al., 2021).

POTENTIAL COMPLICATIONS
A. Pulmonary edema.
B. Renal insufficiency.

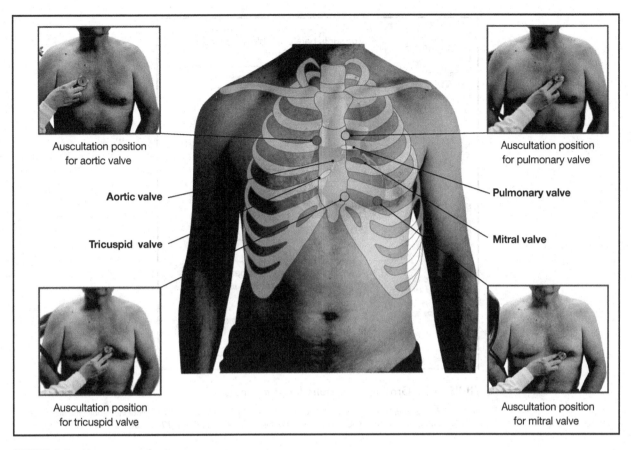

FIGURE 9.1   Heart auscultation.

C. Cerebral insufficiency.
D. Myocardial infarction.
E. Cardiac dysrhythmias (Brashers, 2019; Sommers, 2019).

DISEASE-MODIFYING TREATMENTS
A. Treatment depends on type of heart failure (left or right sided; see Table 9.3).

PALLIATIVE INTERVENTIONS/SYMPTOM MANAGEMENT
A. See Appendix Table 9A.2 for listing of palliative interventions and symptom management.
B. See Appendix D-3 for overview of common symptoms.

PROGNOSIS
A. For men, life expectancy after a diagnosis of heart failure is approximately 1.7 years.
B. For women, life expectancy after a diagnosis of heart failure is approximately 3.2 years.
C. Roughly 75% of patients die within 5 years of diagnosis.
D. Sudden death accounts for about 50% of heart failure mortality (Severino et al., 2019).

NURSING INTERVENTIONS
A. Provide education on disease process and symptom management.
B. Teach patient to take all medications as prescribed.
C. Maintain nutritional status.
D. Encourage smoking cessation (see Appendices B-10 and C-9).
E. Provide spiritual support.
F. Assess caregiver fatigue/burnout.
G. Encourage completion of advance directives.
H. Educate patient and family regarding availability of palliative care.
I. Educate patient and family regarding availability of hospice services (when appropriate).
J. Provide referral to community support groups, as needed.

LEFT HEART FAILURE (CONGESTIVE HEART FAILURE)

DEFINITION/CHARACTERISTICS
A. A type of heart failure manifested by:
    1. Decreased (<40%) ejection fraction (also called systolic heart failure or HFrEF).
    2. Preserved ejection fracture (also called diastolic heart failure or FFpEF).
B. Systolic and diastolic heart failure can occur concomitantly or singularly.

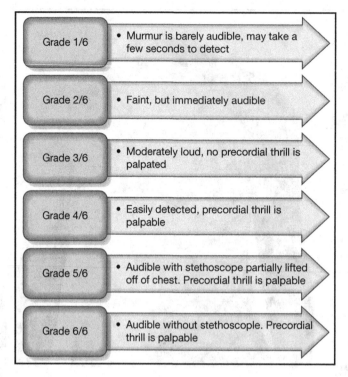

FIGURE 9.2   Grading of systolic heart murmurs.

Source: Adapted from Freeman, A. R., & Levine, S. A. (1933). The clinical significance of the systolic murmur: A study of 1000 consecutive "non-cardiac" cases. *Annals of Internal Medicine, 6*(11), 1371–1385.

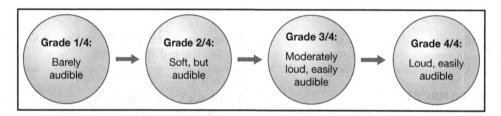

FIGURE 9.3   Grading of diastolic heart murmurs.

Source: Adapted from Patnaik, A. N. (2019). The diastolic murmurs. *Indian Journal of Cardiovascular Disease in Women-WINCARS, 4*(04), 228–232. https://www.thieme-connect.com/products/ejournals/pdf/10.1055/s-0039-3402692.pdf

C. Isolated systolic heart failure occurs when the heart is unable to generate adequate cardiac output and perfusion.

D. Isolated diastolic heart failure involves pulmonary congestion in the presence of normal cardiac output and stroke volume (Brashers, 2019).

INCIDENCE AND PREVALENCE

A. Heart failure affects about 6.2 million adults in the United States; left-sided heart failure is most common.

B. Roughly 600,000 Americans ≥ age 20 have advanced heart failure.

C. Heart failure affects approximately 10% of American seniors.

D. Roughly 550,000 cases of left-sided heart failure are diagnosed each year.

E. Almost 1.4 million people who have left-sided heart failure are under the age of 60.

F. More than 5% of persons ages of 60 to 69 have left-sided heart failure (American Heart Association, 2022; Centers for Disease Control and Prevention, 2022a; Emory Healthcare, 2022).

ETIOLOGY

A. Systolic heart failure.
 1. Myocardial infarction.
 2. Myocarditis.
 3. Cardiomyopathies.
B. Diastolic heart failure.
 1. Hypertension-induced myocardial hypertrophy.
 2. Myocardial ischemia with resultant ventricular remodeling.
 3. Aortic valvular disease.
 4. Mitral valve disease.
 5. Pericardial diseases.
 6. Cardiomyopathies (Brashers, 2019).

PATHOPHYSIOLOGY

A. Progressive cardiac dysfunction occurs due to:
 1. Decreased contractility of the heart muscle.
 2. Ventricular hypertrophy.
 3. Myocyte apoptosis.
 4. Abnormal fibrin deposition.
B. Cardiac dysfunction progressively results in:
 1. Cardiac muscle remodeling (see Figure 9.4).
 2. Venous congestion.
 3. Worsening renal function and/or pulmonary edema (Brashers, 2019).

PREDISPOSING FACTORS

A. Systolic heart failure.
 1. Coronary artery disease (CAD).
 2. Diabetes.
 3. Hypertension.
 4. Valvular heart disease (VHD).
 5. Arrythmias.
 6. Myocarditis.
 7. Illicit drug use.
 8. Alcohol abuse.
 9. Iatrogenic events (including medications).
B. Diastolic heart failure.
 1. Age.
 2. Insulin resistance.
 3. Hypertension.
 4. CAD.
 5. Diabetes.
 6. Obesity.
 7. History of atrial fibrillation (Del Buono et al., 2020; Dumitru, 2020; Obokata et al., 2020; Sorrentino, 2019).

SUBJECTIVE DATA

A. Systolic heart failure.
 1. Orthopnea.
 2. Fatigue.

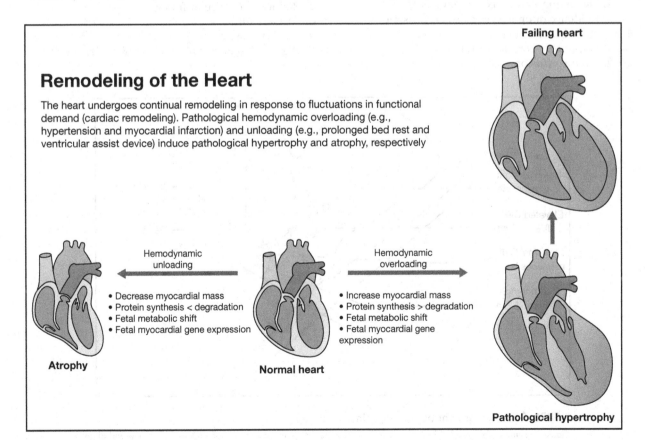

Remodeling of the Heart

The heart undergoes continual remodeling in response to fluctuations in functional demand (cardiac remodeling). Pathological hemodynamic overloading (e.g., hypertension and myocardial infarction) and unloading (e.g., prolonged bed rest and ventricular assist device) induce pathological hypertrophy and atrophy, respectively

Failing heart

Hemodynamic unloading

Hemodynamic overloading

- Decrease myocardial mass
- Protein synthesis < degradation
- Fetal metabolic shift
- Fetal myocardial gene expression

- Increase myocardial mass
- Protein synthesis > degradation
- Fetal metabolic shift
- Fetal myocardial gene expression

Atrophy

Normal heart

Pathological hypertrophy

FIGURE 9.4 Cardiac remodeling.

3. Dyspnea.
4. Reduced exercise tolerance.
5. Early satiety.
6. Abdominal bloating.
B. Diastolic heart failure.
    1. Dyspnea (especially exertional).
    2. Fatigue.
    3. Dizziness.
    4. Exercise intolerance (Brashers, 2019; Del Buono et al., 2020; Murphy et al., 2020).

OBJECTIVE DATA

A. Systolic heart failure.
    1. S_3 gallop on auscultation (see Figure 9.1).
    2. Hypotension or hypertension.
    3. Cyanosis.
    4. Edema.
    5. Cough with frothy sputum.
    6. Oliguria.
    7. Decreased oxygen saturation.
    8. Orthopnea.
    9. Paroxysmal nocturnal dyspnea.
    10. Abdominal distention.
    11. Bendopnea.
    12. Jugular vein distention (see Figure 9.5).
    13. Hepatojugular reflux (see Table 9.1).
    14. Evidence of underlying CAD is possible.
B. Diastolic heart failure.
    1. Inspiratory crackles or rales.
    2. Pleural effusion.

3. Pulmonary hypertension.
4. Right ventricular failure.
5. Left ventricular hypertrophy.
6. Pulmonary congestion with cardiomegaly. (Brashers, 2019; Del Buono et al., 2020; Murphy et al., 2020).

DIAGNOSTIC TESTS

A. See Appendix Table 9A.1 for listing of common diagnostic tests.

DIFFERENTIAL DIAGNOSES

A. Valvular disease.
B. Atrial myxoma.
C. Pericardial disease.
D. Acute coronary syndrome complicated by pulmonary disease.
E. Respiratory distress.
F. Chronic obstructive pulmonary disease (COPD).
G. Nephrotic syndrome.
H. Hypothyroidism.
I. Arteriovenous fistula (Tawil & Gelzini, 2020).

POTENTIAL COMPLICATIONS

A. Decreased myocardial compliance.
B. Reduced ventricular filling.
C. Arterial stiffness.
D. Hypertension.
E. Right-sided heart failure (Tawil & Gelzini, 2020).

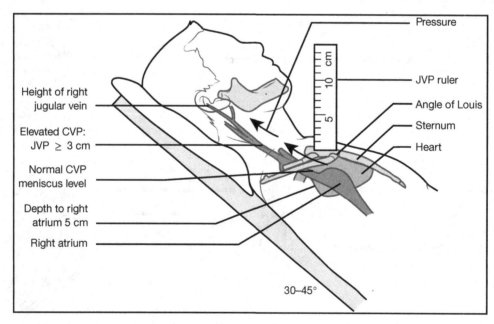

FIGURE 9.5 Assessment of jugular vein distention.

Note: Measurement of JVP. To obtain a patient's JVP, locate the oscillation point in the internal jugular IJ and align the bottom of a ruler with the sternal angle. Then note the vertical distance of the pulsation.

CVP, central venous pressure; JVP, jugular venous pulse.

DISEASE-MODIFYING TREATMENTS

A. Pharmacological interventions for heart failure (see Table 9.2 and Appendix D-1).

B. Supplemental oxygen.

C. Intravenous inotropic medications such as dobutamine and milrinone.

D. Intravenous administration of recombinant B-type natriuretic peptide (BNP).

TABLE 9.2 PHARMACOLOGICAL INTERVENTIONS FOR HEART FAILURE

CATEGORY	ACTION	EXAMPLES
Aldosterone-blocking agents (also called aldosterone receptor antagonists or antimineralocorticoids)	Inhibit the sodium-retaining effects of aldosterone and increase the excretion of hydrogen and potassium, which leads to decreased blood pressure and a decrease in pericardial fluid.	Eplerenone (Inspra) Spironolactone (Aldactone)
Anxiolytics	Used to prevent and treat anxiety, which is common in patients who have heart failure.	Alprazolam (Xanax) Diazepam (Valium) Lorazepam (Ativan) Escitalopram (Lexapro)
ACE inhibitors	Reduce blood pressure by preventing the production of angiotensin, which constricts blood vessels. The overall effect is vasodilation (Note: these drug names all end with "pril").	Benazepril (Lotensin) Captopril Enalapril (Vasotec) Fosinopril Lisinopril (Prinivil, Zestril) Moexipril Perindopril (Aceon) Quinapril (Accupril) Ramipril (Altace) Trandolapril (Mavik)
ARBs	Block the vasoconstrictive effects of angiotensin II. They are used to treat hypertension and heart failure. They are also used in the prevention of renal disease in patients who have type 2 diabetes and to prevent stroke (note: these drugs end with "sartan").	Azilsartan (Edarbi) Candesartan (Atacand) Eprosartan (Teveten) Irbesartan (Avapro) Telmisartan (Micardis) Valsartan (Diovan) Losartan (Cozaar) Olmesartan (Benicar)
Antiarrhythmics	Antiarrhythmics are used to prevent and treat abnormal cardiac impulses or abnormal conduction of impulses. There are four classes of antiarrhythmics, each with its own mechanism of action.	Class I: sodium channel blockers/blockage drugs (e.g., quinidine, lidocaine, propafenone) Class II: beta-blockers (e.g., atenolol, metoprolol, propranolol, carvedilol) Class III: potassium channel blockers (e.g., sotalol, amiodarone) Class IV: calcium channel blockers (e.g., amlodipine, diltiazem, verapamil)
Anticoagulants	Drugs that interfere with any step of the coagulation process and prolong clotting time. There are four types of anticoagulants.	Betrixaban Coumarins and indandiones (e.g., warfarin) Factor Xa inhibitors (rivaroxaban, apixaban, fondaparinux, edoxaban, betrixaban) Heparins (e.g., enoxaparin, dalteparin, tinzaparin, danaparoid) Thrombin inhibitors (e.g., dabigatran, bivalirudin, lepirudin, desirudin)

(continued)

TABLE 9.2   PHARMACOLOGICAL INTERVENTIONS FOR HEART FAILURE (*CONTINUED*)

CATEGORY	ACTION	EXAMPLES
Antiplatelet drugs	These drugs reduce the ability of platelets to stick together and aggregate on a vessel wall.	Abciximab (ReoPro) Anagrelide (Agrylin) Aspirin (generic) Cilostazol (Pletal) Clopidogrel (Plavix) Dipyridamole (Persantine) Eptifibatide (Integrilin) Prasugrel (Effient) Ticagrelor (Brilinta) Ticlopidine (generic) Tirofiban (Aggrastat) Vorapaxar (Zontivity)
Cardiac glycosides	These drugs increase cardiac output and decrease heart rate, and ultimately improve ejection fraction by inhibiting sodium/potassium ATPase.	Digoxin (Lanoxin) Digitoxin
Diuretics	Diuretics decrease cardiac workload by increasing water excretion. Loop diuretics act on the loop of Henle to decrease sodium and water reabsorption.	Bumetanide (Bumex, Burinex) Furosemide (Lasix) Torsemide (Demadex)
NEP inhibitors	Used to treat heart failure with reduced ejection fraction.	Sacubitril/valsartan
Nitrates	Used to treat or prevent angina. Nitrates reduce vascular resistance, decrease left ventricular filling pressure, and increase cardiac output.	Nitroglycerin (Nitrostat, Nitromist, Nitro-Bid) Isosorbide mononitrate or dinitrate (Isordil, Dilatrate SR)
PDE-5 inhibitors	By inhibiting the action of PDE-5, these drugs promote pulmonary vessel dilation. Thus, they are used to treat pulmonary hypertension.	Sildenafil (Viagra, Revatio) Tadalafil (Adcirca)
Statins	Used to prevent and treat atherosclerotic disease. Statin drugs inhibit HMG-CoA reductase, which ultimately leads to a decreased cholesterol synthesis in the liver.	Atorvastatin (Lipitor), Fluvastatin (Lescol), Lovastatin (Mevacor, Altocor) Pravastatin (Pravachol), Simvastatin (Zocor) Rosuvastatin (Crestor)
Renin inhibitors	Block the effects of renin, which causes vasodilation leading to lowered blood pressure.	Aliskiren (Tekturna)

ACE, angiotensin-converting enzyme; ARBs, angiotensin II receptor blockers; ATPase, adenosine triphosphate synthase; HMG-CoA, 3-hydroxy-3-methylglutaryl coenzyme A; 3-hyrdoxy-3-methylglutaryl coenzyme A; NEP, neprilysin; PDE-5, phosphodiesterase 5.

Sources: Epocrates. (2022). *Drugs.* https://online.epocrates.com/drugs; Karch, A. M. (2019). *Focus on nursing pharmacology.* Lippincott Williams & Wilkins; Revuelta-López, E., Núñez, J., Gastelurrutia, P., Cediel, G., Januzzi, J. L., Ibrahim, N. E., Emdin, M., VanKimmenade, R., Pascual-Figal, D., Núñez, E., Gommans, F., Lupón, J., & Bayés-Genís, A. (2020). Neprilysin inhibition, endorphin dynamics, and early symptomatic improvement in heart failure: A pilot study. *ESC Heart Failure, 7*(2), 559–566. https://doi.org/10.1002/ehf2.12607; Wright, P. M. (2019). *Certified hospice and palliative nurse (CHPN) exam review: A study guide with review questions.* Springer Publishing Company.

E. Intra-aortic balloon pump (IABP; see www.youtube.com/watch?v=mADxD7C8jBw).
F. Left ventricular assist device (LVAD).
G. Implementation of cardiac diet.
H. Implanted pacemaker and/or defibrillator (see Figures 9.6 and 9.7).
I. Coronary bypass.
J. Percutaneous coronary intervention (PCI).
K. Heart transplant.

PALLIATIVE INTERVENTIONS/SYMPTOM MANAGEMENT

A. See Appendix Table 9A.2 for listing of palliative interventions and symptom management.
B. SeeSee Appendix D-3 for overview of common symptoms.

PROGNOSIS

A. The 5-year survival rate after hospitalization for left-sided heart failure symptoms is 24.7%.
B. See www.predict-hf.com/, an online tool for determining prognosis for heart failure (Murphy et al., 2020).

NURSING INTERVENTIONS

A. Use and teach patient and family infection control measures.
B. Provide education on disease process and symptom management.
C. Teach patient to take all medications as prescribed.
D. Teach patient to engage in aerobic physical activity as tolerated, alternating periods of activity with periods of rest.
E. Encourage smoking cessation (see Appendices B-10 and C-9).
F. Maintain nutritional status.
G. Assess caregiver fatigue/burnout.
H. Encourage completion of advance directives.
I. Educate patient and family regarding availability of palliative care.
J. Educate patient and family regarding availability of hospice services (when appropriate).
K. Provide referral to community support groups, as needed.

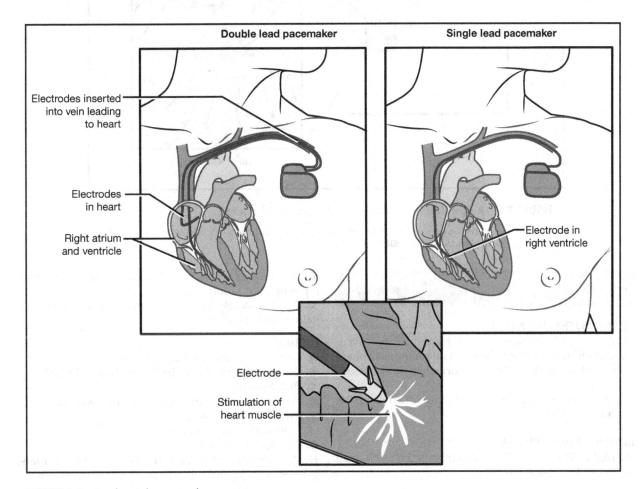

FIGURE 9.6 Implanted pacemaker.

Source: Adapted from National Heart, Lung, and Blood Institute. (2013). *Implantable pacemaker.*

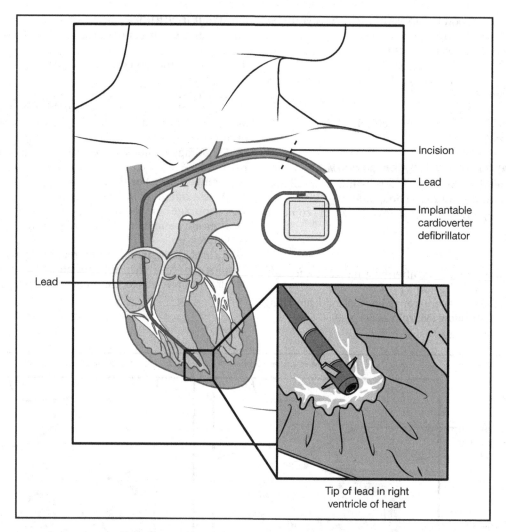

FIGURE 9.7 Automated implantable cardioverter-defibrillator.

Source: Adapted from Blausen.com staff. (2014). Medical gallery of Blausen Medical 2014. *WikiJournal of Medicine, 1*(2).https://doi.org/10.15347/wjm/2014.010.

RIGHT HEART FAILURE (ALSO KNOWN AS COR PULMONALE)

DEFINITION/CHARACTERISTICS
A. A type of heart failure characterized by right ventricular failure, leading to inadequate pulmonary blood flow and circulation despite normal central venous pressure.

B. Often related to pulmonary disease (Brashers, 2019; Workman, 2021).

INCIDENCE AND PREVALENCE
A. Right-sided heart failure accounts for 5% to 7% of all types of heart disease in adults

B. Right-sided heart failure accounts for 25% of all types of heart failure.

C. Approximately 15 million adults have cor pulmonale (Sommers, 2019).

ETIOLOGY
A. Left heart failure (most common).

B. Chronic obstructive pulmonary disease (COPD).

C. Emphysema.

D. Adult respiratory distress syndrome (ARDS).

E. Pulmonary embolism (PE).

F. Ventricular myocardial infarction.

G. Cardiomyopathies.

H. Pulmonic valvular disease (Brashers, 2019; Sommers, 2019; Stromberg, 2021; Workman, 2021).

PATHOPHYSIOLOGY

A. Pulmonary hypertension causes vascular restriction within the lung tissue, which restricts blood flow from the right side of the heart.

B. In response to the increased pressure and workload, cardiac hypertrophy occurs.

C. As the right side of the heart becomes weaker, it loses its ability to overcome the vascular restriction within the lungs, resulting in venous congestion (Stromberg, 2021; Workman, 2021).

PREDISPOSING FACTORS

A. Smoking.

B. Age over 40 years.

C. Male sex.

D. Cystic fibrosis.

E. Hemosiderosis.

F. Upper airway obstruction.

G. Scleroderma.

H. Extensive bronchiectasis.

I. Neurological diseases that affect respiratory muscles (Sommers, 2019).

SUBJECTIVE DATA

A. Dyspnea.

B. Fatigue.

C. Nausea.

D. Anorexia.

E. Anxiety related to dyspnea.

F. Restlessness.

G. Confusion.

H. Irritability (Sommers, 2019; Stromberg, 2021; Workman, 2021).

OBJECTIVE DATA

A. Jugular vein distention (see Figure 9.5).

B. Peripheral edema.

C. Hepatosplenomegaly.

D. Use of accessory muscles with breathing (see www.youtube.com/watch?v=r7pzHhSbjN0).

E. Cyanosis.

F. Weight gain (related to edema).

G. Right ventricular enlargement.

H. Hypoxia.

I. Metabolic and respiratory acidosis.

J. Pulmonary hypertension.

K. Right upper quadrant tenderness.

L. Clubbing of fingers and toes.

M. Rales.

N. Polycythemia.

O. Lifts or heaves in the area of the precordium.

P. S_3 or S_4 gallop.

Q. Increased blood viscosity (Sommers, 2019; Stromberg, 2021; Workman, 2021).

DIAGNOSTIC TESTS

A. See Appendix Table 9A.1 for listing of common diagnostic tests.

DIFFERENTIAL DIAGNOSES

A. Disorders that cause increased blood viscosity, such as:

   1. Left-sided heart failure.

   2. Pericarditis.

   3. Primary pulmonic stenosis.

   4. Right-sided heart failure due to right ventricular infarction or congenital heart disease.

   5. Ventricular septal defect (Leong, 2017).

PALLIATIVE INTERVENTIONS/SYMPTOM MANAGEMENT

A. See Appendix Table 9A.2 for listing of palliative interventions and symptom management.

B. See Appendix D-3 for overview of common symptoms.

POTENTIAL COMPLICATIONS

A. Biventricular heart failure.

B. Hepatomegaly.

C. Pleural effusion.

D. Thromboembolism related to polycythemia (Sommers, 2019).

DISEASE-MODIFYING TREATMENTS

A. Treatment of underlying cause(s), such as:

   1. Left heart failure (see section on Left Heart Failure).

   2. COPD.

   3. Cystic fibrosis.

   4. Primary arterial hypertension.

B. Management of intravascular volume.

C. Assisting right ventricular contractions.

D. Pharmacological interventions (see Table 9.2).

   1. Vasodilators.

   2. Vasopressors.

   3. Calcium channel blockers.

   4. Bronchodilators.

E. Mechanical ventilation.

F. High-flow oxygen if underlying cause of embolism.

G. Correct acid–base imbalances.

H. Correct fluid and electrolyte imbalances.

I. Fluid loading.

J. Single or double lung transplant (Brashers, 2019; Sommers, 2019).

PROGNOSIS

A. Median survival rate from first hospitalization is 5 years.

B. Indicators of poor prognosis include:

   1. Class IV, New York Heart Association (see Table 9.3).

   2. Weight loss.

   3. Cachexia.

   4. Advanced age.

   5. Repeated hospital admissions.

   6. Hyponatremia.

   7. Hypotension.

   8. Frailty.

   9. Declining functional status.

   10. Comorbidities:

      a. COPD.

      b. End-stage renal disease (Pandey et al., 2019; Pantilat et al., 2021).

TABLE 9.3 NEW YORK HEART ASSOCIATION FUNCTIONAL CLASSIFICATION

FUNCTIONAL CAPACITY	OBJECTIVE ASSESSMENT
Class I: Patients with cardiac disease but without resulting limitation on physical activity. Ordinary physical activity does not cause undue fatigue, palpitation, dyspnea, or anginal pain.	A. No objective evidence of cardiovascular disease
Class II: Patients with cardiac disease resulting in slight limitation of physical activity. They are comfortable at rest. Ordinary physical activity results in fatigue, palpitation, dyspnea, or anginal pain.	B. Objective evidence of minimal cardiovascular disease
Class III: Patients with cardiac disease resulting in marked limitation of physical activity. They are comfortable at rest. Less than ordinary activity causes fatigue, palpitation, dyspnea, or anginal pain.	C. Objective evidence of moderately severe cardiovascular disease
Class IV: Patients with cardiac disease resulting in inability to carry on any physical activity without discomfort. Symptoms of heart failure or angina may be present even at rest. If any physical activity is undertaken, discomfort is increased.	D. Objective evidence of severe cardiovascular disease

Source: The Criteria Committee of the New York Heart Association. (1994). Nomenclature and criteria for diagnosis of diseases of the heart and great vessels (9th ed., pp. 253–256). Little, Brown & Co.

NURSING INTERVENTIONS

A. Individualize plan of care to patient's age and lifestyle needs.
B. Provide teaching regarding treatments and treatment side effects.
C. Encourage small, frequent meals and high-calorie snacks.
D. Teach patient to take medications as prescribed.
E. Encourage smoking cessation (see Appendices B-10 and C-9).
F. Offer reputable online resources.
G. Provide spiritual support.
H. Assess caregiver fatigue/burnout.
I. Encourage completion of advance directives.
J. Educate patient and family regarding availability of palliative care.
K. Educate patient and family regarding availability of hospice services (when appropriate).
L. Provide referral to community support groups, as needed.

CORONARY ARTERY DISEASE

DEFINITION/CHARACTERISTICS

A. A condition in which the cardiac muscle is progressively deprived of oxygen and nutrients due to restricted blood flow secondary to atherosclerosis (Centers for Disease Control and Prevention, 2022b).

INCIDENCE AND PREVALENCE

A. Coronary artery disease (CAD) is the number one cause of death in the United States.
B. Roughly 370,000 people die each year from CAD.
C. About one million adults (20 years or older) have CAD (Brashers & Huether, 2019; Centers for Disease Control and Prevention, 2022c).

ETIOLOGY

A. CAD develops secondary to atherosclerosis that causes narrowing of the cardiac vessels, which reduces blood flow to the cardiac muscle (Centers for Disease Control and Prevention, 2022b).

PATHOPHYSIOLOGY

A. Hypercholesteremia contributes to atherosclerosis.
B. Development of atherosclerotic plaques narrows the cardiac vessels, impeding cardiac vascularization (Bergheanu et al., 2017).

PREDISPOSING FACTORS

A. Advanced age.
B. Male gender or postmenopausal female.
C. Genetic predisposition.
D. Dyslipidemia.
E. Hypertension.
F. Cigarette smoking.
G. Diabetes and/or insulin resistance.
H. Obesity.
I. Atherogenic diet (Brashers & Huether, 2019; Centers for Disease Control and Prevention, 2022b).

SUBJECTIVE DATA
A. Angina.
B. Weakness.
C. Dyspnea.
D. Dizziness.
E. Syncope (Brashers, 2019; Centers for Disease Control and Prevention, 2022b).

OBJECTIVE DATA
A. Hypercholesterolemia.
B. Arrythmias (Centers for Disease Control and Prevention, 2022b).

DIAGNOSTIC TESTS
A. See Appendix Table 9A.1 for listing of common diagnostic tests.

TABLE 9.4   DISORDERS OF IMPULSE FORMATION

TYPE	ELECTROCARDIOGRAM	EFFECT	PATHOPHYSIOLOGY	TREATMENT
Sinus bradycardia	P rate 60 or less PR interval normal QRS for each P	Increased preload Decreased mean arterial pressure	Hyperkalemia: slows depolarization Vagal hyperactivity: unknown Digoxin toxicity: common Late hypoxia: lack of ATP	If hypotensive, treat cause and support Follow with sympathomimetics, cardiotonics, and pacer Vagolytics
Simple sinus tachycardia	P rate 100–150 PR interval normal QRS for each P	Decreased filling times Decreased mean arterial pressure Increased myocardial demand	Catecholamines; rise in resting potential, calcium influx Fever: unknown Early failure and lung disease: hypoxic cell metabolism Hypercalcemia	Oxygen, bed rest Calcium channel blockers
PACs or beats	Early P waves that may have changed morphology PR interval normal QRS for each P	Occasional decreased filling time and mean arterial pressure	Electrolyte disturbances: decrease in all phases Hypoxia and elevated preload: cell membrane disturbances Hypercalcemia	Treat underlying cause Digoxin
Sinus dysrhythmias	Rate varies P-P regularly irregular, short with inspiration, long with exhalation PR interval normal QRS for each P	Variable filling times Variable mean arterial pressures Variable oxygen demand	Unknown Common in young children and young adults	None
Atrial tachycardia (includes premature atrial tachycardia if onset is abrupt)	P rate 151–250; morphology may differ from sinus PPR interval normal P:QRS ratio variable	Decreased filling time Decreased mean arterial pressure Increased myocardial demand	Same as PACs: leads to increased atrial automaticity, atrial reentry Digoxin toxicity: common	Control ventricular rate Digoxin, calcium channel blockers, vagus stimulation Pace to override

(continued)

TABLE 9.4   DISORDERS OF IMPULSE FORMATION (*CONTINUED*)

TYPE	ELECTROCARDIOGRAM	EFFECT	PATHOPHYSIOLOGY	TREATMENT
Atrial flutter[a]	P rate 251–300; morphology may vary from sinus P PR interval usually not observable P:QRS ratio variable	Decreased filling time Decreased mean arterial pressure	Same as atrial tachycardia Aging	Same as atrial tachycardia Synchronous cardioversion
Atrial fibrillation[a]	P rate >300 and usually not observable No PR interval QRS rate variable and rhythm irregular	Same as atrial flutter	Same as atrial tachycardia Aging	Same as atrial tachycardia
Idiojunctional rhythm	P absent or independent QRS normal, rate 41–59, regular	Decreased cardiac output from loss of atrial contribution to ventricular preload Decreased mean atrial pressure as a result of bradycardia	Atrial and sinus bradycardia, standstill, or block	Same as sinus bradycardia
Junctional bradycardia	P absent or independent QRS normal, rate 40 or less	Same as idiojunctional rhythm	Same as idiojunctional rhythm Vagal hyperactivity	Same as sinus bradycardia
PJCs or beats	Early beats without P waves QRS morphology normal	Decreased cardiac output from loss of atrial contribution to ventricular preload for that beat	Hyperkalemia (6–5.4 mEq/L) Hypercalcemia, hypoxia, and elevated preload (see PACs)	Same as PACs
Accelerated junctional rhythm	P absent or independent QRS morphology normal, rate 60–99	Decreased cardiac output from loss of atrial contribution to ventricular preload	Same as PJCs	Same as PACs
Junctional tachycardia	P absent or independent QRS morphology normal, rate 100 or more	Decreased cardiac output from loss of atrial contribution to ventricular preload Increased myocardial demand because of tachycardia	Same as PJCs	Same as PACs

(*continued*)

TABLE 9.4   DISORDERS OF IMPULSE FORMATION (*CONTINUED*)

TYPE	ELECTROCARDIOGRAM	EFFECT	PATHOPHYSIOLOGY	TREATMENT
Idioventricular rhythm[b]	P absent or independent QRS >0.11 and rate 20–39	Same as idiojunctional rhythm	Sinus, atrial, and junctional bradycardia, standstill, or block	Same as sinus bradycardia
Ventricular bradycardia[b]	P absent or independent QRS >0.11 and rate 60–21	Same as idiojunctional rhythm	Same as idiojunctional rhythm	Same as sinus bradycardia
Agonal rhythm/ electromechanical dissociation[b]	P absent or independent QRS >0.11 and rate 20 or less	Absent or barely present cardiac output and pulse Not compatible with life	Depolarization and contraction not coupled: electrical activity present with little or no mechanical activity Usually caused by profound hypoxia	Vigorous pharmacology aimed at restoring rate and force Usually ineffective May attempt to pace
Ventricular standstill or asystole[b]	P absent or independent QRS absent	No cardiac output Not compatible with life	Profound ischemia, hyperkalemia, acidosis	Same as agonal rhythm, including electrical defibrillation
PVCs or depolarizations[a]	Early beats with P waves QRS occasionally opposite in deflection from usual QRS	Same as PJCs	Same as PJCs, including aging and induction of anesthesia Impulse originates in cell outside normal conduction system and spreads through intercalated disks	Pharmacology to change thresholds, refractory periods; reduce myocardial demand, increase supply Removal of cause
Accelerated ventricular rhythm	P absent or independent QRS >0.11 and rate 41–99	Same as accelerated junctional rhythm	Same as PVCs	Same as PVCs
Ventricular tachycardia[b]	P absent or independent QRS >0.11 and rate 100 or more	Same as junctional tachycardia	Same as PVCs	Same as PVCs, including electrical cardioversion
Ventricular fibrillation[b]	P absent QRS >300 and usually not observable	Same as ventricular standstill	Same as PVCs rapid infusion of potassium	Same as PVCs including electrical defibrillation

[a]Most common in adults. [b]Life threatening in adults.

ATP, adenosine triphosphate; PACs, premature atrial contractions; PJCs, premature junctional contractions; PVCs, premature ventricular contractions.

Source: Brashers, V. L. (2019). Alterations in cardiovascular function. In K. L. McCance & S. E. Huether (Eds.), *Pathophysiology: The biologic basis for disease in adults and children* (8th ed., pp. 1058–1690). Elsevier. Used with permission.

TABLE 9.5   DISORDERS OF IMPULSE CONDUCTION

TYPE	ELECTROCARDIOGRAM	EFFECT	PATHOPHYSIOLOGY	TREATMENT
Sinus block	Occasionally absent P, with loss of QRS for that beat	Occasional decrease in cardiac output Increase in preload for the following beat	Local hypoxia, scarring of intra-atrial conduction pathways, electrolyte imbalances Increased atrial preload	Conservative Usually do not progress in severity Pharmacological treatment includes vagolytics, sympathomimetics, and pacing
First-degree block[a]	PR interval >0.2	None	Same as sinus block Hyperkalemia (>7 mEq/L) Hypokalemia (<3.5 mEq/L) Formation of myocardial abscesses in endocarditis	Conservative Discovery and correction of cause
Second-degree block, Mobitz I, or Wenckebach[a]	Progressive prolongation of PR interval until one QRS is dropped Pattern of prolongation resumes	Same as sinus block	Hypokalemia (<3.5 mEq/L) Faulty cell metabolism in AV node Severity increases as heart rate increases Supports theory that AV node is fatiguing Digoxin toxicity, beta-blockade CAD, MI, hypoxia, increased preload, valvular surgery and disease, diabetes	Same as sinus block
Second-degree block or Mobitz II	Same as sinus block	Same as sinus block	Hypokalemia (<3.5 mEq/L) Faulty cell metabolism below AV node Antidysrhythmics, cyclic antidepressants CAD, MI, hypoxia, increased preload, valvular surgery and disease, diabetes	More aggressive than Mobitz I because block can progress to type III Pacemaker after pharmacological treatment
Third-degree block[b]	P waves present and independent of QRS No observed relationship between P and QRS Always AV dissociation	Same as idiojunctional rhythm	Hypokalemia (<3.5 mEq/L) Faulty cell metabolism low in bundle of His MI, especially inferior wall, as nodal artery interrupted; results in ischemia of AV node	Pharmacological until pacemaker inserted Temporary pacing if caused by inferior MI because ischemia usually resolves
Atrioventricular dissociation	P waves present and independent of QRS, but not always because of block (e.g., ventricular tachycardia) AV dissociation not always third-degree block	Decreased cardiac output from loss of atrial contribution to ventricular preload Variable effect on myocardial demand, depending on ventricular rate	May result from third-degree block or accelerated junctional or ventricular rhythm, or be caused by sinus, atrial, and junctional bradycardias	Treat according to cause Pacemaker or reducing rate of AV or ventricular discharge, or increasing rate of sinus or AV node discharge

TYPE	ELECTROCARDIOGRAM	EFFECT	PATHOPHYSIOLOGY	TREATMENT
Ventricular block	QRS >0.11 R-S-R' in V_1, V_2, V_5, V_6	None	Faulty cell metabolism in right and left bundle branches RBBB more common than LBBB because of dual blood supply to left bundle branch Congestive heart failure, mitral regurgitation, especially anterior MI, because of infarct of fascicles Left anterior hemiblock more common than left posterior hemiblock, since posterior fascicles have dual blood supply	Isolated RBBB or LBBB or hemiblock not treated If acute and/or associated with acute anterior MI, treated with permanent pacer and vigorous pharmacology
Aberrant conduction	QRS >0.11	None unless ventricular rate abnormalities present	Conduction of impulse through intercalated disks because conduction system transiently blocked because of hypoxia, electrolyte imbalances, digoxin toxicity, excessively rapid rates of discharge	Correct underlying cause
Preexcitation syndromes (Wolff–Parkinson–White and Lown–Ganong–Levine)	P present with QRS for each P PR interval >0.12 and QRS >0.11 because of presence of delta wave in PR interval	None	Congenital presence of accessory pathways (bundle of Kent and fiber of Mahaim) that conduct very rapidly and bypass the AV node, causing early ventricular depolarization in relation to atrial depolarization Prone (reason unknown) to tachycardias and atrial fibrillation that can result in very rapid ventricular rates	Aimed at lining up refractory periods of accessory pathway and AV node to prevent reentry May slow rate with pharmacology May surgically cut pathways

[a]Most common in adults. [b]Life threatening in adults.

AV, atrioventricular; CAD, coronary artery disease; LBBB, left bundle branch block; MI, myocardial infarction; RBBB, right bundle branch block.

Source: Brashers, V. L. (2019). Alterations in cardiovascular function. In K. L. McCance & S. E. Huether (Eds.), *Pathophysiology: The biologic basis for disease in adults and children* (8th ed., pp. 1058–1690). Elsevier. Used with permission.

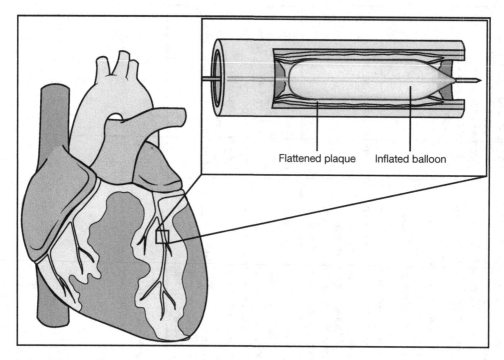

Flattened plaque   Inflated balloon

FIGURE 9.8 Balloon angioplasty.

Source: Adapted from Blausen Medical Communications, Inc. (n.d.). *Angioplasty balloon inflated.*

DIFFERENTIAL DIAGNOSES
A. Pericarditis.
B. Dilated cardiomyopathy.
C. Hypertensive heart disease.
D. Myocarditis.
E. Pulmonary embolism (PE).
F. Left ventricular infarction.
G. Unstable angina (Shah, 2021).

POTENTIAL COMPLICATIONS
A. Arrythmias or dysrhythmias.
B. Heart failure.
C. Angina.
D. Myocardial infarction (Mayo Clinic, 2022b).

DISEASE-MODIFYING TREATMENTS
A. Medical management (see Table 9.2):
    1. Statin therapy.
    2. Cholesterol absorption inhibitors.
    3. Bile acid sequestrants.
    4. Proprotein convertase subtilisin kexin type-9 inhibitors.
    5. Fibrates.
    6. N-3 fatty acids.
    7. Cholesteryl ester transfer protein (CETP) inhibitors.
B. Management of dysrhythmias (see Tables 9.4 and 9.5).
C. Supplemental oxygen.
D. Cardiac revascularization.
E. Coronary artery bypass graft (CABG)
F. Percutaneous coronary intervention (PCI).
    1. Balloon angioplasty (see Figure 9.8).
    2. Angioplasty with stent (see Figure 9.9).
    3. Rotational atherectomy.
    4. Impella-supported PCI (Bergheanu et al., 2017; Ramadan et al., 2018).

PALLIATIVE INTERVENTIONS/SYMPTOM MANAGEMENT
A. See Appendix Table 9A.2 for listing of palliative interventions and symptom management.
B. See Appendix D-3 for overview of common symptoms.

PROGNOSIS
A. The risk of a major adverse cardiovascular event is greatly elevated in those with CAD.
B. The 10-year mortality rate for CAD is 21% (Zeitouni et al., 2020).

NURSING INTERVENTIONS
A. Teach patient to report palpitations, dizziness, or fainting.
B. Teach patient to monitor for and report symptoms of heart failure such as:
    1. Weight gain of >3 pounds in 1 week.
    2. Decreased exercise tolerance lasting more than 2 to 3 days.
    3. Cough lasting more than 3 to 5 days.
    4. Nocturia.
    5. Development or worsening of dyspnea on exertion or unstable angina.

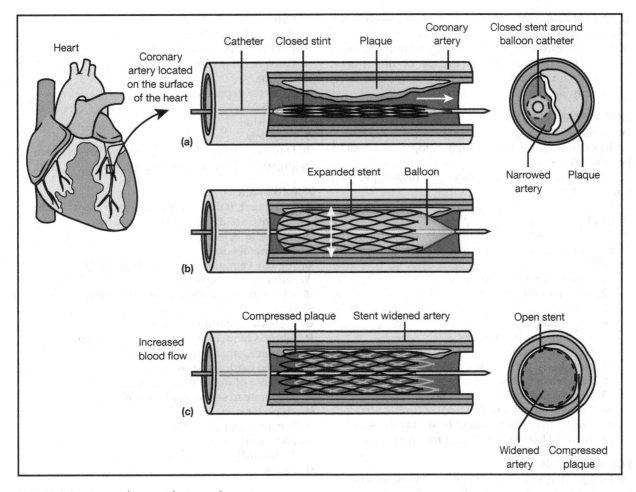

FIGURE 9.9 Angioplasty with stent placement.

Source: Adapted from National Institutes of Health. (2006). *Diagram of coronary angioplasty and stent placement.* https://www.nhlbi.nih.gov/health/heart-treatments-procedures

C. Teach patient to take all medications as prescribed, modify diet and fluid intake as recommended, and implement recommended lifestyle changes.

D. Encourage smoking cessation (see Appendices B-10 and C-9).

E. Provide spiritual support.

F. Teach patient to modify diet for cardiac health.

G. Encourage exercise as tolerated.

H. Assess caregiver fatigue/burnout.

I. Encourage completion of advance directives.

J. Educate patient and family regarding availability of palliative care.

K. Educate patient and family regarding availability of hospice services (when appropriate).

L. Provide referral to community support groups, as needed.

DILATED CARDIOMYOPATHY

DEFINITION/CHARACTERISTICS

A. A progressive, usually irreversible cardiac disease involving structural abnormality of the heart characterized by:
  1. Extensive damage to the myofibrils.
  2. Altered myocardial metabolism.
  3. Ventricular dilation and hypertrophy.
  4. Atrial enlargement.
  5. Stasis of blood in the left ventricle.
  6. Decreased cardiac contractility.

B. Cardiomyopathy is classified as:
  1. Primary (cause unknown).
  2. Secondary (resulting from another disease process).

C. Dilated cardiomyopathy is the most common type of cardiomyopathy.

D. Dilated cardiomyopathy is one of the most common causes of heart failure.

E. Dilated cardiomyopathy most commonly manifests in the third or fourth decade of life (Burke, 2015; Dechant & Heimgartner, 2021; Sommers, 2019; Stromberg, 2021).

INCIDENCE AND PREVALENCE

A. Prevalence is roughly 1 in 2,500.

B. Incidence discovered through autopsy is 4.5 cases per 100,000 per year.

C. Clinical incidence is 2.45 cases per 100,000 per year (Burke, 2015).

ETIOLOGY

A. May be unknown in certain cases, but certain conditions are known to cause dilated cardiomyopathy, including:

  1. Ischemic heart disease.
  2. Valvular disease.
  3. Diabetes.
  4. Renal failure.
  5. Alcohol or drug toxicity.
  6. Hyperthyroidism.
  7. Nutritional deficiencies.
  8. Systemic infection.
  9. Genetic disorders.
  10. Chronic inflammation.
  11. Connective tissue disorder(s) (Brashers, 2019; Dechant & Heimgartner, 2021; Stromberg, 2021).

PATHOPHYSIOLOGY

A. Increased cardiac workload and hypertrophy of heart chambers lead to diminished cardiac performance.

B. Dilated cardiomyopathy is progressive and leads to heart failure if left untreated (Sommers, 2019; Stromberg, 2021).

PREDISPOSING FACTORS

A. Alcohol abuse.
B. Cocaine use.
C. Anesthesia agents.
D. Chemotherapy.
E. Systemic infection.
F. Chronic inflammation.
G. Poor nutrition.
H. Male sex.
I. Genetic predisposition.
J. Occurs most often in middle age (Dechant & Heimgartner, 2021; Sommers, 2019; Stromberg, 2021).

SUBJECTIVE DATA

A. Dyspnea on exertion.
B. Fatigue.
C. Lower extremity edema.
D. Decreased exercise capacity.
E. Palpitations.
F. Generalized weakness.
G. Orthopnea.
H. Activity intolerance.
I. Dizziness and/or syncope.
J. Paroxysmal nocturnal dyspnea.
K. Angina.
L. Anxiety/depression.
M. Restlessness.
N. Confusion.
O. Insomnia.
P. Difficulty concentrating (Brashers, 2019; Dechant & Heimgartner, 2021; Sommers, 2019; Stromberg, 2021).

OBJECTIVE DATA

A. Left heart failure or biventricular heart failure is characteristic of dilated cardiomyopathy.

B. S_3 and/or S_4 gallop.
C. Peripheral edema.
D. Jugular vein distention (see Figure 9.5).
E. Pulmonary congestion.
F. Dysrhythmias including atrial fibrillation and heart block.
G. Systemic or pulmonary emboli.
H. Fibrosis of myocardium and endocardium.
I. Displaced apical pulse.
J. Dilated cardiac chambers.
K. Presence of mural wall thrombi.
L. Moderate to severe cardiomegaly.
M. Hypertension.
N. Narrow pulse pressure.
O. Pleural effusions.
P. Tachycardia.
Q. Pallor.
R. Cyanosis.
S. Ascites.
T. Hepatojugular reflux (see Table 9.1).
U. Hepatomegaly.
V. Crackles on auscultation.
W. Bounding or alternating strength peripheral pulses.
X. Valvular murmurs (see Figures 9.1, 9.2, and 9.3; Brashers, 2019; Dechant & Heimgartner, 2021; Sommers, 2019; Stromberg, 2021).

DIAGNOSTIC TESTS

A. See Appendix Table 9A.1 for listing of common diagnostic tests.

DIFFERENTIAL DIAGNOSES

A. Differential diagnoses in cases of dilated cardiomyopathy are used to exclude secondary causes such as:

  1. Chronic hypertension.
  2. Valvular disease.
  3. Severe coronary disease (Burke, 2015).

POTENTIAL COMPLICATIONS

A. Arrythmias or dysrhythmias.

B. Heart failure with decreased ejection fraction (Brashers, 2019; Stromberg, 2021).

DISEASE-MODIFYING TREATMENTS

A. Treatment is focused on management of underlying cause.

B. Medical management (see Table 9.2):

1. Vasodilators.
2. Diuretics.
3. Cardiac glycosides.
4. Beta-blockers.
5. Digoxin.
6. Antiarrhythmics.
7. Anticoagulants.
8. Antihypertensives.
9. Angiotensin-converting enzyme (ACE) inhibitors.

C. Management of dysrhythmias.

D. Supplemental oxygen.

E. Fluid and electrolyte management.

F. Cardiac resynchronization therapy (biventricular pacing).

G. Implanted pacemaker or implantable cardioverter-defibrillator (see Figures 9.6 and 9.7).

H. Left ventricular assist device (LVAD) as destination or bridge therapy (see Figure 9.10).

I. Heart transplant is required in severe cases (Brashers, 2019; Dechant & Heimgartner, 2021; Sommers, 2019; Stromberg, 2021).

PALLIATIVE INTERVENTIONS/SYMPTOM MANAGEMENT

A. See Appendix Table 9A.2 for listing of palliative interventions and symptom management.

B. See Appendix D-3 for overview of common symptoms.

PROGNOSIS

A. Severe dilated cardiomyopathy can be rapidly fatal.

B. In the late stages, right heart failure develops and is associated with poor prognosis.

C. Heart transplants are often necessary; 99% of all heart transplants are due to dilated cardiomyopathy.

D. Prognosis of less than 5 years in most patients.

E. Survival rate is less than 50% at 10 years (Burke, 2015; Dechant & Heimgartner, 2021; Sommers, 2019: Stromberg, 2021).

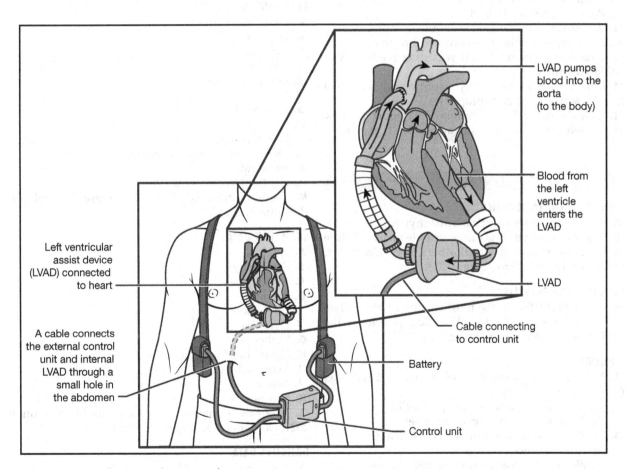

FIGURE 9.10 Left ventricular assist device.

Source: Adapted from National Heart Lung and Blood Institute. (2013). *Implantable VLAD.*

NURSING INTERVENTIONS

A. Use and teach patient and family infection control measures.

B. Teach patient to report palpitations, dizziness, or fainting.

C. Teach patient to avoid alcohol use.

D. Teach patient to monitor for and report symptoms of heart failure such as:

    1. Weight gain of >3 pounds in 1 week.

    2. Decreased exercise tolerance lasting more than 2 to 3 days.

    3. Cough lasting more than 3 to 5 days.

    4. Nocturia.

    5. Development or worsening of dyspnea on exertion or unstable angina.

E. Educate patient on prevention of exacerbations.

F. Teach patient to take all medications as prescribed, modify diet and fluid intake as recommended, and implement recommended lifestyle changes.

G. Encourage smoking cessation (see Appendices B-10 and C-9).

H. Maintain nutritional status.

I. Provide spiritual support.

J. Assess caregiver fatigue/burnout.

K. Encourage completion of advance directives.

L. Educate patient and family regarding availability of palliative care.

M. Educate patient and family regarding availability of hospice services (when appropriate).

N. Provide referral to community support groups, as needed (Dechant & Heimgartner, 2021; Sommers, 2019).

DYSRHYTHMIAS

DEFINITION/CHARACTERISTICS

A. Alterations in the heart's normal rhythm.

B. Chronic dysrhythmias can contribute to heart failure or can cause sudden death (Brashers, 2019; Dechant & Heimgartner, 2021; Stromberg, 2021).

INCIDENCE AND PREVALENCE

A. Atrial fibrillation is the most common type of dysrhythmia, affecting 2.7 to 6.1 million people in the United States (Dechant & Heimgartner, 2021).

ETIOLOGY

A. There are two main causes of cardiac dysrhythmias (see Tables 9.4 and 9.5):

    1. Abnormal rate of impulse generation.

    2. Abnormal conduction of impulses.

B. Cardiac dysthymias can result from a variety of underlying conditions such as:

    1. Electrolyte disturbances, especially potassium and magnesium.

    2. Vagal hyperactivity.

    3. Drug toxicity.

    4. Hypoxia.

    5. Catecholamines.

    6. Pulmonary disease.

    7. Ischemia.

    8. Acidosis.

    9. Abnormalities of the cardiac electrical conduction system.

    10. Cardiac autonomic neuropathy.

    11. Myocardial infarction.

    12. Hypovolemia.

    13. Anxiety (Brashers, 2019; Dechant & Heimgartner, 2021).

PATHOPHYSIOLOGY

A. The electrical signal generated by the sinoatrial (SA) node causes atrial and ventricular contraction and relaxation at a rate sufficient to provide tissue oxygenation at various levels of physical activity.

B. When electrical signal conduction is impaired by nerve or tissue dysfunction, dysrhythmias occur (Brashers, 2019).

PREDISPOSING FACTORS

A. Older age.

B. Hypertension.

C. Obesity.

D. Diabetes.

E. European ancestry.

F. Heart failure.

G. Ischemic heart disease.

H. Hyperthyroidism.

I. Chronic kidney disease.

J. Moderate to heavy alcohol use.

K. Smoking.

L. Cardiac hypertrophy.

M. Chronic stress (Center for Disease Control and Prevention, 2021).

SUBJECTIVE DATA

A. Angina.

B. Restlessness.

C. Nervousness.

D. Anxiety.

E. Confusion.

F. Dyspnea.

G. Orthopnea.

H. Generalized weakness.

I. Extreme fatigue.

J. Nausea.

K. Syncope.

L. Dizziness (Centers for Disease Control & Prevention, 2021; Dechant & Heimgartner, 2021)

OBJECTIVE DATA

A. Pulse deficit.

B. Change in pulse strength, rate, or rhythm.

C. Tachypnea.

D. Pulmonary crackles.

▶

E. S_3 or S_4 sounds.
F. Jugular vein distention (see Figure 9.5).
G. Pale, cool skin.
H. Diaphoresis.
I. Vomiting.
J. Oliguria.
K. Delayed capillary filling.
L. Hypotension (Dechant & Heimgartner, 2021).

DIAGNOSTIC TESTS
A. See Appendix Table 9A.1 for listing of common diagnostic tests.

DIFFERENTIAL DIAGNOSES
A. Anxiety.
B. Menopause.
C. Thyroid dysfunction.
D. Atrial flutter.
E. Atrial tachycardia.
F. Atrioventricular nodal reentry tachycardia.
G. Multifocal atrial tachycardia.
H. Paroxysmal supraventricular tachycardia.
I. Wolf–Parkinson–White syndrome (Rosenthal, 2019).

POTENTIAL COMPLICATIONS
A. Stroke.
B. Sudden death.
C. Heart failure (Mayo Clinic, 2022a).

DISEASE-MODIFYING TREATMENTS
A. Pharmacological management.
B. Cardioversion.
C. Implanted pacemaker (see Figure 9.6).
D. Automated implantable cardioverter-defibrillator (AICD; see Figure 9.7).
E. Left ventricular assist device (LVAD) if heart failure occurs (see Figure 9.10).
F. Ablation therapy (Mayo Clinic, 2022a).

PALLIATIVE INTERVENTIONS/SYMPTOM MANAGEMENT
A. See Appendix Table 9A.2 for listing of palliative interventions and symptom management.
B. See Appendix D-3 for overview of common symptoms.

NURSING INTERVENTIONS
A. Use and teach patient and family infection control measures.
B. Teach patient to take all medications as prescribed.
C. Maintain nutritional status.
D. Auscultate heart sounds noting abnormal rhythms or murmurs (see Figures 9.1, 9.2, and 9.3).
E. Provide spiritual support.
F. Encourage smoking cessation (see Appendices B-10 and C-9).
G. Assess caregiver fatigue/burnout.
H. Encourage completion of advance directives.
I. Educate patient and family regarding availability of palliative care.

J. Educate patient and family regarding availability of hospice services (when appropriate).
K. Provide referral to community support groups, as needed.

INFECTIVE ENDOCARDITIS

DEFINITION/CHARACTERISTICS
A. A general term used to describe infection and inflammation of the endocardium, especially the cardiac valves.
B. Formerly called bacterial endocarditis.
C. Infectious agent can be bacterial, fungal, or viral.
D. Aortic valve is the most commonly affected (Brashers, 2019; Dechant & Heimgartner, 2021; Stromberg, 2021).

INCIDENCE AND PREVALENCE
A. There are 13 cases per 100,000 annually (Sommers, 2019).

ETIOLOGY
A. The most common infective agents are *Streptococcus viridans* and *Streptococcus aureus.*
B. Infective endocarditis can also be caused by:
   1. Enterococci.
   2. Viruses.
   3. Fungi.
   4. Rickettsia.
   5. Parasites.
C. Portals of entry for infectious agents include:
   1. Injection drug use.
   2. Valve replacement.
   3. Systemic infection secondary to skin, genitourinary, and/or gastrointestinal infections.
   4. Oral cavity (particularly after dental procedures).
   5. Skin lesions, abscesses, or rashes.
   6. Surgery or other invasive medical procedures, including intravenous catheter placement.
   7. Gastrointestinal, urinary, or respiratory tract (Brashers, 2019; Dechant & Heimgartner, 2021; Stromberg, 2021).

PATHOPHYSIOLOGY
A. Inflammatory responses to endocardial infections result in endocardial damage.
B. Blood-borne pathogens adhere to the damaged endocardium (vegetation).
C. Vegetation activates a clotting cascade and can result in the formation of fibrin clots.
D. The fibrin clots protect the growing colonies, making the infection and inflammation challenging to control and reverse (Brashers, 2019; Dechant & Heimgartner, 2021; Liesenborghs et al., 2020).

PREDISPOSING FACTORS
A. Prosthetic heart valves.
B. Congenital heart disease.
C. Ventricular septal defects.

▶

D. Mitral valve prolapse.
E. Intravenous drug use.
F. Long-term use of intravenous catheters.
G. Implanted cardiac pacemaker and/or automated implantable cardioverter-defibrillator (AICD; see Figures 9.6 and 9.7).
H. Heart transplant with defective valve.
I. Trauma.
J. Valvular heart disease (VHD).
K. Structural cardiac defects.
L. Rheumatic fever.
M. Dental work (within past 3–6 months), especially in those with preexisting cardiac abnormalities.
N. Asymmetric septal hypertrophy.
O. Marfan syndrome.
P. Previous episode of infective endocarditis.
Q. Skin, bone, or pulmonary infection.
R. Immune deficiency.
S. Male sex.
T. Age over 45 years (Brashers, 2019; Dechant & Heimgartner, 2021; Stromberg, 2021; Sommers, 2019).

SUBJECTIVE DATA
A. Symptoms usually occur within 2 weeks of infection.
B. Diagnosis may be difficult as symptoms are often vague.
C. Chills.
D. Night sweats.
E. Malaise.
F. Fatigue.
G. Anorexia.
H. Muscle aches.
I. Headache.
J. Sharp, stabbing chest pain.
K. Joint pain.
L. Dyspnea.
M. Cough.
N. Night sweats (Brashers, 2019; Dechant & Heimgartner, 2021; Stromberg, 2021).

OBJECTIVE DATA
A. Signs usually occur within 2 weeks of infection.
B. Splinter hemorrhages.
C. Janeway lesions (non-painful lesions on the palms and soles).
D. New or worsening murmur (see Figures 9.1–9.3).
E. Osler nodes (painful, erythematous nodules on the pads of the fingers and toes).
F. Weight loss.
G. Heart failure.
H. Central nervous system, splenic, renal, pulmonary, coronary, or ocular emboli.
I. Petechial lesions of the skin, conjunctiva, and oral mucosa.
J. Recurrent fevers (temperatures of 99°F to 103°F/37.2°C to 39.4°C). Note: As a result of physiological changes of aging, older adults may be afebrile.

K. Roth spots (retinal hemorrhaging).
L. Positive blood cultures.
M. S_3 or S_4 sounds.
N. Splenomegaly.
O. Patient appears acutely ill.
P. Dry mucosal membranes (Brashers, 2019; Dechant & Heimgartner, 2021; Stromberg, 2021).

DIAGNOSTIC TESTS
A. See Appendix Table 9A.1 for listing of common diagnostic tests.

DIFFERENTIAL DIAGNOSES
A. Antiphospholipid syndrome.
B. Atrial myxoma.
C. Infective endocarditis.
D. Lyme disease.
E. Systemic lupus erythematosus (SLE).
F. Polymyalgia rheumatica.
G. Primary cardiac neoplasms.
H. Reactive arthritis (Brusch, 2021).

POTENTIAL COMPLICATIONS
A. Heart failure (most common).
B. Arterial embolism (up to 50% of cases).
C. Splenic infarction.
D. Neurological complications.
E. Thromboembolism leading to:
　1. Stroke.
　2. Myocardial infarction.
　3. Cardiac valve insufficiency.
　4. Myocardial abscess.
　5. Arthritis.
　6. Myositis.
F. Pulmonary complications.
G. Dysrhythmias.
H. Endocardial scarring.
I. Valvular stenosis (especially mitral and aortic; Dechant & Heimgartner, 2021; Stromberg, 2021; Sommers, 2019).

DISEASE-MODIFYING TREATMENTS
A. Antimicrobial therapy (particularly penicillin).
B. Valve replacement or repair.
C. Left ventricular assist device (LVAD; see Figure 9.10) if heart failure has developed.
D. Surgical interventions:
　1. Valve repair/replacement.
　2. Repair/removal of congenital shunt.
　3. Drainage of cardiac abscess.
E. Mechanical ventilation if pulmonary complications occur.
F. Antiarrhythmics (Dechant & Heimgartner, 2021; Stromberg, 2021).

PALLIATIVE INTERVENTIONS/SYMPTOM MANAGEMENT
A. See Appendix Table 9A.2 for listing of palliative interventions and symptom management.

▶

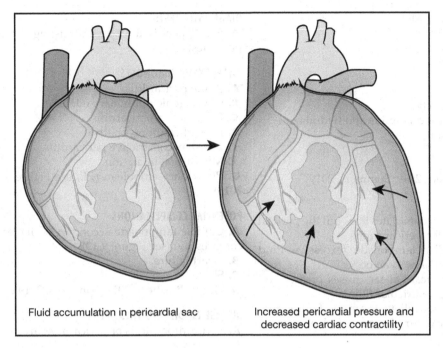

Fluid accumulation in pericardial sac

Increased pericardial pressure and decreased cardiac contractility

FIGURE 9.11 Pericardial effusion.

Source: Adapted from Scientific Animations. (2018). *Inflammation of the pericardium membrane causing pericardial effusion.* www.scientificanimations.com.

B. See Appendix D-3 for overview of common symptoms.

PROGNOSIS

A. Prognosis for acute infective endocarditis is 6 weeks, untreated.

B. Prognosis for subacute infective endocarditis is up to 1 year, untreated (Sommers, 2019).

NURSING INTERVENTIONS

A. Use and teach patient and family infection control measures.

B. Teach patient to take all medications as prescribed.

C. Educate patient and family on disease trajectory and possible interventions.

D. Maintain/address nutritional status.

E. Encourage smoking cessation (see Appendices B-10 and C-9).

F. Provide spiritual support.

G. Assess caregiver fatigue/burnout.

H. Encourage completion of advance directives.

I. Educate patient and family regarding availability of palliative care.

J. Educate patient and family regarding availability of hospice services (when appropriate).

K. Provide referral to community support groups, as needed.

PERICARDIAL EFFUSION

DEFINITION/CHARACTERISTICS

A. Gradual accumulation of fluid in the pericardial cavity (see Figure 9.11).

B. The pericardium slowly stretches and can accommodate more than 1 L of fluid.

C. Generally indicative of biventricular failure (Dechant & Heimgartner, 2021; Stromberg, 2021; Sommers, 2019).

INCIDENCE AND PREVALENCE

A. On general autopsy, pericardial effusion was found in 3.4% of cases.

B. Pericardial effusion is found in 21% of patients with malignancy.

C. Pericardial effusion is found in 5% to 43% of patients with human immunodeficiency syndrome (Strimel, 2018).

ETIOLOGY

A. Between 26% and 86% of cases are idiopathic.

B. Causes can include:

1. Neoplasm.
2. Infection.
3. Acute pericarditis.
4. Heart surgery.
5. Chemotherapy.
6. Radiation treatments.

7. Autoimmune disorders.

8. Left heart failure.

9. Overhydration.

10. Hypoproteinemia.

11. Tuberculosis.

12. Uremia

13. Myocardial infarction.

14. Drugs such as procainamide and hydralazine.

15. Aortic aneurysm.

16. Sarcoidosis.

17. Myxedema.

18. Trauma (Brashers, 2019; Sommers, 2019).

PATHOPHYSIOLOGY

A. Occurs when fluid accumulates between the parietal and visceral layers of the pericardium.

B. If untreated, cardiac tamponade (excessive fluid buildup in the pericardial sac) can occur.

C. The fluid in the pericardial sac causes pressure on the ventricles, limiting ventricular filling.

D. If the pressure is not relieved, cardiac failure and, ultimately, death can occur (Dechant & Heimgarten, 2021; Stromberg, 2021).

PREDISPOSING FACTORS

A. Rheumatoid arthritis.

B. Systemic lupus erythematosus (SLE).

C. Immunosuppression.

D. Cardiac surgery.

E. Kidney failure.

F. Cancer.

G. Radiation therapy (Sommers, 2019).

SUBJECTIVE DATA

A. Dyspnea.

B. Precordial or retrosternal pain.

C. Chest pain relieved by sitting up and leaning forward.

D. Malaise.

E. Fatigue.

F. Restlessness.

G. Anxiety.

H. Confusion (Brashers, 2019; Sommers, 2019; Stromberg, 2021).

OBJECTIVE DATA

A. Tachycardia.

B. Jugular vein distention (see Figure 9.5).

C. Cardiomegaly.

D. Pulsus paradoxus.

E. Distant or muffled heart sounds.

F. Poorly palpable apical pulse.

G. Fever.

H. Pericardial friction rub.

I. Hypotension.

J. Tachypnea (Brashers, 2019).

DIAGNOSTIC TESTS

A. See Appendix Table 9A.1 for listing of common diagnostic tests.

DIFFERENTIAL DIAGNOSES

A. Acute pericarditis.

B. Cardiogenic pulmonary edema.

C. Constrictive pericarditis.

D. Dilated cardiomyopathy.

E. Effusive–constrictive pericarditis.

F. Myocardial infarction.

G. Pulmonary embolism (PE; see Figure 9.12; Strimel, 2018).

POTENTIAL COMPLICATIONS

A. Cardiac tamponade secondary to increased cardiac compression (see Figure 9.13).

B. Heart failure.

C. Shock.

D. Death (Brashers, 2019; Sommers, 2019).

DISEASE-MODIFYING TREATMENTS

A. Pericardiocentesis or pericardiotomy.

B. Surgery.

C. Surgical creation of a pericardial window.

D. Sclerosing agents (Brashers, 2019; Sommers, 2019).

PALLIATIVE INTERVENTIONS/SYMPTOM MANAGEMENT

A. See Appendix Table 9A.2 for listing of palliative interventions and symptom management.

B. See Appendix D-3 for overview of common symptoms.

PROGNOSIS

A. If left untreated, pericardial effusion can be fatal.

B. Chronic pericardial effusion carries a higher rate of mortality due to repeated invasive procedures such as pericardiotomy (Sommers, 2019).

NURSING INTERVENTIONS

A. Individualize plan of care to patient's age and lifestyle needs.

B. Encourage small, frequent meals and high-calorie snacks.

C. Teach patient to take medications as prescribed.

D. Implement interventions for pain and symptom management.

E. Splint cough with pillows to reduce chest pain.

F. Offer reputable online resources.

G. Encourage smoking cessation (see Appendices B-10 and C-9).

H. Provide spiritual support.

I. Assess caregiver fatigue/burnout.

J. Encourage completion of advance directives.

K. Educate patient and family regarding availability of palliative care.

▶

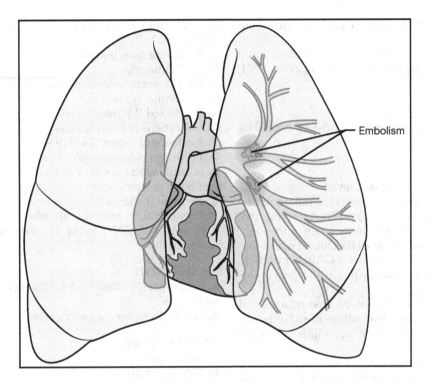

FIGURE 9.12   Pulmonary embolism.

Source: Adapted from Scientific Animations. (2020). *3D medical animation still shot showing pulmonary embolism in human lungs.* www.scientificanimations.com

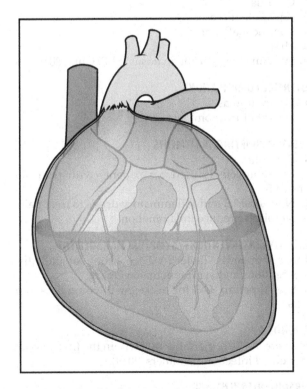

FIGURE 9.13   Cardiac tamponade.

Source: Adapted from Blausen.com staff. (2014). *Cardiac tamponade.* Blausen Medical.

L. Educate patient and family regarding availability of hospice services (when appropriate).

M. Provide referral to community support groups, as needed.

RHEUMATIC HEART DISEASE

DEFINITION/CHARACTERISTICS

A. Also called rheumatic carditis or rheumatic endocarditis.

B. An autoimmune disorder that follows upper respiratory infection with group A beta-hemolytic streptococci (GABHS).

C. Manifested as scarring and deformities of heart valves occurs as a result of rheumatic fever.

D. Formation of Aschoff bodies is a hallmark finding of rheumatic heart disease (RHD).

E. RHD is usually preventable when appropriate antibiotic therapy is initiated within 9 days of onset of rheumatic fever (Brashers, 2019; Dechant & Heimgarten, 2021; Sommers, 2019).

INCIDENCE AND PREVALENCE

A. Only 3% of those who are infected with pharyngeal GABHS infection will develop RHD.

B. Occurs most often in children ages 5 to 15 years; mean age is 12.

C. Rarely occurs in those >30 years.

D. RHD occurs in 50% to 60% of patients with rheumatic fever.

E. Approximately 10% of rheumatic fever cases result in RHD (Brashers, 2019; Dechant & Heimgarten, 2021; Sommers, 2019).

ETIOLOGY

A. Rheumatic fever, an inflammatory disease caused by GABHS (Brashers, 2019).

PATHOPHYSIOLOGY

A. RHD is a sequela of rheumatic fever.

B. Rheumatic fever leads to systemic inflammation and proliferation of exudative lesions in the connective tissues, especially in the heart, joints, brain, and skin.

C. If rheumatic fever results in RHD, clinical manifestations will occur within 1 to 6 weeks of GABHS infection.

D. RHD initially manifests as carditis in all layers of cardiac tissues.

E. As RHD progresses, heart valves become inflamed and less elastic, and valve leaflets may adhere to each other.

F. Diffuse cellular infiltrates develop, which may result in heart failure.

G. The pericardium thickens and is covered in exudate, which may lead to a serosanguinous pericardial effusion.

H. Hemorrhagic and fibrous lesions form on the inflamed heart valves, causing stenosis and regurgitation of the mitral and aortic valves.

I. More likely to damage mitral valve in females, aortic valves in males.

J. Damage to tricuspid and pulmonic valves is rare (Brashers, 2019; Dechant & Heimgarten, 2021; Johns Hopkins Medicine, 2022; Sommers, 2019).

PREDISPOSING FACTORS

A. Pharyngeal GABHS infection.

B. Genetic predisposition.

C. Skin infections.

D. Environmental factors such as overcrowding and poor sanitation (Sommers, 2019).

SUBJECTIVE DATA

A. Nausea.

B. Abdominal pain.

C. Chest pain.

D. Dyspnea.

E. Joint and/or muscle pain (Brashers, 2019; Johns Hopkins Medicine, 2022; Sommers, 2019).

OBJECTIVE DATA

A. Fever.

B. Lymphadenopathy.

C. Arthralgia.

D. Vomiting.

E. Epistaxis.

F. Tachycardia.

G. Carditis.

H. Acute migratory arthralgia.

I. Chorea.

J. Erythema marginatum.

K. Cardiomegaly.

L. New-onset or worsening murmurs.

M. Pericardial friction rub.

N. Prolonged P-R interval on EKG.

O. Indications of heart failure.

P. Evidence of recent GABHS infection.

Q. Erythema marginatum.

R. Subcutaneous nodules (<1 cm) on skin, especially over bony prominences.

S. Peripheral edema.

T. Polyarticular arthritis (Brashers, 2019; Dechant & Heimgarten, 2021; Johns Hopkins Medicine, 2022; Sommers, 2019).

DIAGNOSTIC TESTS

A. See Appendix Table 9A.1 for listing of common diagnostic tests.

B. See Table 9.6 for diagnostic criteria.

DIFFERENTIAL DIAGNOSES

A. Sarcoidosis.

B. Valvular insufficiency.

C. Dilated cardiomyopathy.

D. Glomerular nephritis.

E. Heart failure.

F. Carditis.

G. Kawasaki disease.

H. Cardiac malignancy.

I. HIV.

J. Systemic lupus erythematosus (SLE; Chin, 2019).

POTENTIAL COMPLICATIONS

A. Dysrhythmias.

B. Heart failure (Sommers, 2019).

DISEASE-MODIFYING TREATMENTS

A. Penicillin.

B. Erythromycin is used for patients with penicillin sensitivity.

C. Nonsteroidal anti-inflammatory drugs to treat pain

D. Steroids to reduce inflammation.

PALLIATIVE INTERVENTIONS/SYMPTOM MANAGEMENT

A. See Appendix Table 9A.2 for listing of palliative interventions and symptom management.

B. See Appendix D-3 for overview of common symptoms.

PROGNOSIS

A. There is a 20% mortality rate within the first 10 years after initial infection (Sommers, 2019).

NURSING INTERVENTIONS

A. Use and teach patient and family infection control measures.

▶

TABLE 9.6 JONES CRITERIA FOR DIAGNOSIS OF RHEUMATIC FEVER

When supported by evidence of recent GABHS infection, presence of two major criteria OR 1 major criteria and 2 minor criteria indicate a high probability of rheumatic fever

MAJOR CRITERIA	MINOR CRITERIA
<ul><li>Carditis</li><li>Polyarthritis</li><li>Subcutaneous nodules (Aschoff bodies)</li><li>Erythema marginatum</li><li>Chorea</li></ul>	<ul><li>Polyarthralgia</li><li>Fever (≥101.3°F/38.5°C)</li><li>Eosinophil sedimentation rate ≥60 mm in first hour ***and/or*** C-reactive protein ≥3 mg/dL</li><li>Prolonged PR interval on electrocardiogram</li></ul>

Note: Evidence of recent GABHS infection includes positive throat culture/positive rapid streptococcal test or elevated/rising antibody titer.

Source: Gewitz, M. H., Baltimore, R. S., Tani, L. Y., Sable, C. A., Shulman, S. T., Carapetis, J., Remenyi, B., Taubert, K. A., Bolger, A. F., Beerman, L., Mayosi, B. M., Beaton, A., Pandian, N. G., & Kaplan, E. L. (2015). Revision of the Jones Criteria for the diagnosis of acute rheumatic fever in the era of Doppler echocardiography: A scientific statement from the American Heart Association. *Circulation, 131*(20), 1806–1818. https://www.ahajournals.org/doi/full/10.1161/cir.0000000000000205

B. Teach patient to take all medications as prescribed.

C. If patient has history of RHD, reinforce teaching that prophylactic antibiotic therapy is required prior to invasive interventions.

D. Maintain nutritional status.

E. Encourage smoking cessation (see Appendices B-10 and C-9).

F. Provide spiritual support

G. Assess caregiver fatigue/burnout

H. Encourage completion of advance directives.

I. Educate patient and family regarding availability of palliative care.

J. Educate patient and family regarding availability of hospice services (when appropriate).

K. Provide referral to community support groups, as needed.

VALVULAR HEART DISEASE

DEFINITION/CHARACTERISTICS

A. Disorders involving insufficiency, incompetence, abnormalities, or stiffness of cardiac valves that result in altered filling or emptying of the chambers of the heart.

B. Clinical manifestations are related to the specific valve affected and the type of irregularity (see Table 9.7).

C. There are two main types of cardiac valvular disorders:

    1. Valvular stenosis.

        a. Constriction of the valvular orifice resulting in diminished blood flow and increased effort of the chamber closest to the affected valve.

        b. Results in myocardial hypertrophy.

    2. Valvular regurgitation.

        a. Also called valvular insufficiency or valvular incompetence.

        b. Insufficient closure of the valvular leaflet or cusps resulting in leakage of blood back into the chamber most proximal to the affected valve.

        c. Results in audible murmur on auscultation (Brashers, 2019).

INCIDENCE AND PREVALENCE

A. Roughly 2% of the population in United States has valvular heart disease (VHD).

B. More common in older adults.

C. VHD deaths are more commonly associated with aortic valve disease.

D. Bicuspid aortic valve occurs in 1% to 2% of the population and is more common in males (Centers for Disease Control & Prevention, 2019).

ETIOLOGY

A. Congenital heart valve disease.

B. Rheumatic heart disease (RHD).

C. Endocarditis.

D. Heart failure.

E. Atherosclerosis.

F. Thoracic aortic aneurysm.

G. Hypertension.

H. Myocardial infarction.

I. Marfan syndrome

J. Systemic lupus erythematosus (SLE; Centers for Disease Control & Prevention, 2019).

PATHOPHYSIOLOGY

A. Increased cardiac workload secondary to increased blood volume in the affected chamber leads to chamber dilation and cardiac hypertrophy.

▶

TABLE 9.7 CARDIAC VALVE DISORDERS

VALVULAR STENOSIS	ETIOLOGY	CLINICAL MANIFESTATIONS
Aortic valve stenosis	• Congenital bicuspid valve • Rheumatic fever • Age-related valvular calcification	• Left ventricular hypertrophy • Left heart failure • Decreased coronary blood flow leading to myocardial infarction • Pulmonary edema • Dyspnea on exertion • Syncope • Angina pectoris • Systolic murmur at right parasternal intercostal space radiating to the neck
Mitral valve stenosis	• Rheumatic heart disease	• Left atrial hypertrophy and dilation with fibrillation leading to right heart failure • Dyspnea on exertion • Orthopnea • Paroxysmal nocturnal orthopnea • Nocturnal orthopnea • Frequent respiratory infections • Hemoptysis • Pulmonary hypertension • Edema • Emboli • Atypical chest pain • Low rumbling diastolic murmur appreciated at the apex and radiating to the axilla with accentuated heart sounds and opening snap
VALVULAR REGURGITATION	**ETIOLOGY**	**CLINICAL MANIFESTATIONS**
Aortic regurgitation	• Infective endocarditis • Aortic root disease • Marfan syndrome • Dilation of the aortic root secondary to hypertension and/or angina	• Left ventricular hypertrophy and dilation leading to heart failure • Pulmonary edema • Syncope • Angina pectoris • Diastolic murmur appreciated at the right parasternal second intercostal space and radiating to the neck
Mitral regurgitation	• Myxomatous degeneration (mitral valve collapse)	• Left atrial hypertrophy and dilation followed by left heart failure • Pulmonary edema with dyspnea on exertion • Atypical chest pain • Holosystolic murmur appreciated at the apex and radiating to the axilla
Tricuspid regurgitation	Congenital	• Right heart failure • Dyspnea • Palpitations • Holosystolic murmur best heard at lower sternal border

Source: Adapted from Brashers, V. L. (2019). Alterations in cardiovascular function. In K. L. McCance & S. E. Huether (Eds.), *Pathophysiology: The biologic basis for disease in adults and children* (8th ed., pp. 1058–1690). Elsevier.

B. Eventually, myocardial contractility is diminished, ejection fraction is reduced, and diastolic pressure increases as the affected chamber fails from overload.

PREDISPOSING FACTORS
A. Hypertension.
B. Diabetes mellitus.
C. Hyperlipidemia.
D. Genetic predisposition (Otto et al., 2021).

SUBJECTIVE DATA
A. Dyspnea.
B. Angina.
C. Fatigue.
D. Dizziness.
E. Syncope (Centers for Disease Control & Prevention, 2019).

OBJECTIVE DATA
A. Heart murmur.
B. Rapid weight gain.
C. Dysrhythmias.
D. Fever (Brashers, 2019; Centers for Disease Control & Prevention, 2019).

DIAGNOSTIC TESTS
A. See Appendix Table 9A.1 for listing of common diagnostic tests.
B. See Table 9.8 for staging of VHD.

DIFFERENTIAL DIAGNOSES
A. Aortic valve insufficiency.
B. Mitral valve prolapse.
C. RHD.
D. Aortic stenosis.
E. Ventricular septal defect.
F. Turner syndrome.
G. Williams syndrome (Bayne, 2016).

POTENTIAL COMPLICATIONS
A. Heart failure.
B. Stroke.
C. Thrombi.
D. Infective endocarditis.
E. Thrombotic endocarditis (Cruz-Flores, 2014).

DISEASE-MODIFYING TREATMENTS
A. Valvular repair or replacement.
B. Anticoagulation therapy.
C. Prophylaxis for endocarditis, as needed.
D. Lifestyle modification.
E. Diuretics.
F. Angiotensin-converting enzyme (ACE) inhibitors.
G. Angiotensin receptor blockers (ARBs).
H. Aldosterone antagonists.
I. Sacubitril/valsartan.
J. Biventricular pacing (Brashers, 2019; Otto et al., 2021).

PALLIATIVE INTERVENTIONS/SYMPTOM MANAGEMENT
A. See Appendix Table 9A.2 for listing of palliative interventions and symptom management.
B. See Appendix D-3 for overview of common symptoms.

PROGNOSIS
A. When VHD is associated with aortic stenosis, prognosis is 3 years after onset of symptoms.
B. About 80% of those with mitral valve stenosis live 10 or more years after diagnosis.
C. Mortality increases when symptoms become pronounced.
D. If pulmonary hypertension develops, prognosis is less than 3 years (Uttekar, 2020).

NURSING INTERVENTIONS
A. Individualize plan of care to patient's age and lifestyle needs.

TABLE 9.8 STAGES OF VALVULAR HEART DISEASE

STAGE	DETAIL
A	Patient is at risk for VHD.
B	Patient has progressive VHD and is asymptomatic or has only mild or moderate symptoms.
C	Patient is asymptomatic but has severe VHD with either compensation or decompensation of left or right ventricle.
D	Patient is symptomatic and has severe VHD.

VHD, valvular heart disease.

Source: Otto, C. M., Nishimura, R. A., Bonow, R. O., Carabello, B. A., Erwin III, J. P., Gentile, F., Jneid, H., Krieger, E. V., Mack, M., McLeod, C., O'Gara, P. T., Rigolin, V. H., Sundt, T. M., Thompson, A., & Toly, C. (2021). 2020 ACC/AHA guideline for the management of patients with valvular heart disease: A report of the American College of Cardiology/American Heart Association Joint Committee on Clinical Practice Guidelines. *Journal of the American College of Cardiology, 77*(4), e25–e197. https://www.ahajournals.org/doi/epub/10.1161/CIR.0000000000000923

B. Encourage small, frequent meals and high-calorie snacks.

C. Teach patient to take medications as prescribed.

D. Implement interventions for pain and symptom management.

E. Encourage smoking cessation (see Appendices B-10 and C-9).

F. Offer reputable online resources.

G. Provide spiritual support.

H. Assess caregiver fatigue/burnout.

I. Encourage completion of advance directives.

J. Educate patient and family regarding availability of palliative care.

K. Educate patient and family regarding availability of hospice services (when appropriate).

L. Provide referral to community support groups, as needed.

REFERENCES

Abt, D., Bywater, M., Engeler, D. S., & Schmid, H. P. (2013). Therapeutic options for intractable hematuria in advanced bladder cancer. *International Journal of Urology*, 20(7), 651–660. https://doi.org/10.1111/iju.12113

American Heart Association. (2022). *Advanced heart failure.* https://www.heart.org/en/health-topics/heart-failure/living-with-heart-failure-and-managing-advanced-hf/advanced-heart-failure#:~:text=What%20is%20advanced%20heart%20failure,percent%20have%20advanced%20heart%20failure

Bayne, E. J. (2016). *Bicuspid aortic valve differential diagnoses.* https://emedicine.medscape.com/article/893523-differential

Bergheanu, S. C., Bodde, M. C., & Jukema, J. W. (2017). Pathophysiology and treatment of atherosclerosis. *Netherlands Heart Journal*, 25(4), 231–242. https://www.ncbi.nlm.nih.gov/pmc/articles/PMC5355390/pdf/12471_2017_Article_959.pdf

Blausen.com staff. (2014). Medical gallery of Blausen Medical 2014. *WikiJournal of Medicine*, 1(2). https://doi.org/10.15347/wjm/2014.010. ISSN 2002-4436.

Brashers, V. L. (2019). Alterations in cardiovascular function. In K. L. McCance & S. E. Huether (Eds.), *Pathophysiology: The biologic basis for disease in adults and children* (8th ed., pp. 1058–1690). Elsevier.

Brashers, V. L., & Huether, S.E. (2019). Alterations in pulmonary function. In K. L. McCance & S. E. Huether (Eds.), *Pathophysiology: The biologic basis for disease in adults and children* (8th ed., pp. 1163–1201). Elsevier.

Brusch, J. L. (2021, January 21). *Infective endocarditis differential diagnoses.* https://emedicine.medscape.com/article/216650-differential

Burke, A. P. (2015). *Dilated cardiomyopathy pathology.* https://emedicine.medscape.com/article/2017823-overview#a1

Centers for Disease Control & Prevention. (2019). *Valvular heart disease.* https://www.cdc.gov/heartdisease/valvular_disease.htm#:~:text=About%202.5%25%20of%20the%20U.S.,1943%20have%20valvular%20heart%20disease

Centers for Disease Control & Prevention. (2021). *Atrial fibrillation.* https://www.cdc.gov/heartdisease/atrial_fibrillation.htm

Centers for Disease Control & Prevention. (2022a). *Heart failure.* https://www.cdc.gov/heartdisease/heart_failure.htm

Centers for Disease Control and Prevention. (2022b). *Coronary artery disease.* https://www.cdc.gov/heartdisease/coronary_ad.htm

Centers for Disease Control and Prevention. (2022c). *Heart disease facts.* https://www.cdc.gov/heartdisease/facts.htm

Chin, T. K. (2019). *Pediatric rheumatic heart disease differential diagnoses.* https://emedicine.medscape.com/article/891897-differential

Cleveland Clinic. (2022). *Ventricular arrhythmias.* https://my.clevelandclinic.org/health/diseases/21854-ventricular-arrhythmia

Cruz-Flores, S. (2014). Neurologic complications of valvular heart disease. In J. Biller & J. M. Ferro (Eds.), *Handbook of Clinical Neurology, 119* (pp. 61–73). Elsevier. https://www.sciencedirect.com/science/article/abs/pii/B9780702040863000060?casa_token=_WPk4WU5nXsAAAAA:Fv-CwCcIdJfKzkM5jG_T39CytyRwCxwDB6TfEIPGtUJufOXEK-PCXTjL1MbxecwkLNLVWYXEFw

Dechant, L. M., & Heimgartner, N. M. (2021). Concepts of care for patients with cardiac problems. In D. D. Ignatavicius, M. L. Workman, C. Rebar, & N. M. Heimgarten (Eds.), *Medical-surgical nursing* (10th ed., pp. 665–696). Elsevier.

Del Buono, M. G., Iannaccone, G., Scacciavillani, R., Carbone, S., Camilli, M., Niccoli, G., Borlaug, B. A., Lavie, C. J., Arena, R., Crea, F., & Abbate, A. (2020). Heart failure with preserved ejection fraction diagnosis and treatment: An updated review of the evidence. *Progress in cardiovascular diseases*, 63(5), 570–584. https://doi.org/10.1016/j.pcad.2020.04.011

Dumitru, I. (2020). *What are the underlying causes of systolic heart failure?* https://www.medscape.com/answers/163062-86163/what-are-the-underlying-causes-of-systolic-heart-failure

Dumitru, I. (2022). *Heart failure differential diagnosis.* https://emedicine.medscape.com/article/163062-differential

Emory Healthcare. (2022). *Heart failure statistics.* https://www.emoryhealthcare.org/centers-programs/heart-vascular-center/wellness/heart-failure-statistics.html

Epocrates. (2022). *Drugs.* https://online.epocrates.com/drugs

Freeman, A. R., & Levine, S. A. (1933). The clinical significance of the systolic murmur: A study 1000 consecutive "non-cardiac" cases. *Annals of Internal Medicine*, 6(11), 1371–1385. https://doi.org/10.7326/0003-4819-6-11-1371

Gewitz, M. H., Baltimore, R. S., Tani, L. Y., Sable, C. A., Shulman, S. T., Carapetis, J., Remenyi, B., Taubert, K. A., Bolger, A. F., Beerman, L., Mayosi, B. M., Beaton, A., Pandian, N. G., & Kaplan, E. L. (2015). Revision of the Jones Criteria for the diagnosis of acute rheumatic fever in the era of Doppler echocardiography: A scientific statement from the American Heart Association. *Circulation*, 131(20), 1806–1818. https://www.ahajournals.org/doi/full/10.1161/cir.0000000000000205

Guyer, D. L., Almhanna, K., & McKee, K. Y. (2020). Palliative care for patients with esophageal cancer: A narrative review. *Annals of Translational Medicine*, 8(17). https://doi.org/10.21037/atm-20-3676

Johns Hopkins Medicine. (2022). *Rheumatic heart disease.* https://www.hopkinsmedicine.org/health/conditions-and-diseases/rheumatic-heart-disease

Karch, A. M. (2019). *Focus on nursing pharmacology.* Lippincott Williams & Wilkins.

Leong, D. (2017). *Which conditions are in the differentials for cor pulmonale?* https://www.medscape.com/answers/154062-69195/which-conditions-are-in-the-differentials-for-cor-pulmonale

Liesenborghs, L., Meyers, S., Vanassche, T., & Verhamme, P. (2020). Coagulation: At the heart of infective endocarditis. *Journal of Thrombosis and Haemostasis*, 18(5), 995–1008. https://doi.org/10.1111/jth.14736

Mailk, A., Brito, D., Vaqar, S., & Chhabra, L. (2021). *Congestive heart failure.* https://www.ncbi.nlm.nih.gov/books/NBK430873/#_NBK430873_pubdet_

Mayo Clinic. (2022a). *Heart arrythmias.* https://www.mayoclinic.org/diseases-conditions/heart-arrhythmia/diagnosis-treatment/drc-20350674

Mayo Clinic. (2022b). *Coronary artery disease.* https://www.mayoclinic.org/diseases-conditions/coronary-artery-disease/symptoms-causes/syc-20350613

Murphy, S. P., Ibrahim, N. E., & Januzzi, J. L. (2020). Heart failure with reduced ejection fraction: A review. *JAMA, 324*(5), 488–504. https://doi.org/10.1001/jama.2020.10262

National Heart, Lung, and Blood Institute. (2013). *Implantable pacemaker.* https://commons.wikimedia.org/wiki/File:Pacemaker_NIH.jpg

Obokata, M., Reddy, Y. N., & Borlaug, B. A. (2020). Diastolic dysfunction and heart failure with preserved ejection fraction: Understanding mechanisms by using noninvasive methods. *JACC: Cardiovascular Imaging, 13*(1 Part 2), 245–257. https://www.sciencedirect.com/science/article/pii/S1936878X1930347X?via%3Dihub

Otto, C. M., Nishimura, R. A., Bonow, R. O., Carabello, B. A., Erwin, III, J. P., Gentile, F., Jneid, H., Krieger, E. V., Mack, M., McLeod, C., O'Gara, P. T., Rigolin, V. H., Sundt, T. M., Thompson, A., & Toly, C. (2021). 2020 ACC/AHA guideline for the management of patients with valvular heart disease: A report of the American College of Cardiology/American Heart Association Joint Committee on Clinical Practice Guidelines. *Journal of the American College of Cardiology, 77*(4), e25–e197. https://www.ahajournals.org/doi/epub/10.1161/CIR.0000000000000923

Pandey, A., Kitzman, D., & Reeves, G. (2019). Frailty is intertwined with heart failure: Mechanisms, prevalence, prognosis, assessment, and management. *JACC: Heart Failure, 7*(12), 1001–1011. https://doi.org/10.1016/j.jchf.2019.10.005

Pantilat, S., Davidson, P., & Psotka, M. (2021). Advanced heart failure. In N. I. Cherny, M. T. Fallon, S. Kassa, R. K. Portenoy, & D. C. Currow (Eds.), *Oxford textbook of palliative care* (6th ed., pp. 976–986). Oxford University Press.

Patnaik, A. N. (2019). The diastolic murmurs. *Indian Journal of Cardiovascular Disease in Women-WINCARS, 4*(04), 228–232. https://www.thieme-connect.com/products/ejournals/pdf/10.1055/s-0039-3402692.pdf

Ramadan, R., Boden, W. E., & Kinlay, S. (2018). Management of left main coronary artery disease. *Journal of the American Heart Association, 7*(7), e008151. https://www.ahajournals.org/doi/full/10.1161/jaha.117.008151

Revuelta-López, E., Núñez, J., Gastelurrutia, P., Cediel, G., Januzzi, J. L., Ibrahim, N. E., Emdin, M., VanKimmenade, R., Pascual-Figal, D., Núñez, J., Gommans, F., Lupón, J., & Bayés-Genís, A. (2020). Neprilysin inhibition, endorphin dynamics, and early symptomatic improvement in heart failure: A pilot study. *ESC Heart Failure, 7*(2), 559–566. https://doi.org/10.1002/ehf2.12607

Rosenthal, L. (2019). *Atrial fibrillation differential diagnoses.* https://emedicine.medscape.com/article/151066-differential

Severino, P., Mather, P. J., Pucci, M., D'Amato, A., Mariani, M. V., Infusino, F., Birtolo, L. I., Maestrini, V., Mancone, M., & Fedele, F. (2019). Advanced heart failure and end-stage heart failure: Does a difference exist. *Diagnostics, 9*(4), 170. https://doi.org/10.3390/diagnostics9040170

Shah, S. (2021). *Coronary artery atherosclerosis: Differential diagnoses.* https://emedicine.medscape.com/article/153647-differential

Sinibaldi, V. J., Pratz, C. F., & Yankulina, O. (2018). Kidney cancer: Toxicity management, symptom control, and palliative care. *Journal of Clinical Oncology, 36*(36), 3632–3638. https://doi.org/10.1200/JCO.2018.79.0188

Sommers, M. S. (2019). *Davis's diseases and disorders: A nursing therapeutics manual.* F.A. Davis. https://www.fadavis.com/product/nursing-fundamentals-med-surg-diseases-disorders-nursing-therapeutics-manual-sommers-6

Sorrentino, M. J. (2019). The evolution from hypertension to heart failure. *Heart failure clinics, 15*(4), 447–453. https://doi.org/10.1016/j.hfc.2019.06.005

Strimel, W. J. (2018). *Pericardial effusion.* https://emedicine.medscape.com/article/157325-overview#a1

Stromberg, H. (2021). *DeWit's Medical-surgical nursing: Concepts and practice* (4th ed.). Elsevier.

Tawil, J., & Gelzini, T. A. (2020). Differential diagnosis and clinical management of diastolic heart failure: Current best practice. *Research Reports in Clinical Cardiology, 7*, 117–135. https://www.dovepress.com/getfile.php?fileID=32707

Topan, A., Carstina, D., Slavcovici, A., Rancea, R., Capalneanu, R., & Lupse, M. (2015). Assessment of the Duke criteria for the diagnosis of infective endocarditis after twenty-years. An analysis of 241 cases. *Clujul Medical, 88*(3), 321. https://www.ncbi.nlm.nih.gov/pmc/articles/PMC4632890/pdf/cm-88-321.pdf

Tsao, C. W., Aday, A. W., Almarzooq, Z. I., Alonso, A., Beaton, A. Z., Bittencourt, M. S., ... & American Heart Association Council on Epidemiology and Prevention Statistics Committee and Stroke Statistics Subcommittee. (2022). Heart disease and stroke statistics—2022 update: a report from the American Heart Association. *Circulation, 145*(8), e153–e639.

Uttekar, P. S. (2020). *How long can you live with heart valve disease?* https://www.medicinenet.com/how_long_can_you_live_with_heart_valve_disease/article.htm

Workman, M. L. (2021). Concepts of care for patients with noninfectious lower respiratory problems. In D. D. Ignatavicius, M. L. Workman, C. Rebar & N. M. Heimgarten (Eds.), *Medical-surgical nursing* (10th ed., pp. 532–565). Elsevier.

Wright, P. M. (2019). *Certified hospice and palliative nurse (CHPN) exam review: A study guide with review questions.* Springer Publishing Company.

Zeitouni, M., Clare, R. M., Chiswell, K., Abdulrahim, J., Shah, N., Pagidipati, N. P., Shah, S. H., Roe, M. T., Patel, M. P., & Jones, W. S. (2020). Risk factor burden and long-term prognosis of patients with premature coronary artery disease. *Journal of the American Heart Association, 9*(24), e017712. https://www.ahajournals.org/doi/10.1161/JAHA.120.017712

APPENDIX

TABLE 9A.1   DIAGNOSTIC TESTS FOR CARDIAC DISEASE

TYPE	NOTES
Physical examination	• Thorough medical exam with focused pulmonary and cardiac assessments • See Figures 9.1, 9.2, and 9.3
Imaging	• Echocardiogram (advanced and end stage heart failure, left heart failure [congestive heart failure], right heart failure [cor pulmonale], coronary artery disease, dilated cardiomyopathy, dysrhythmias, infectious endocarditis, pericardial effusion, valvular heart disease) • Multigated blood pool imaging (advanced and end-stage heart failure) • Chest x-ray (left heart failure [congestive heart failure], right heart failure [cor pulmonale], coronary artery disease, dilated cardiomyopathy, pericardial effusion, RHD, valvular heart disease) • Cardiac catheterization (as indicated; left heart failure [congestive heart failure], coronary artery disease, dilated cardiomyopathy, valvular heart disease) • Cardiac MRI (left heart failure [congestive heart failure], coronary artery disease, dilated cardiomyopathy, dysrhythmias, infectious endocarditis, pericardial effusion, RHD, valvular heart disease) • PET scan (left heart failure [congestive heart failure], valvular heart disease) • Tc-99m PYP scintigraphy (left heart failure [congestive heart failure]) • CT Scan (coronary artery disease, dilated cardiomyopathy, infective endocarditis, pericardial effusion, RHD, valvular heart disease) • Exercise stress test (coronary artery disease, dysrhythmias, valvular heart disease) • Coronary angiogram, coronary artery calcium scan (coronary artery disease) • EKG (dilated cardiomyopathy, dysrhythmias, infective endocarditis, pericardial effusion, RHD) • Holter monitor (dysrhythmias, valvular heart disease) • Implantable loop recorder, tilt table test (dysrhythmias) • TEE, TTE (infective endocarditis, valvular heart disease) • Two-dimensional cardiac ultrasound Doppler (infective endocarditis)
Laboratory tests	• BNP (advanced and end-stage heart failure, left-sided heart failure, right-sided heart failure [cor pulmonale], RHD) • Serum BNP (left heart failure [congestive heart failure], right-sided heart failure [cor pulmonale], coronary artery disease, dilated cardiomyopathy, dysrhythmias) • Soluble suppression of tumorigenicity-2 (left heart failure [congestive heart failure]) • CBC (left heart failure [congestive heart failure], right heart failure [cor pulmonale], coronary artery disease, dilated cardiomyopathy, dysrhythmias, infective endocarditis, pericardial effusion, RHD) • BMP (left heart failure [congestive heart failure], right heart failure [cor pulmonale], coronary artery disease, dilated cardiomyopathy, dysrhythmias) • Liver function tests, hemoglobin A1C (left heart failure [congestive heart failure]) • Lipid panel (left heart failure [congestive heart failure], coronary artery disease) • Iron levels (left heart failure [congestive heart failure]) • Thyroid function studies (left heart failure [congestive heart failure, dysrhythmias]) • Genetic testing (coronary artery disease, dilated cardiomyopathy, dysrhythmias) • Sedimentation rate (infective endocarditis, pericardial effusion, RHD) • C-reactive protein test (infective endocarditis, pericardial effusion, RHD) • Leukocyte count, rheumatoid factor (infective endocarditis) • Blood cultures (infective endocarditis, RHD) • ASO titer, rapid antigen test, throat culture for GABHS (RHD) • Biomarkers (valvular heart disease)

(continued)

TABLE 9A.1 DIAGNOSTIC TESTS FOR CARDIAC DISEASE (*CONTINUED*)

TYPE	NOTES

Pathology	• Endocardial biopsy (left heart failure [congestive heart failure])
	• Myocardial biopsy (to exclude secondary causes; coronary artery disease, dilated cardiomyopathy)
	• Pericardial fluid analysis (pericardial effusion)
	• Jones criteria is used to make a diagnosis of rheumatic fever (see Table 9.6; RHD)
	• Heart failure is staged using the New York Heart Association criteria (see Table 9.3)
	• Valvular lesions are staged as 1–4 with 1 = at risk, 2 = progressive, 3 =asymptomatic but severe, and 4 = symptomatic (valvular heart disease)
	• Valvular heart disease is classified as Stage A, B, C, or D (see Table 9.8)
	• Diagnosis is made using the Duke Criteria (see also https://www.mdcalc.com/duke-criteria-infective-endocarditis#use-cases; infective endocarditis)
	   ▪ Major criteria (if both are present, the diagnosis is confirmed. If only one major criterion is present, then three minor criteria must be present): positive blood culture drawn at least 12 hours apart and evidence of endocardial involvement (echocardiography)
	   ▪ Minor criteria include fever, evidence of vascular involvement (Janeway lesions), evidence of immunologic involvement (Osler nodes), and microbiologic and echocardiogram evidence that do not fulfill major criteria

ASO, antistreptolysin O; BMP, basic metabolic profile; BNP, B-type natriuretic peptide; CBC, complete blood count; RHD, rheumatic heart disease; Tc-99m PYP, technetium-99m pyrophosphate; TEE, transesophageal echocardiography; TTE, transthoracic echocardiography; GABHS, group A beta-hemolytic streptococci.

Sources: Brashers, V. L. (2019). Alterations in cardiovascular function. In K. L. McCance & S. E. Huether (Eds.), *Pathophysiology: The biologic basis for disease in adults and children* (8th ed., pp. 1058–1690). Elsevier; Burke, A. P. (2015). *Dilated cardiomyopathy pathology.* https://emedicine.medscape.com/article/2017823-overview#a1; Centers for Disease Control and Prevention. (2022b). *Coronary artery disease.* https://www.cdc.gov/heartdisease/coronary_ad.htm; Dechant, L. M. & Heimgartner, N. M. (2021). Concepts of care for patients with cardiac problems. In D. D. Ignatavicius, M. L. Workman, C. Rebar, & N. M. Heimgarten (Eds.), *Medical-surgical nursing.* (10th ed., pp. 665–696). Elsevier; Mayo Clinic. (2022a). *Heart arrythmias.* https://www.mayoclinic.org/diseases-conditions/heart-arrhythmia/diagnosis-treatment/drc-20350674; Murphy, S. P., Ibrahim, N. E., & Januzzi, J. L. (2020). Heart failure with reduced ejection fraction: A review. *JAMA, 324*(5), 488–504. https://doi:10.1001/jama.2020.10262; Otto, C. M., Nishimura, R. A., Bonow, R. O., Carabello, B. A., Erwin III, J. P., Gentile, F., Jneid, H., Krieger, E. V., Mack, M., McLeod, C., O'Gara, P. T., Rigolin, V. H., Sundt, T. M., Thompson, A., & Toly, C. (2021). 2020 ACC/AHA guideline for the management of patients with valvular heart disease: A report of the American College of Cardiology/American Heart Association Joint Committee on Clinical Practice Guidelines. *Journal of the American College of Cardiology, 77*(4), e25–e197. https://www.ahajournals.org/doi/epub/10.1161/CIR.0000000000000923; Sommers, M. S. (2019). *Davis's diseases and disorders: A nursing therapeutics manual.* F.A. Davis. https://www.fadavis.com/product/nursing-fundamentals-med-surg-diseases-disorders-nursing-therapeutics-manual-sommers-6; Stromberg, H. (2021). *DeWit's Medical-surgical nursing: Concepts and practice* (4th ed.). Elsevier; Topan, A., Carstina, D., Slavcovici, A., Rancea, R., Capalneanu, R., & Lupse, M. (2015). Assessment of the Duke criteria for the diagnosis of infective endocarditis after twenty-years. An analysis of 241 cases. *Clujul Medical, 88*(3), 321. https://www.ncbi.nlm.nih.gov/pmc/articles/PMC4632890/pdf/cm-88-321.pdf; Workman, M. L. (2021). Concepts of care for patients with non-infectious lower respiratory problems. In D. D. Ignatavicius, M. L. Workman, C. Rebar & N. M. Heimgarten (Eds.), *Medical-surgical nursing* (10th ed., pp. 532–565). Elsevier.

TABLE 9A.2 PALLIATIVE INTERVENTIONS/SYMPTOM MANAGEMENT FOR CARDIAC DISEASE

SYMPTOM	INTERVENTION
Angina (stable/typical)	• Encourage rest • Administer nitroglycerin as prescribed • Offer small, frequent meals • Reduction of emotional stress
Anorexia	• Use of appetite stimulants (see Appendix D-1) • Offer small, frequent meals and snacks • Offer nutritional supplements
Anxiety and depression (see Appendix D)	• Antidepressants, anxiolytics, or benzodiazepines as indicated by patient's condition, age, and life expectancy (see Appendix D) • Non-pharmacological interventions

(continued)

TABLE 9A.2 PALLIATIVE INTERVENTIONS/SYMPTOM MANAGEMENT FOR CARDIAC DISEASE (CONTINUED)

SYMPTOM	INTERVENTION
Caregiver burden	• Support of interdisciplinary hospice or palliative team • Non-pharmacological interventions for caregivers (see Appendix D-2; valvular heart disease)
Dyspnea (see Appendix D)	• Corticosteroids for reducing inflammation • Opioids to reduce inspiratory effort and tachypnea • Bronchodilators for opening airways (mechanism of action of relaxation of muscular bands that surround bronchi, thus widening the airway) • Diuretics to reduce systemic congestion • Anticholinergics to reduce secretions, especially at the end of life • Use of fans • Lower temperature in the room

Dysrhythmias	• Treatment depends on underlying cause (see section on dysrhythmias)
	• Possible interventions include (see Appendix D-1):
	  ▪ Medications (e.g., adenosine, atropine, beta-blockers, calcium channel blockers, epinephrine, amiodarone, anticoagulants, lidocaine)
	  ▪ Pacemaker placement
	  ▪ Cardioversion (as indicated by patient preference and disease progression)

Edema	• Use of diuretics as indicted (see Appendix D-1) • Elevation of extremity • Compression (left-sided heart failure [congestive heart failure], right-sided heart failure [cor pulmonale], infectious endocarditis, rheumatic heart disease)
Fatigue and somnolence	• Alternate periods of rest with periods of activity • Utilize energy conversation techniques • Psychostimulants (see Appendix D)
Fever	• Address underlying cause, when possible (RHD) • Use of antipyretics (RHD) • Application of cool compresses (RHD) • Increase fluids to address dehydration, if applicable (RHD)
Hypoxia	• Elevate head of bed • Use deep breathing and coughing techniques • Provide supplemental oxygen as indicated • Use opioids or bronchodilators as indicated • Address underlying anxiety and depression (advanced and end-stage heart failure, left heart failure [congestive heart failure], right heart failure [cor pulmonale], dilated cardiomyopathy, infective endocarditis)
Inflammation	• NSAIDS (pericardial effusion) • Corticosteroids (see Appendix D; pericardial effusion)

(continued)

TABLE 9A.2   PALLIATIVE INTERVENTIONS/SYMPTOM MANAGEMENT FOR CARDIAC DISEASE (CONTINUED)

SYMPTOM	INTERVENTION
Insomnia (see Appendix D)	• Use of benzodiazepines, antidepressants, or antihistaminic agents, as indicated by patient's condition, age, and life expectancy (dilated cardiomyopathy, infective endocarditis, valvular heart disease) • Provide proper sleep hygiene (dilated cardiomyopathy, infective endocarditis, valvular heart disease) • Use non-pharmacological interventions for relaxation (dilated cardiomyopathy, infective endocarditis, valvular heart disease)
Nausea	• Antiemetics (see Appendix D-1; advanced and end-stage heart failure, left heart failure [congestive heart failure], right heart failure [cor pulmonale], dilated cardiomyopathy) • Non-pharmacological interventions (see Appendix D-2; advanced and end-stage heart failure, left heart failure [congestive heart failure], right heart failure [cor pulmonale], dilated cardiomyopathy)
Pain management	• See Appendix E
Wound care (for slow-healing wounds)	• See Appendix F

NSAIDS, nonsteroidal anti-inflammatory drugs; RHD, rheumatic heart disease.

Sources: Abt, D., Bywater, M., Engeler, D. S., & Schmid, H. P. (2013). Therapeutic options for intractable hematuria in advanced bladder cancer. *International Journal of Urology, 20*(7), 651–660. https://doi.org/10.1111/iju.12113; American Cancer Society. (2022). *Supportive treatments for patients with multiple myeloma.* https://www.cancer.org/cancer/multiple-myeloma/treating/supportive.html. Brashers, V. L. (2019). Alterations in cardiovascular function. In K. L. McCance & S. E. Huether (Eds.), *Pathophysiology: The biologic basis for disease in adults and children.* (8th ed., pp. 1058–1690). Elsevier; Center to Advance Palliative Care. (2021). *Disease types and palliative care.* https://getpalliativecare.org/whatis/disease-types/; Cornish, L. (2019). Holistic management of malignant wounds in palliative patients. *British Journal of Community Nursing, 24*(Sup9), S19–S23. https://www.magonlinelibrary.com/toc/bjcn/current; Guyer, D. L., Almhanna, K., & McKee, K. Y. (2020). Palliative care for patients with esophageal cancer: A narrative review. *Annals of Translational Medicine, 8*(17). https://doi.org/10.21037/atm-20-3676; Hubert, R. J. & VanMeter, K. C. (2018). *Gould's pathophysiology for the health professions* (6th ed). Elsevier Inc.; Moffitt Cancer Center. (2018). *Stages of leukemia.* https://moffitt.org/cancers/leukemia/diagnosis/stages/; Sinibaldi, V. J., Pratz, C. F., & Yankulina, O. (2018). Kidney cancer: Toxicity management, symptom control, and palliative care. *Journal of Clinical Oncology, 36*(36), 3632–3638. doi:https://doi.org/10.1200/JCO.2018.79.0188; Sommers, M. S. (2019). *Davis's diseases and disorders: A nursing therapeutics manual.* F.A. Davis. https://www.fadavis.com/product/nursing-fundamentals-med-surg-diseases-disorders-nursing-therapeutics-manual-sommers-6; Wright, P. M. (2019). *Certified hospice and palliative nurse (CHPN) exam review: A study guide with review questions.* Springer Publishing Company.

CHAPTER 10

DEMENTIA

ALZHEIMER–TYPE DEMENTIA

DEFINITION/CHARACTERISTICS
A. Also referred to as dementia of Alzheimer type (DAT).
B. Alzheimer-type dementia accounts for 60% to 80% of all cases of dementia.
C. There are three forms:
   1. Nonhereditary or late onset (70%–90% of cases).
   2. Early onset familial.
   3. Early onset (very rare; Alzheimer's Association, 2022a; Boss & Huether, 2019; Wright, 2019).

INCIDENCE AND PREVALENCE
A. Alzheimer dementia is the leading cause of severe cognitive dysfunction in older adults.
B. Roughly 6.5 million adults in the United States have been diagnosed with Alzheimer dementia (see Figure 10.1).
C. About 73% of those who have been diagnosed with Alzheimer dementia are over the age 75 or older (see Figure 10.2).
D. About 10% of adults aged 65 and older have been diagnosed with dementia.
E. Women are disproportionately affected, accounting for two thirds of all diagnosed cases.
F. Alzheimer is often underdiagnosed in the primary care setting.
G. The estimated lifetime risk for developing Alzheimer dementia at age 45 is approximately 1 in 5 for women and 1 in 10 for men; risk increases at the age of 65 (Alzheimer's Association, 2022a; Boss & Huether, 2019; Wright, 2019).

ETIOLOGY
A. The exact cause of Alzheimer dementia is not known (Alzheimer's Association, 2022a; Boss & Huether, 2019).

PATHOPHYSIOLOGY
A. Amyloid deposits (amyloid plaques) within cerebral arteries reduce cerebral blood flow, causing amyloid angiopathy.
B. The development of neurofibrillary tangles leads to neurodegeneration.

C. Amyloid deposits outside of the neurons combined with the neurofibrillary tangles inside of the neurons leads to atrophy of the brain tissue.
D. An inflammatory immune response may be launched within the body in response to the changes in the brain (Alzheimer's Association, 2022a; Boss & Huether, 2019).

PREDISPOSING FACTORS
A. Advanced age.
B. Genetic predisposition.
C. Adult-onset diabetes.
D. Hyperlipidemia.
E. Midlife hypertension.
F. Midlife obesity.
G. Smoking.
H. Depression.
I. Cognitive inactivity.
J. Female sex.
K. Estrogen deficiency at the time of menopause.
L. Physical inactivity.
M. Head trauma.
N. Neuroinflammation.
O. Down syndrome.
P. Social isolation.
Q. Critical illness with hospitalization (Alzheimer's Association, 2022a; Boss & Huether, 2019; Wright, 2019).

SUBJECTIVE DATA
A. Memory loss that interferes with activities of daily living.
B. Progressive memory loss.
C. Disorientation.
D. Confusion.
E. Emotional lability.
F. Loss of executive functions (Alzheimer's Association, 2022a; Boss & Huether, 2019).

OBJECTIVE DATA
A. Difficulty completing familiar tasks.
B. Word searching.
C. Progressive loss of executive functions.
D. Dyspraxia.
E. Mental status changes.
F. Behavioral changes.
G. Muscular rigidity.
H. Flexion posturing.

▶

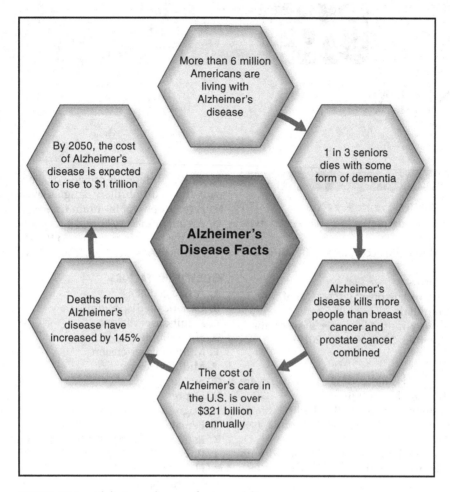

FIGURE 10.1   Alzheimer disease facts and figures.

Source: Adapted from Alzheimer's Association. (2022). *2022 Alzheimer's disease facts and figures.* https://www.alz.org/media/Documents/alzheimers-facts-and-figures-infographic.pdf

I. Weight loss.

J. Dysgraphia.

K. Poor judgment and decision–making.

L. Social withdrawal

M. Personality changes (Alzheimer's Association, 2022a; Boss & Huether, 2019).

DIAGNOSTIC TESTS

A. See Appendix Table 10A.1 for listing of common diagnostic tests.

DIFFERENTIAL DIAGNOSES

A. Vascular dementia.

B. Mixed dementia.

C. Lewy body dementia.

D. Parkinson disease.

E. Frontotemporal dementia.

F. Creutzfeldt–Jakob disease.

G. Normal pressure hydrocephalus.

H. Huntington disease.

I. Korsakoff syndrome (Alzheimer's Association, 2022b).

POTENTIAL COMPLICATIONS

A. Immobility.

B. Thromboembolism.

C. Sepsis.

D. Aspiration pneumonia.

E. Malnutrition and/or dehydration.

F. Restlessness and agitation.

G. Incontinence.

H. Depression.

I. Unsteady gait leading to falls (Alzheimer's Association, 2022a; Legg, 2017).

DISEASE-MODIFYING TREATMENTS

A. There are no Federal Drug Administration (FDA)-approved treatments to prevent or cure Alzheimer disease.

B. Some medications may be used to slow the progression of the disease, such as:

    1. Cholinesterase inhibitors.

    2. *N*-methyl-*D*-aspartate (NMDA) receptor antagonists (Alzheimer's Association, 2022a; Boss & Huether, 2019).

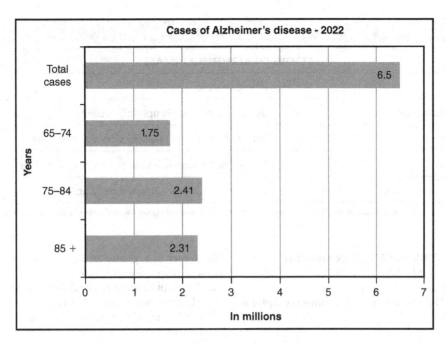

FIGURE 10.2   Age ranges of those diagnosed with Alzheimer disease.

Source: Adapted from Alzheimer's Association. (2022). *Special report, more than normal aging: Understanding mild cognitive impairment.* https://doi.org/10.1002/alz.12638.

TABLE 10.1   SYMPTOMS ASSOCIATED WITH TYPES OF DEMENTIA

TYPE OF DEMENTIA	SYMPTOMS
Alzheimer	• Short-term memory loss, forgetfulness, difficulty with new skills, decreased attention span, word searching, decreased recognition of persons, places, and things. • Characterized by its insidious onset and slow progression. Deterioration occurs over 6 to 8 years and is punctuated with periods of acute exacerbation of underlying diseases.
Frontotemporal	• Disinhibition, aphasia, emotional distancing, obstinacy, apathy, egocentric behaviors, motor disturbances, decreased facial recognition. • Frontotemporal dementia is an umbrella term for cognitive and physical deterioration caused by nerve cell damage. Progression of symptoms is dependent on the underlying cause of the damage.
Huntington	• Symptoms are related to mood, concentration, executive function, and physical function affecting gait, swallowing, speech, and so on. • Associated with slow, progressive decline. Prognosis is 10 to 30 years from time of onset.
Lewy body	• Variations in cognitive ability, visual hallucinations, parkinsonian movements, sleep disturbances, sensitivity to neuroleptics, numerous falls, autonomic disorders, systematic delusions. • Results from abnormal deposits of the alpha-synuclein protein in the brain. Symptoms are progressive and include changes in memory and cognition, movement disorders, and/or neurocognitive changes.
Vascular	• Impaired executive function, motor deficits, decreased recall, aphasia, decreased problem-solving abilities. • Involves irregular variability of symptoms accompanied by a stepwise decline. Onset of symptoms generally corresponds to transient ischemic attack or a cerebrovascular accident, or cerebral infarct.

Note: Mixed-type dementia includes features of both Alzheimer-type and vascular.

Source: Modified from Wright, P. M. (2019). *Certified Hospice and Palliative Nurse (CHPN) exam review.* Springer Publishing Company.

TABLE 10.2 ALZHEIMER DISEASE CONTINUUM

STAGES OF ALZHEIMER DISEASE	
Preclinical	Asymptomatic
Mild cognitive impairment	Symptoms do not disrupt daily activities
Mild dementia	Symptoms begin to interfere with daily activities
Moderate dementia	Symptoms frequently interfere with daily activities
Severe dementia	Symptoms interfere with most daily activities

Source: Adapted from from Alzheimer's Association. (2022). *Special report, more than normal aging: Understanding mild cognitive impairment.* https://doi.org/10.1002/alz.12638.

PALLIATIVE INTERVENTIONS/SYMPTOM MANAGEMENT
A. See Appendix Table 10A.2 for listing of palliative interventions and symptom management.
B. See Appendix D-3 for overview of common symptoms.

PROGNOSIS
A. The trajectory of Alzheimer disease is lengthy; time from diagnosis to death is typically 6 to 8 years or more (see Appendix C-1 and Table 10.2).
B. The most common causes of death that result as complications of Alzheimer disease include aspiration pneumonia and other infections, dehydration, or malnutrition (Mayo Clinic, 2022a).

NURSING INTERVENTIONS
A. Provide education on disease process and symptom management.
B. Teach patient to take all medications as prescribed.
C. Maintain nutritional and fluid status.
D. Address immobility and limb contractures.
E. Provide incontinence and skin care.
F. Encourage smoking cessation (see Appendices B-10 and C-9).
G. Provide spiritual support.
H. Assess caregiver fatigue/burnout.
I. Encourage completion of advance directives.
J. Discuss wishes regarding withholding or withdrawing of life-sustaining interventions in late stage of disease with patient (if possible) and/or primary caregiver (see Appendices C-2, C-3, and C-4).
K. Educate patient and family regarding availability of palliative care.
L. Educate patient and family regarding availability of hospice services (when appropriate).
M. Provide referral to community support groups, as needed.

FRONTOTEMPORAL DEMENTIA

DEFINITION/CHARACTERISTICS
A. Formerly referred to as Pick syndrome.
B. Refers to a group of disorders characterized by the area of neurodegeneration.
C. Types of frontotemporal dementia include:
  1. Behavioral variant (frontal lobe).
  2. Primary Progressive Aphasia (PPA; temporal lobe).
    a. Non-fluent/agrammatic.
    b. Semantic (Alzheimer's Association, 2022c; Boss & Huether, 2019; Weder et al., 2007).

INCIDENCE AND PREVALENCE
A. Frontotemporal dementia is one of the less common forms of dementia.
B. Roughly 50,000 to 60,000 people are affected by frontotemporal dementia.
C. Age of onset is generally between 35 and 75.
D. The majority of those affected are between 45 and 65 years old.
E. The incidence of frontotemporal dementia is 2.2/100,000 for those between 40 and 49 years of age, 3.3/100,000 for those between the ages of 50 to 59, and 8.9/100,000 for those between 60 and 69 years.
F. Mean age at the time of presentation is 59 years.
G. Frontotemporal dementia is more common among males (Alzheimer's Association, 2022c; Boss & Huether, 2019; Khan & De Jesus, 2022).

ETIOLOGY
A. The exact cause of frontotemporal dementia is not known (Alzheimer's Association, 2022c; Boss & Huether, 2019).

PATHOPHYSIOLOGY
A. Frontotemporal dementia is characterized by aggregation of abnormal proteins (such as tau) in the frontal or temporal regions of the brain.
B. The development of the protein aggregates leads to neurodegeneration, microvacuoles, and astrocytosis.
C. The location of the neuronal damage correlates to the signs and symptoms exhibited (Alzheimer's Association, 2022c; Boss & Huether, 2019, Khan & De Jesus, 2022).

PREDISPOSING FACTORS
A. Genetic predisposition (Alzheimer's Association, 2022c; Boss & Huether, 2019).

SUBJECTIVE DATA
A. Behavioral.
    1. Change in food preferences (toward sweet foods).
    2. Apathy.
    3. Change in appetite.
    4. Progressive attention deficit.
    5. Loss of emotional awareness and empathy.
B. Non-fluent/agrammatic.
    1. Behavior changes may occur in late stages.
C. Semantic.
    1. Compulsivity.
    2. Emotional disturbances.
    3. Mental fixation.
    4. Changes in clothing preferences.
    5. Altered pain threshold (may be heightened or lowered).
    6. Decreased capacity to show fear (Alzheimer's Association, 2022c; Boss & Huether, 2019).

OBJECTIVE DATA
A. Behavioral.
    1. Personality changes.
    2. Loss of judgment.
    3. Loss of executive function.
    4. Antisocial behaviors/social withdrawal.
    5. Disinhibition.
    6. Repeated use of "catch phrases."
    7. Poor abstraction.
B. Non-fluent/agrammatic.
    1. Expressive and receptive aphasia.
    2. Dysgraphia.
    3. Word searching.
C. Semantic.
    1. Abnormality of language.
    2. Word searching.
    3. Loss of memory for words or meaning of words.
    4. Loss of ability to recognize faces, objects, or sensory stimuli.
    5. Working memory and autobiographical memory often remain intact (Alzheimer's Association, 2022c; Weder et al., 2007).

DIAGNOSTIC TESTS
A. See Appendix Table 10A.1 for listing of common diagnostic tests.
B. See Figure 10.3 for staging.

DIFFERENTIAL DIAGNOSES
A. Cerebrovascular accident (CVA).
B. Parkinson disease.
C. Huntington disease.
D. Hypothyroidism.
E. HIV.
F. Substance abuse (primarily alcohol).
G. Motor neuron disease.
H. Corticobasal degeneration.
I. Progressive supranuclear palsy.
J. Often misdiagnosed as Alzheimer dementia (Alzheimer's Association, 2022c).

POTENTIAL COMPLICATIONS
A. Immobility.
B. Thromboembolism.
C. Sepsis.

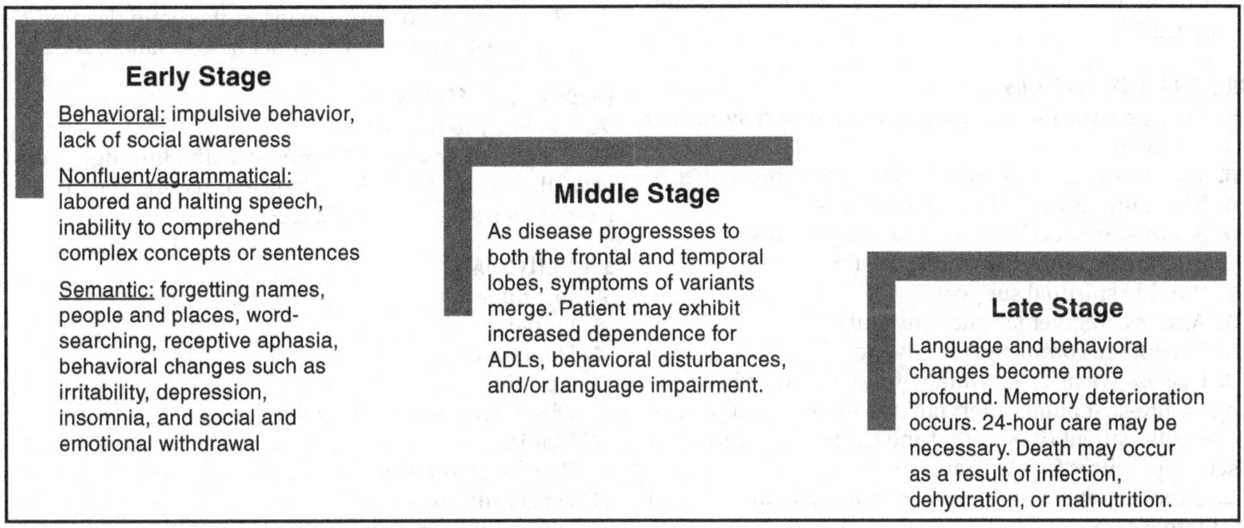

Early Stage

Behavioral: impulsive behavior, lack of social awareness

Nonfluent/agrammatical: labored and halting speech, inability to comprehend complex concepts or sentences

Semantic: forgetting names, people and places, word-searching, receptive aphasia, behavioral changes such as irritability, depression, insomnia, and social and emotional withdrawal

Middle Stage

As disease progressses to both the frontal and temporal lobes, symptoms of variants merge. Patient may exhibit increased dependence for ADLs, behavioral disturbances, and/or language impairment.

Late Stage

Language and behavioral changes become more profound. Memory deterioration occurs. 24-hour care may be necessary. Death may occur as a result of infection, dehydration, or malnutrition.

FIGURE 10.3 Stages of frontotemporal dementia.

ADLs, activities of daily living.

Source: Adapted from Ellison, J. M. (2021). *What are the stages of frontotemporal dementia?* https://www.brightfocus.org/alzheimers/article/what-are-stages-frontotemporal-dementia

D. Aspiration pneumonia.

E. Malnutrition and/or dehydration.

F. Restlessness and agitation.

G. Incontinence.

H. Depression.

I. Unsteady gait leading to falls (Alzheimer's Association, 2022c; National Institute of Neurological Disorders and Stroke, 2022).

DISEASE-MODIFYING TREATMENTS

A. There are no Federal Drug Administration (FDA)-approved treatments to prevent or cure frontotemporal dementia.

B. Some medications may be used to control symptoms including:

1. Selective serotonin reuptake inhibitors.
2. Trazodone.
3. Antipsychotics.

C. Speech therapy, physical therapy, and occupational therapy may help to maintain or prolong function (Alzheimer's Association, 2022c; Boss & Huether, 2019).

PALLIATIVE INTERVENTIONS/SYMPTOM MANAGEMENT

A. See Appendix Table 10A.2 for listing of palliative interventions and symptom management.

B. See Appendix D-3 for overview of common symptoms.

PROGNOSIS

A. The prognosis for frontotemporal dementia is poor, ranging from 2 to 10 years depending on rapidity of decline.

B. 24-hour care may be required for patient safety.

C. Common causes of death include aspiration pneumonia and other infections, dehydration, or malnutrition (National Institute of Neurological Disorders and Stroke, 2022).

NURSING INTERVENTIONS

A. Provide education on disease process and symptom management.

B. Teach patient to take all medications as prescribed.

C. Maintain nutritional and fluid status.

D. Address immobility and limb contractures.

E. Provide incontinence and skin care.

F. Provide spiritual support.

G. Assess caregiver fatigue/burnout.

H. Encourage completion of advance directives.

I. Discuss wishes regarding withholding or withdrawing of life-sustaining interventions in late stage of disease with patient (if possible) and/or primary caregiver (see Appendices C-2, C-3, and C-4).

J. Educate patient and family regarding availability of palliative care.

K. Educate patient and family regarding availability of hospice services (when appropriate).

L. Provide referral to community support groups, as needed.

HUNTINGTON DISEASE

DEFINITION/CHARACTERISTICS

A. Rare, genetic disease characterized by neurodegeneration resulting in impaired movements, cognition, and emotional regulation.

B. The striatum is the most commonly affected area of the brain (Alzheimer's Association, 2022d; Huntington's Disease Society of America, 2022; Mayo Clinic, 2022b).

INCIDENCE AND PREVALENCE

A. Commonly diagnosed between the ages of 35 and 45.

B. When diagnosed in those younger than 20 years, the condition is referred to as juvenile Huntington disease.

C. One in every 10,000 persons has Huntington disease.

D. Nearly 30,000 people in the United States have Huntington disease.

E. Juvenile Huntington accounts for about 16% of all cases.

F. Huntington disease is not prevalent within any particular population.

G. All races and ethnic groups and both sexes are affected (Alzheimer's Society, 2022; Center for Neurological Treatment & Research, 2023; Mayo Clinic, 2022b; Yohrling et al., 2020).

ETIOLOGY

A. Autosomal dominant genetic disorder inherited from a parent (Huntington's Disease Society of America, 2022; Mayo Clinic, 2022b).

PATHOPHYSIOLOGY

A. Mutations in the HTT gene (the gene that encodes the huntingtin protein) cause:

1. Abnormal protein synthesis.
2. Accumulation of proteins in the brain, leading to neurodegeneration (Alzheimer's Association, 2022d).

PREDISPOSING FACTORS

A. Genetic predisposition.

B. If a parent has been diagnosed with Huntington disease, their child has a 50% chance of having the disease (Alzheimer's Association, 2022c).

SUBJECTIVE DATA

A. Insomnia.

B. Lethargy.

C. Depression.

D. Apathy.

E. Obsessive-compulsive behaviors.

F. Mania.

G. Poor concentration.

H. Forgetfulness.

I. Difficulty organizing tasks.

J. Poor impulse control.

K. Impaired mentation.

L. Lack of awareness of one's own actions.

M. Suicidal ideation.

N. Social withdrawal (Alzheimer's Society, 2022; Huntington's Disease Society of America, 2022; Mayo Clinic, 2022b).

OBJECTIVE DATA
A. Impaired voluntary muscle movements (jerky or writhing).
B. Ataxia.
C. Diminished executive function.
D. Inability to recognize emotions in others.
E. Dysphagia.
F. Dysarthria.
G. Muscle rigidity or contractions.
H. Frequent falls or clumsiness (Alzheimer's Society, 2022; Huntington's Disease Society of America, 2022; Mayo Clinic, 2022b).

DIAGNOSTIC TESTS
A. See Appendix Table 10A.1 for listing of common diagnostic tests.
B. See Figure 10.4 for stages.

DIFFERENTIAL DIAGNOSES
A. Pantothenate kinase-associated neurodegeneration (PKAN).
B. Neuroacanthocytosis syndrome.
C. Metal accumulation disorders.
D. Friedreich ataxia.
E. McLeod syndrome (males only).
F. Oculomotor apraxia.
G. Lesch–Nyhan syndrome (Martino et al., 2013).

POTENTIAL COMPLICATIONS
A. Progressively diminished functionality.
B. Progressive dependence.
C. Immobility (Mayo Clinic, 2022b).

DISEASE-MODIFYING TREATMENTS
A. There are no Federal Drug Administration (FDA)-approved treatments to prevent or cure Huntington disease.
B. Some medications may be used to control symptoms including:
  1. Vesicular monoamine transporter 2 (VMAT2) inhibitors.
  2. Selective serotonin reuptake inhibitors.
  3. Antipsychotics.
  4. Anticonvulsants.
C. Speech therapy, physical therapy, and occupational therapy may help to maintain or prolong function.
D. Counseling may help with emotional disturbances (Alzheimer's Association, 2022d; Huntington's Disease Society of America, 2022).

PALLIATIVE INTERVENTIONS/SYMPTOM MANAGEMENT
A. See Appendix Table 10A.2 for listing of palliative interventions and symptom management.
B. See Appendix D-3 for overview of common symptoms.

PROGNOSIS
A. The prognosis is 10 to 30 years from the time of symptom onset.
B. The disease involves a slow, progressive declinatory trajectory (see Appendix C-1).
C. 24-hour care may be required for patient safety.
D. Common causes of death include aspiration pneumonia and other infections, dehydration, or malnutrition (Alzheimer's Society, 2022; Mayo Clinic, 2022b).

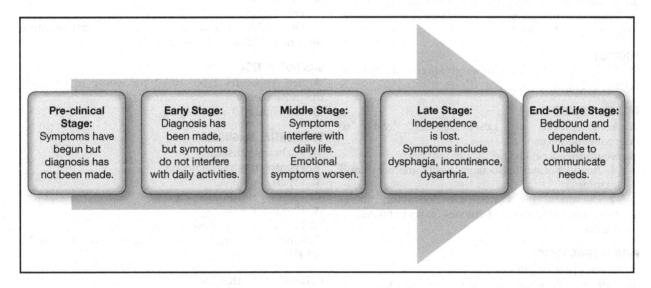

FIGURE 10.4   Stages of Huntington disease.

Source: Adapted from Shaikh, J. (2020). *What are the 5 stages of Huntington's disease?* https://www.medicinenet.com/what_are_the_5_stages_of_huntingtons_disease/article.htm

NURSING INTERVENTIONS

A. Provide education on disease process and symptom management.

B. Teach patient to take all medications as prescribed.

C. Maintain nutritional and fluid status.

D. Address immobility and limb contractures.

E. Provide incontinence and skin care.

F. Provide spiritual and emotional support.

G. Assess caregiver fatigue/burnout.

H. Encourage completion of advance directives.

I. Discuss wishes regarding withholding or withdrawing of life-sustaining interventions in late stage of disease with patient (if possible) and/or primary caregiver (see Appendices C-2, C-3, and C-4).

J. Educate patient and family regarding availability of palliative care.

K. Educate patient and family regarding availability of hospice services (when appropriate).

L. Provide referral to community support groups, as needed.

LEWY BODY DEMENTIA

DEFINITION/CHARACTERISTICS

A. A neurodegenerative disorder characterized by:

1. Abnormal aggregation of alpha-synuclein (Lewy bodies) in the brain.

2. Disrupted production of acetylcholine and dopamine (National Institute on Aging, 2021a; Taylor et al., 2020).

INCIDENCE AND PREVALENCE

A. Lewy body dementia is one of the most common forms of dementia.

B. It affects over 1 million adults in the United States.

C. Symptoms usually begin at age 50 or older (National Institute on Aging, 2021a).

ETIOLOGY

A. The exact cause is unknown (National Institute on Aging, 2021a).

PATHOPHYSIOLOGY

A. Accumulation of Lewy bodies leads to neurodegeneration.

B. Neurodegeneration specifically reduces:

1. Acetylcholine (associated with memory and learning).

2. Dopamine (associated with behavior, movement, mood, and sleep; National Institute on Aging, 2021a).

PREDISPOSING FACTORS

A. Genetic predisposition.

B. History of Parkinson disease (see Figure 10.5).

C. Sleep disorders.

D. Genetic predisposition (National Institute on Aging, 2021a; Walker et al., 2015).

SUBJECTIVE DATA

A. Insomnia.

B. Impaired cognition.

C. Visual hallucinations.

D. Lethargy.

E. Diminished attention span.

F. Memory loss.

G. Fatigue.

H. Depression.

I. Apathy.

J. Anxiety.

K. Delusions.

L. Paranoia (National Institute on Aging, 2021a; Taylor et al., 2020).

OBJECTIVE DATA

A. Muscle rigidity and stiffness.

B. Shuffling gait.

C. Slow movements.

D. Frozen gait.

E. Resting tremor.

F. Poor balance.

G. Repeated falls.

H. Stooped posture.

I. Flat affect.

J. Dysphagia.

K. Restless leg syndrome.

L. Postural hypotension.

M. Incontinence.

N. Loss of sense of smell.

O. Gastroparesis.

P. Behavioral changes.

Q. Decreased alertness.

R. Poor judgment.

S. Disorientation.

T. Dysarthria.

U. Diminished executive function (National Institute on Aging, 2021a; Taylor et al., 2020).

DIAGNOSTIC TESTS

A. See Appendix Table 10A.1 for listing of common diagnostic tests.

B. See Figure 10.6 for staging.

DIFFERENTIAL DIAGNOSES

A. Alzheimer disease.

B. Frontotemporal dementia.

C. Hydrocephalus.

D. Lacunar syndrome.

E. Parkinson disease.

F. Prion-related diseases.

G. Progressive supranuclear palsy (Crystal & Chawla, 2019).

POTENTIAL COMPLICATIONS

A. Severe dementia.

B. Aggressive behavior.

C. Depression.

▶

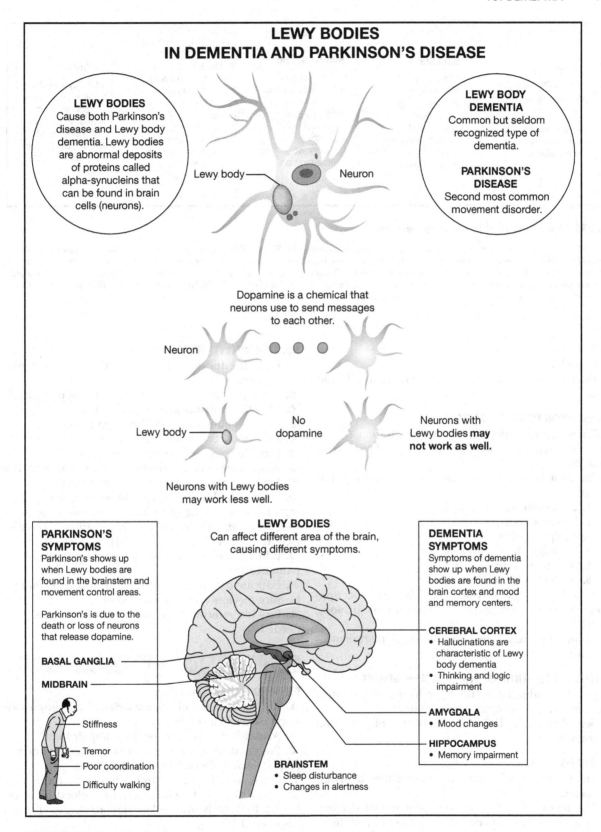

FIGURE 10.5 Lewy body dementia.

Source: Adapted from National Library of Medicine. (2019). *Lewy bodies dementia.* https://magazine.medlineplus.gov/multimedia/lewy-bodies-dementia

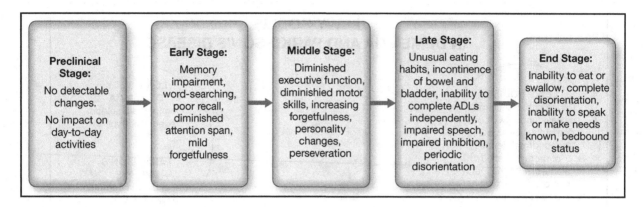

FIGURE 10.6 Stages of Lewy body dementia.

Sources: Adapted from Crystal, H. A., & Chawla, J. (2019). *Lewy body dementia: Differential diagnoses.* https://emedicine.medscape.com/article/1135041-differential; MeasurAbilities. (2023). *7 stages of Lewy body dementia.* https://measurabilities.com/7-stages-of-lewy-body-dementia/; National Institute on Aging. (2021a). *What is Lewy body dementia? Causes, symptoms, and treatments.* https://www.nia.nih.gov/health/what-lewy-body-dementia-causes-symptoms-and-treatments; Walker, Z., Possin, K. L., Boeve, B. F., & Aarsland, D. (2015). Lewy body dementias. *The Lancet, 386*(10004), 1683–1697. https://doi.org/10.1016/S0140-6736(15)00462-6

D. Risk for falls or injury.

E. Immobility.

F. Progressive parkinsonian symptoms (Mayo Clinic, 2022c).

DISEASE-MODIFYING TREATMENTS

A. There are no Federal Drug Administration (FDA)-approved treatments to prevent or cure Lewy body dementia.

B. Some medications may be used to control symptoms including:

  1. Cholinesterase inhibitors.

  2. Psychostimulants.

  3. Antipsychotics.

  4. Decarboxylase inhibitors.

  5. Antidepressants.

  6. Antiepileptic medications.

C. Speech therapy, physical therapy, and occupational therapy may help to maintain or prolong function.

D. Counseling may help with emotional disturbances (National Institute on Aging, 2021b).

PALLIATIVE INTERVENTIONS/SYMPTOM MANAGEMENT

A. See Appendix Table 10A.2 for listing of palliative interventions and symptom management.

B. See Appendix D-3 for overview of common symptoms.

PROGNOSIS

A. The prognosis is 5 to 8 years from the time of symptom onset.

B. The disease involves a slow, progressive declinatory trajectory (see Appendix C-1; National Institute on Aging, 2021a).

NURSING INTERVENTIONS

A. Provide education on disease process and symptom management.

B. Teach patient to take all medications as prescribed.

C. Maintain nutritional and fluid status.

D. Address immobility and limb contractures.

E. Provide incontinence and skin care.

F. Provide spiritual and emotional support.

G. Assess caregiver fatigue/burnout (see Appendix B-5).

H. Encourage completion of advance directives.

I. Discuss wishes regarding withholding or withdrawing of life-sustaining interventions in late stage of disease with patient (if possible) and/or primary caregiver (see Appendices C-2, C-3, and C-4).

J. Educate patient and family regarding availability of palliative care.

K. Educate patient and family regarding availability of hospice services (when appropriate).

L. Provide referral to community support groups, as needed.

VASCULAR DEMENTIA

DEFINITION/CHARACTERISTICS

A. A form of dementia characterized by a progressive, stepwise declinatory trajectory.

B. Also called "vascular cognitive impairment."

C. Presentation of deficits may be in only one domain (e.g., speech is affected but not cognition).

D. Often results from stroke but can result from any condition that reduces cerebral blood flow (see Figure 10.7; Alzheimer's Association, 2022e; Hinkle & Cheever, 2018).

Understanding Vascular Dementia

A Form of Dementia

- Dementia is a loss of brain function that affects reasoning, memory, and behavior, and which interferes with everyday life.
- There are many different forms of dementia, each with unique symptoms caused by microscopic changes in the brain.

Vascular Dementia

- Vascular dementia is considered the second-most common form of dementia after Alzheimer's disease.
- It results from injuries to the vessels supplying blood to the brain, often after a major stroke or series of smaller strokes.
- Symptoms can be similar to Alzheimer's disease, and both conditions can occur at the same time.

Symptoms (vary)

1. Confusion
2. Issues with organization and problem solving
3. Memory impairment
4. Difficulty with speech
5. Mood changes; depression
6. Difficulty with movement and balance

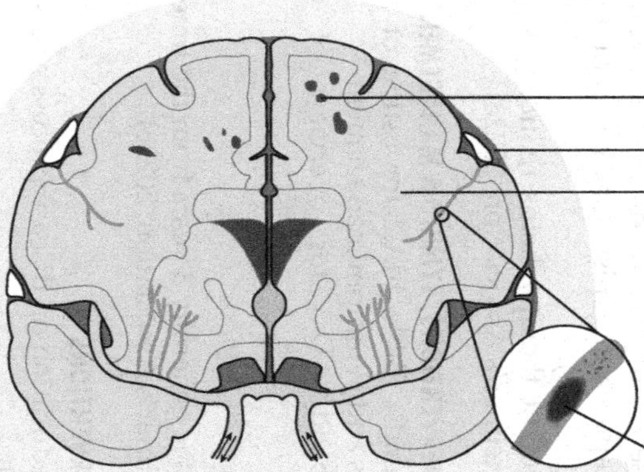

Causes

- Vascular dementia occurs when not enough nutrients and oxygen get to the brain because their supply is cut off. This happens when blood vessels in and around the brain get damaged. Blood vessels are tube-like structures that carry blood through tissues and organs. Without a blood supply, brain cells die, causing the symptoms of dementia that impact daily life.
- Many cases of vascular dementia develop after a stroke or series of strokes. Strokes occur when the blood supply to a certain part of your brain is interrupted. This can be because a blood vessel is blocked, or it is damaged enough to leak or burst.
- Strokes are considered a medical emergency because, without oxygen and nutrients, brain tissue begins to die within minutes. Whether the stroke symptoms are obvious, or the stroke is silent, risk of vascular dementia increases proportionally with the number of strokes that occur over time.
- Vascular dementia can also be caused by brain hemorrhages - ruptured blood vessels leaking and putting damaging pressure on surrounding brain cells. Other chronic conditions can cause narrowed or damaged brain vessels that, in turn, increase the risk of vascular dementia.

Small Strokes

Blood Vessels

White Matter
White matter is the paler, deep tissue of the brain containing nerve fibers (axons), which are extensions of brain cells. It enables the relay of information between brain regions.

Blood Clot
A blood clot is one way a blood vessel can become blocked. Disruption to the brain's blood flow can lead to a series of mini strokes.

Blood Flow

Types of Vascular Dementia

Mixed Dementia
Mixed dementia occurs when vascular dementia and Alzheimer's disease coexist.

Subcortical Vascular Dementia
Binswanger's disease, or subcortical vascular dementia is a disease of small blood vessels that lie deep within the brain. Many of these blood vessels develop thick walls, become still, twisted, and damaged. This causes damage to the brain's white matter (deep tissue of the brain).

Multi-Infarct Dementia
Muti-infarct dementia is more common than single-infarct dementia and is a result of a series of mini strokes. Unlike major strokes that permanently cut off blood supply, mini strokes last no more than 24 hours. In multi-infarct dementia, a series of mini strokes causes multiple infarcts (areas of dead tissue resulting from failed blood supply) and leads to vascular dementia.

Risk Factors

1. **Aging:** The risk of developing Vascular Dementia doubles every 5 years over the age of 65.
2. **History of Stroke:** Loss of oxygen to the brain causes brain damage and increases risk of dementia.
3. **Blood Pressure:** High blood pressure puts stress on blood vessels, causing vessels to be damaged or burst.
4. **High Cholesterol:** Higher levels of low-density lipoprotein increases risk of vascular dementia.
5. **Smoking:** Smoking directly damages blood vessels.
6. **Obesity:** Obesity can cause vascular disease and increase risk of vascular dementia.
7. **Heart Disease:** History of heart attack or atrial fibrillation increases risk of vascular dementia.

FIGURE 10.7 Vascular dementia.

Source: Adapted from Miller, N. (2021). *Understanding vasulcar dementia.* https://pennmemorycenter.org/education-and-support-resources/understanding-my-diagnosis/ed-vascular-dementia/

INCIDENCE AND PREVALENCE

A. The second most common form of dementia; it accounts for 15% to 20% of cases in North America and Europe.

B. Vascular dementia is commonly found as an aspect of mixed dementia.

C. Only 5% to 10% of all cases present as vascular dementia alone (Alzheimer's Association, 2022e; Hinkle & Cheever, 2018; Wolters & Ikram, 2019).

ETIOLOGY

A. Caused by any condition that impedes blood flow to the brain (Alzheimer's Association, 2022e; National Institute on Aging, 2021b).

PATHOPHYSIOLOGY

A. Diminished cerebral blood flow is secondary to stroke or any other condition that reduces cerebral circulation.

B. Inadequate blood flow to the brain causes neuronal death (Alzheimer's Association, 2022e).

PREDISPOSING FACTORS

A. History of stroke.

B. Cerebral hemorrhage.

C. Atherosclerosis.

D. Obesity.

E. Atrial fibrillation.

F. Hypertension.

G. Cardiovascular disease.

H. Hypercholesterolemia.

I. Smoking.

J. Diabetes.

K. Advancing age (Alzheimer's Association, 2022e; Hinkle & Cheever, 2018; Mayo Clinic, 2022d).

SUBJECTIVE DATA

A. Confusion.

B. Disorientation.

C. Depression.

D. Difficulty concentrating.

E. Diminished cognition.

F. Apathy.

G. Difficulty organizing tasks (Alzheimer's Association, 2022e; Hinkle & Cheever, 2018; Mayo Clinic, 2022d; see Table 10.1 and Figure 10.7).

OBJECTIVE DATA

A. Word searching.

B. Receptive or expressive aphasia.

C. Impaired mobility.

D. Poor balance.

E. Hemiparesis.

F. Unsteady gait.

G. Dysphagia (Alzheimer's Association, 2022e; Hinkle & Cheever, 2018; Mayo Clinic, 2022d; see Table 10.1 and Figure 10.7).

DIAGNOSTIC TESTS

A. See Appendix Table 10A.1 for listing of common diagnostic tests.

DIFFERENTIAL DIAGNOSES

A. Alzheimer disease.

B. Brain tumor.

C. Creutzfeldt–Jakob disease.

D. Neurosyphilis.

E. Normal pressure hydrocephalus.

F. Frontotemporal dementia.

G. Lewy body dementia (Alzheimer's Association, 2022e).

POTENTIAL COMPLICATIONS

A. Immobility.

B. Thromboembolism.

C. Stroke.

D. Heart disease.

E. Malnutrition and/or dehydration.

F. Opportunistic infections.

G. Incontinence.

H. Depression.

I. Unsteady gait leading to falls (Alzheimer's Association, 2022e; National Library of Medicine, 2020b).

DISEASE-MODIFYING TREATMENTS

A. Lifestyle modifications are recommended to prevent vascular disease or further deterioration.

B. Medications used to treat Alzheimer disease (i.e., cholinesterase inhibitors and *N*-methyl-*D*-aspartate (NMDA) receptor antagonists may be useful in slowing disease progression).

C. Anticoagulant therapy helps reduce risk of future strokes (Alzheimer's Association, 2022e).

PALLIATIVE INTERVENTIONS/SYMPTOM MANAGEMENT

A. See Appendix Table 10A.2 for listing of palliative interventions and symptom management.

B. See Appendix D-3 for overview of common symptoms.

PROGNOSIS

A. Prognosis is generally 3 years from the time of diagnosis (Alzheimer's Association, 2022e).

NURSING INTERVENTIONS

A. Provide education on disease process and symptom management.

B. Teach patient to take all medications as prescribed.

C. Maintain nutritional and fluid status.

D. Address immobility and limb contractures.

E. Provide incontinence and skin care.

F. Encourage smoking cessation (see Appendices B-10 and C-9).

G. Provide spiritual support.

H. Assess caregiver fatigue/burnout.

I. Encourage completion of advance directives.

J. Discuss wishes regarding withholding or withdrawing of life-sustaining interventions in late stage of disease with patient (if possible) and/or primary caregiver (see Appendices C-2, C-3, and C-4).

K. Educate patient and family regarding availability of palliative care.

▶

L. Educate patient and family regarding availability of hospice services (when appropriate).

M. Provide referral to community support groups, as needed.

REFERENCES

Abt, D., Bywater, M., Engeler, D. S., & Schmid, H. P. (2013). Therapeutic options for intractable hematuria in advanced bladder cancer. *International Journal of Urology*, 20(7), 651–660. https://doi.org/10.1111/iju.12113

Alzheimer's Association. (2022a). *2022 Alzheimer's disease facts and figures.* https://www.alz.org/media/Documents/alzheimers-facts-and-figures-infographic.pdf

Alzheimer's Association. (2022b). *Differential diagnoses.* https://www.alz.org/professionals/health-systems-clinicians/dementia-diagnosis/differential-diagnosis

Alzheimer's Association. (2022c). *Frontotemporal dementia.* https://www.alz.org/alzheimers-dementia/what-is-dementia/types-of-dementia/frontotemporal-dementia

Alzheimer's Association. (2022d). *Differential diagnosis of Huntington's disease.* https://www.alz.org/professionals/health-systems-clinicians/dementia-diagnosis/differential-diagnosis/differential_diagnosis_of_huntington_s_disease

Alzheimer's Association. (2022e). *Vascular dementia.* https://www.alz.org/alzheimers-dementia/what-is-dementia/types-of-dementia/vascular-dementia

Alzheimer's Society. (2022). *Huntington's disease.* https://www.alzheimers.org.uk/about-dementia/types-dementia/huntingtonsdisease

Boss, J. B., & Huether, S. E. (2019). Alternations in cognitive hemodynamics and motor function. In K. L. McCance & S. E. Huether (Eds.), *Pathophysiology: The biologic basis for disease in adults and children* (8th ed., pp. 504–549). Elsevier.

Center for Neurological Treatment & Research. (2023). *Huntington's disease overview, incidence and prevalence of HD.* http://www.neurocntr.com/huntingtons-disease

Crystal, H. A., & Chawla, J. (2019). *Lewy body dementia: Differential diagnoses.* https://emedicine.medscape.com/article/1135041-differential

Ellison, J. M. (2021). *What are the stages of frontotemporal dementia?* https://www.brightfocus.org/alzheimers/article/what-are-stages-frontotemporal-dementia

Guyer, D. L., Almhanna, K., & McKee, K. Y. (2020). Palliative care for patients with esophageal cancer: A narrative review. *Annals of Translational Medicine*, 8(17), 1103. https://doi.org/10.21037/atm-20-3676

Hinkle, J. L., & Cheever, K. H. (2018). *Brunner & Siddarth's textbook of medical-surgical nursing* (14th ed., pp. 1377–1427). Wolters Kluwer.

Huether, S. E. (2019a). Alternations in digestive function. In K. L. McCance & S. E. Huether (Eds.), *Pathophysiology: The biologic basis for disease in adults and children* (8th ed., pp. 1321–1372). Elsevier.

Huntington's Disease Society of America. (2022). *Overview of Huntington's disease.* https://hdsa.org/what-is-hd/overview-of-huntingtons-disease/

Khan, I., & De Jesus, O. (2022). *Frontotemporal lobe dementia.* https://www.ncbi.nlm.nih.gov/books/NBK559286/

Legg, T. J. (2017). *Complications of Alzheimer's disease (AD).* https://www.healthline.com/health/alzheimers-disease-complications

Martino, D., Stamelou, M., & Bhatia, K. P. (2013). The differential diagnosis of Huntington's disease-like syndromes: 'Red flags' for the clinician. *Journal of Neurology, Neurosurgery & Psychiatry*, 84(6), 650–656. https://jnnp.bmj.com/content/84/6/650.short

Mayo Clinic. (2022a). *Alzheimer's stages: How the disease progresses.* https://www.mayoclinic.org/diseases-conditions/alzheimers-disease/in-depth/alzheimers-stages/art-20048448

Mayo Clinic. (2022b). *Huntington's disease.* https://www.mayoclinic.org/diseases-conditions/huntingtons-disease/symptoms-causes/syc-20356117

Mayo Clinic. (2022c). *Lewy body dementia.* https://www.mayoclinic.org/diseases-conditions/lewy-body-dementia/symptoms-causes/syc-20352025

Mayo Clinic. (2022d). *Vascular dementia.* https://www.mayoclinic.org/diseases-conditions/vascular-dementia/symptoms-causes/syc-20378793

MeasurAbilities. (2023). *7 stages of Lewy body dementia.* https://measurabilities.com/7-stages-of-lewy-body-dementia/

National Institute on Aging. (2021a). *What is Lewy body dementia? Causes, symptoms, and treatments.* https://www.nia.nih.gov/health/what-lewy-body-dementia-causes-symptoms-and-treatments#:~:text=Lewy%20body%20dementia%20(LBD)%20is,movement%2C%20behavior%2C%20and%20mood

National Institute on Aging. (2021b). *Vascular dementia: Causes, symptoms, and treatments.* https://www.nia.nih.gov/health/vascular-dementia

National Institute of Neurological Disorders and Stroke. (2022). *Frontotemporal dementia.* https://www.ninds.nih.gov/health-information/disorders/frontotemporal-dementia#:~:text=The%20outcome%20for%20people%20with,in%20an%20institutionalized%20care%20setting

National Library of Medicine. (2019a). *Lewy bodies dementia.* https://magazine.medlineplus.gov/multimedia/lewy-bodies-dementia

National Library of Medicine. (2020b). *Vascular dementia.* https://medlineplus.gov/ency/article/000746.htm

Shaikh, J. (2020). *What are the 5 stages of Huntington's disease?* https://www.medicinenet.com/what_are_the_5_stages_of_huntingtons_disease/article.htm

Sommers, M. S. (2019). *Davis's diseases and disorders: A nursing therapeutics manual.* F.A. Davis. https://www.fadavis.com/product/nursing-fundamentals-med-surg-diseases-disorders-nursing-therapeutics-manual-sommers-6

Taylor, J. P., McKeith, I. G., Burn, D. J., Boeve, B. F., Weintraub, D., Bamford, C., Allan, L. M., Thomas, A. J., & O'Brien, J. T. (2020). New evidence on the management of Lewy body dementia. *The Lancet Neurology*, 19(2), 157–169. https://www.sciencedirect.com/science/article/abs/pii/S147444221930153X

U.S. National Library of Medicine. (2022). *Amyotrophic lateral sclerosis (ALS).* https://medlineplus.gov/ency/article/000688.htm

Walker, Z., Possin, K. L., Boeve, B. F., & Aarsland, D. (2015). Lewy body dementias. *The Lancet*, 386(10004), 1683–1697. https://doi.org/10.1016/S0140-6736(15)00462-6

Weder, N. D., Aziz, R., Wilkins, K., & Tampi, R. R. (2007). Frontotemporal dementias: A review. *Annals of General Psychiatry*, 6(1), 1–10. https://annals-general-psychiatry.biomedcentral.com/articles/10.1186/1744-859X-6-15

Wolters, F. J., & Ikram, M. A. (2019). Epidemiology of vascular dementia: Nosology in a time of epidemics. *Arteriosclerosis, Thrombosis, and Vascular Biology*, 39(8), 1542–1549. https://www.ahajournals.org/doi/10.1161/ATVBAHA.119.311908

Wright, P. M. (2019). *Certified hospice and palliative nurse (CHPN) exam review: A study guide with review questions.* Springer Publishing Company.

Yohrling, G., Raimundo, K., Crowell, V., Lovecky, D., Vetter, L., & Seeberger, L. (2020). Prevalence of Huntington's disease in the US (954). *Neurology*, 94(15S), 954. https://n.neurology.org/content/94/15_Supplement/954.abstract

APPENDIX

TABLE 10A.1   DIAGNOSTIC TESTS FOR DEMENTIA

TYPE	NOTES
Physical examination	• Thorough physical examination with focused neurological assessment, mental status evaluation, and neurophysiological testing • Neuropsychometric testing for frontotemporal, HD, and Lewy body dementia
Imaging	• PET scan (Alzheimer-type dementia, Lewy body dementia) • CT scan (Alzheimer-type dementia, Lewy body dementia, vascular dementia) • MRI • FDG-PET scan (frontotemporal dementia) • Testing for sleep apnea (frontotemporal dementia) • Single photon CT scan (Lewy body dementia) • Carotid ultrasound (vascular dementia)
Laboratory tests	• Biomarker testing (Alzheimer-type dementia, Lewy body dementia) • Genetic testing (Alzheimer-type dementia, HD) • Cerebrospinal fluid analysis (Alzheimer-type dementia, frontotemporal dementia) • Complete blood count (frontotemporal dementia, vascular dementia) • Liver function studies (frontotemporal dementia) • Chemistry panel (Lewy body dementia) • Thyroid studies (Lewy body dementia, vascular dementia) • Vitamin B_{12} levels (Lewy body dementia, vascular dementia) • Syphilis, Lyme, or HIV testing, when appropriate (Lewy body dementia) • Lipid profile (vascular dementia) • Complete metabolic profile (vascular dementia)
Pathology	• Alzheimer dementia is a diagnosis of exclusion; confirmation is through autopsy • Alzheimer disease progression is evaluated using the FAST Scale (see Appendix A-5) • Frontotemporal dementia is staged according to level of disease progression: early stage, middle stage, late stage (see Figure 10.3; frontotemporal dementia) • Huntington disease is staged as follows: preclinical stage, early stage, middle stage, late stage, end of life (see Figure 10.4) • Lewy body dementia is staged as follows: preclinical stage, early stage, middle stage, late stage, end of life (see Figure 10.6) • Vascular dementia is staged as early, middle, and late, corresponding to the level of impairment

FAST, Functional Assessment Staging Tool; FDG-PET, fluorodeoxyglucose positron emission tomography; HD, Huntington disease.

Sources: Alzheimer's Association. (2022a). *2022 Alzheimer's disease facts and figures.* https://www.alz.org/media/Documents/alzheimers-facts-and-figures-infographic.pdf, Alzheimer's Association. (2022d). *Differential diagnosis of Huntington's disease.* https://www.alz.org/professionals/health-systems-clinicians/dementia-diagnosis/differential-diagnosis/differential_diagnosis_of_huntington_s_disease; Boss, J. B., & Huether, S. E. (2019). Alternations in cognitive hemodynamics and motor function. In K. L. McCance & S. E. Huether (Eds.), *Pathophysiology: The biologic basis for disease in adults and children* (8th ed., pp. 504–549). Elsevier; Crystal, H. A., & Chawla, J. (2019). *Lewy body dementia: Differential diagnoses.* https://emedicine.medscape.com/article/1135041-differential; MeasurAbilities. (2023). *7 stages of Lewy body dementia.* https://measurabilities.com/7-stages-of-lewy-body-dementia/; National Institute on Aging. (2021a). *What is Lewy body dementia? Causes, symptoms, and treatments.* https://www.nia.nih.gov/health/what-lewy-body-dementia-causes-symptoms-and-treatments#:~:text=Lewy%20body%20dementia%20(LBD)%20is,movement%2C%20behavior%2C%20and%20mood; Walker, Z., Possin, K. L., Boeve, B. F., & Aarsland, D. (2015). Lewy body dementias. *The Lancet, 386*(10004), 1683–1697. https://doi.org/10.1016/S0140-6736(15)00462-6

TABLE 10A.2 PALLIATIVE INTERVENTIONS/SYMPTOM MANAGEMENT FOR DEMENTIA

SYMPTOM	INTERVENTION
Anorexia	• Use of appetite stimulants (see Appendix D-1) • Offer small, frequent meals and snacks • Offer nutritional supplements
Anxiety and depression	• Antidepressants, anxiolytics, or benzodiazepines as indicated by patient's condition, age, and life expectancy (see Appendix D) • Non-pharmacological interventions (see Appendix D-2)
Caregiver burden	• Support of interdisciplinary hospice or palliative team • Non-pharmacological interventions for caregivers (see Appendix D-2)
Communication barriers	• Use nonthreatening body language (place yourself at eye level, use therapeutic touch) • Use a soft tone of voice and use short phrases • Avoid use of hand gestures when speaking as this may seem threatening to the person • Reduce distractions • Offer a limited number of choices • Use a picture board, if needed
Dysphagia	• Dietary modification (puree, thickened liquids, etc.) • Crush medications or use liquid formulations when possible
Dyspnea (see Appendix D)	• Corticosteroids for reducing inflammation (Alzheimer-type dementia, vascular dementia) • Opioids to reduce inspiratory effort and tachypnea (Alzheimer-type dementia, vascular dementia) • Bronchodilators for opening airways (mechanism of action of relaxation of muscular bands that surround bronchi, thus widening the airway; Alzheimer-type dementia, vascular dementia) • Diuretics to reduce systemic congestion (Alzheimer-type dementia, vascular dementia) • Anticholinergics to reduce secretions, especially at the end of life (Alzheimer-type dementia, vascular dementia) • Use of fans (Alzheimer-type dementia, vascular dementia) • Lower temperature in the room (Alzheimer-type dementia, vascular dementia)
Fatigue and somnolence	• Alternate periods of rest with periods of activity • Utilize energy conversation techniques • Psychostimulants (see Appendix D)
Immobility	• Encourage active participation in repositioning, when possible • Implement use of bed mobility devices such as a bed hoist, bed ladder, grab rail, or trapeze bar • Frequently reposition patient to relieve pressure on bony surfaces • Use pillows, cushions, anti-pressure mattresses to alleviate pressure wound risk (see Appendix A) • If patient is at risk for falls, safety measures such as nonskid slippers, shoes, or socks, bed or chair alarms, floor sensor, or fall mat

(continued)

TABLE 10A.2 PALLIATIVE INTERVENTIONS/SYMPTOM MANAGEMENT FOR DEMENTIA (*CONTINUED*)

SYMPTOM	INTERVENTION
Incontinence	• Identify and correct causes of incontinence, if possible (i.e., urinary tract infection, *Clostridium difficile*, etc.) • Use protective pads/undergarments • Utilize urinary diversion devices (indwelling catheter, condom catheter, etc.), as appropriate • Provide meticulous skin care and reposition patient at least every 2 hours • Utilize fecal collection devices as indicated (i.e., external pouch, rectal tubes)
Pain management	• See Appendix E

Sources: Abt, D., Bywater, M., Engeler, D. S., & Schmid, H. P. (2013). Therapeutic options for intractable hematuria in advanced bladder cancer. *International Journal of Urology, 20*(7), 651–660. https://doi.org/10.1111/iju.12113; Guyer, D. L., Almhanna, K., & McKee, K. Y. (2020). Palliative care for patients with esophageal cancer: A narrative review. *Annals of Translational Medicine, 8*(17). https://doi.org/10.21037/atm-20-3676; Sinibaldi, V. J., Pratz, C. F., & Yankulina, O. (2018). Kidney cancer: Toxicity management, symptom control, and palliative care. *Journal of Clinical Oncology, 36*(36), 3632–3638. doi:https://doi.org/10.1200/JCO.2018.79.0188; Sommers, M. S. (2019). *Davis's diseases and disorders: A nursing therapeutics manual.* F.A. Davis. https://www.fadavis.com/product/nursing-fundamentals-med-surg-diseases-disorders-nursing-therapeutics-manual-sommers-6

CHAPTER 11

HEPATIC DISORDERS

CIRRHOSIS

DEFINITION/CHARACTERISTICS
A. A form of chronic liver disease characterized by replacement of healthy liver tissue with fibrotic scar tissue.
B. Classified according to cause (see Table 11.1):
   1. Viral.
   2. Toxin-related.
   3. Autoimmune.
   4. Cholestatic.
   5. Vascular.
   6. Metabolic (hemochromatosis, nonalcoholic steatohepatitis [NASH], Wilson disease, alpha-1 antitrypsin deficiency, cryptogenic cirrhosis).
C. The most common types, accounting for 90% of cases, are:
   1. Alcoholic.
   2. Cryptogenic biliary (Hinkle & Cheever, 2018; Sommers, 2019).

INCIDENCE AND PREVALENCE
A. Cirrhosis is most commonly diagnosed in those ages 40 to 50 years.
B. About 31,000 deaths are attributed to cirrhosis in the United States each year.
C. The prevalence of cirrhosis has increased by 13% in the past two decades.
D. Liver cancer, a main complication of cirrhosis, accounts for 3.5% of deaths worldwide (Hinkle & Cheever, 2018; Moon et al., 2020; Sommers, 2019).

ETIOLOGY
A. Causes vary depending on the type of cirrhosis (see Table 11.1).
B. The most common cause is alcohol abuse (Sommers, 2019).

PATHOPHYSIOLOGY
A. Cirrhosis stems from the destruction of healthy liver cells resulting from an underlying pathology.
B. Damaged liver cells are replaced with fibrotic tissue that does not function as healthy liver tissue.
C. The growth of fibrotic tissue alters lymphatic function, liver structure and, function, and blood circulation.
D. Over time, the amount of scar tissue becomes greater than functioning liver tissue and the liver itself shrinks in size (Sommers, 2019).

PREDISPOSING FACTORS
A. Genetic predisposition.
B. European ancestry.
C. History of alcohol or drug abuse.
D. History of viral liver disease, such as hepatitis C.
E. Exposure to chemicals such as carbon tetrachloride, chlorinated naphthalene, arsenic, or phosphorus.
F. Infectious schistosomiasis.
G. Female sex (Hinkle & Cheever, 2018; Sommers, 2019).

SUBJECTIVE DATA
A. Agitation.
B. Forgetfulness.
C. Disorientation.
D. Fatigue.
E. Drowsiness.
F. Mild tremors.
G. Flu-like symptoms.
H. Changes in bowel habits.
I. Menstrual irregularities.
J. Early morning nausea and vomiting.
K. Anorexia.
L. Indigestion.
M. Weakness.
N. Lethargy.
O. Gastroesophageal reflux disease.
P. Sexual dysfunction.
Q. Abdominal pain (Hinkle & Cheever, 2019; Sommers, 2019).

OBJECTIVE DATA
A. Bruising.
B. Bleeding.
C. Weight loss.
D. Hypotension.
E. Esophageal varices.
F. Ascites.
G. Abdominal pain.
H. Muscle atrophy.
I. Jaundice.
J. Decreased skin turgor.

TABLE 11.1   TYPES OF CIRRHOSIS

TYPE	CAUSES	MANIFESTATIONS
Viral	Hepatitis B, C, or D	Painful hepatomegaly, ascites, and abnormal liver tests
Toxin-related	Alcohol or drug abuse. Can result from other toxins, such as environmental or occupational toxin exposure	Progressive symptoms beginning with vague fatigue and weakness, nausea, anorexia, weight loss, spider angiomas, jaundice, hematemesis, dark urine, clay-colored stools, bleeding or bruising, edema
Autoimmune	Often follows an infection such as measles, herpes simplex, or Epstein–Barr virus. May also be hereditary	Fatigue, myalgias, nausea, anorexia, abdominal pain (upper right quadrant), jaundice, dark urine, clay-colored stools, ascites, pruritis, lower extremity edema
Cholestatic	Often autoimmune or genetic	The classic presentation involves nausea, fatigue, and pruritus, followed by dark urine and jaundice
Vascular	Results from any condition that causes occlusion of the hepatic vascular system, such as embolism, schistosomiasis, Budd–Chiari syndrome, sinusoidal obstruction syndrome, and others	Classic presentation involves painful hepatomegaly, ascites, and abnormal liver tests
Metabolic	Genetic disorders that result in metabolic disturbances such as Wilson disease, α_1 antitrypsin deficiency, hereditary hemachromatosis, and others.	May be asymptomatic but if liver damage occurs, symptoms may include pruritus, jaundice, hypoglycemia, vitamin deficiencies, fatigue, bleeding or bruising, ascites, and abdominal tenderness

Sources: Aqel, B. A. (2010). *Vascular diseases of the liver.* https://doi.org/10.1002/9781444325249.ch26; Le Garf, S., Nègre, V., Anty, R., & Gual, P. (2021). Metabolic fatty liver disease in children: A growing public health problem. *Biomedicines, 9*(12), 1915. https://www.mdpi.com/2227-9059/9/12/1915/htm; National Health Service. (2021). *Overview: Cirrhosis.* https://www.nhs.uk/conditions/cirrhosis/; National Institute of Diabetes and Digestive and Kidney Diseases. (2018). *Symptoms & causes of autoimmune hepatitis.* https://www.niddk.nih.gov/health-information/liver-disease/autoimmune-hepatitis/symptoms-causes; National Institute of Diabetes and Digestive and Kidney Diseases. (2019). *Cholestatic hepatitis.* https://www.ncbi.nlm.nih.gov/books/NBK548914/?report=reader

K. Spider angiomas.
L. Palmer erythema.
M. Gynecomastia.
N. Abdominal distension.
O. Everted umbilicus.
P. Caput medusae.
Q. Asterixis.
R. Splenomegaly.
S. Hepatomegaly.
T. Lower extremity edema.
U. Low-grade fever.
V. Purpura (Hinkle & Cheever, 2019; Sommers, 2019).

DIAGNOSTIC TESTS
A. See Appendix Table 11A.1 for listing of common diagnostic tests.
B. See Table 11.2 for grading scale.

DIFFERENTIAL DIAGNOSES
A. Acute fatty liver disease.
B. Acetaminophen toxicity.

C. Bacillus cereus toxin.
D. Hemolysis, elevated liver enzymes, low platelets (HELLP) of pregnancy.
E. Viral infection (i.e., Ebola, Lassa virus, Marburg virus).
F. Idiopathic drug reaction (Sharma & John, 2021).

POTENTIAL COMPLICATIONS
A. Liver cancer.
B. Ruptured esophageal varices.
C. Encephalopathy.
D. Spontaneous bacterial peritonitis.
E. Hepatorenal syndrome (Sharma & John, 2021; Sommers, 2019; see Figure 11.1).

DISEASE-MODIFYING TREATMENTS
A. Lifestyle changes (alcohol and drug abstinence, weight loss; see Appendix B-6).
B. Placement of peritoneal jugular shunt.
C. Paracentesis.
D. Liver transplantation (see Table 11.3).

▶

TABLE 11.2   MODIFIED CHILD–PUGH CLASSIFICATION FOR GRADING LIVER DISEASE

CLINICAL MANIFESTATION →	ALBUMIN LEVEL	ASCITES	BILIRUBIN LEVEL	ENCEPHALOPATHY	PROTHROMBIN TIME	
1 point →	> 3.5 (1 point)	None (1 point)	≤ 2 mg/dL (1 point)	Absent (1 point)	1–3 sec (1 point)	Total points ↓
2 points →	2.8-3.5 (2 points)	Small amount (2 points)	2–3 mg/dL (2 points)	Slight (2 points)	4–6 secs (2 points)	
3 points →	< 2.8 (3 points)	Moderate amount (3 points)	> 3 mg/dL (3 points)	Moderate (3 points)	> 6 secs (3 points)	
Subtotal points from each column →	↓	↓	↓	↓	↓	
Interpretation of results →	**Total score: 5–6** Grade A 5-year survival rate = 95%		**Total Score: 7–9** Grade B 5-year survival rate = 75%		**Total Score: 10** Grade C 5-year survival rate = 50%	

Sources: Frothingham, S. (2022). *What is the Child-Pugh score?* https://www.healthline.com/health/child-pugh-classification; Hinkle, J. L., & Cheever, K. H. (2018). *Brunner & Siddarth's textbook of medical-surgical nursing* (14th ed., pp. 1377–1427). Wolters Kluwer; Pugh, R. N. H., Murray-Lyon, I. M., Dawson, J. L., Pietroni, M. C., & Williams, R. (1973). Transection of the oesophagus for bleeding oesophageal varices. *British Journal of Surgery, 60*(8), 646–649.

E. Medical management is based on etiology but may include (see Figure 11.2):
  1. Antiviral medications.
  2. Steroids.
  3. Immune suppressant agents.
  4. Ursodeoxycholic acid.
  5. Obeticholic acid.
  6. Copper chelation.
  7. Iron chelation.
  8. Phlebotomy (Sharma & John, 2021; Sommers, 2019).

PALLIATIVE INTERVENTIONS/SYMPTOM MANAGEMENT
A. See Appendix Table 11A.2 for listing of palliative interventions and symptom management.
B. See Appendix D-3 for overview of common symptoms.

PROGNOSIS
A. Onset is usually insidious.
B. The trajectory is lengthy, sometimes as long as 30 years (see Appendix C-1).
C. Death often follows a somewhat brief period of rapid decline.
D. The 10-year survival rate in patients with compensated cirrhosis is 47%.
E. If decompensation occurs, the 10-year survival rate drops to 16% (Hinkle & Cheever, 2018; Sharma & John, 2021).

NURSING INTERVENTIONS
A. Provide education on disease process and symptom management.
B. Teach patient to take all medications as prescribed.
C. Provide high-calorie (2,500–3,000 calories/day) diet with moderate to high protein, low fat, low sodium and supplemental vitamins, and folic acid.
D. Administer vitamin K injections as prescribed.
E. Limit fluid intake to 500 to 1,000 mL daily as prescribed.
F. Monitor intake and output.
G. Measure and record abdominal girth.
H. Assess ascites (see Figure 11.3).
I. Assess bowel sounds.
J. Encourage ambulation and activity to prevent muscle wasting.
K. Provide spiritual support.
L. Assess caregiver fatigue/burnout.
M. Encourage completion of advance directives.
N. Discuss wishes regarding withholding or withdrawing of life-sustaining interventions in late stage of disease with patient (if possible) and/or primary caregiver (see Appendices C-2, C-3, and C-4).
O. Educate patient and family regarding availability of palliative care.
P. Educate patient and family regarding availability of hospice services (when appropriate).
Q. Provide referral to community support groups, as needed.

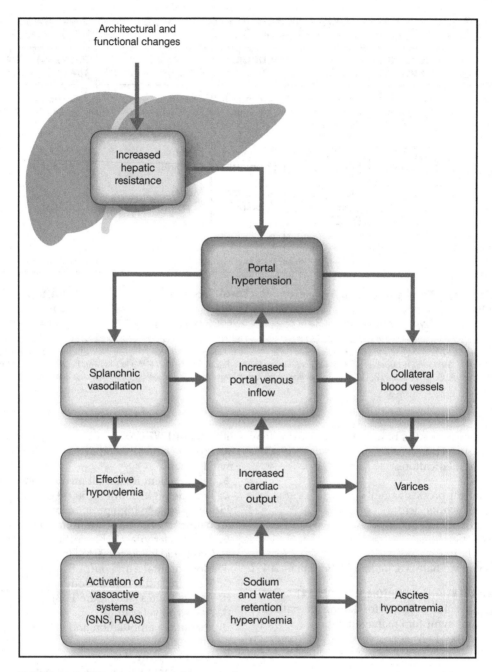

FIGURE 11.1 Consequences of liver dysfunction.

CHRONIC VIRAL HEPATITIS

DEFINITION/CHARACTERISTICS
A. A viral infection that primarily affects the liver, causing hepatitis.
B. Hepatitis viruses B (HBV), C (HCV), and D (HDV) can result in chronic hepatitis (Huether, 2018).

INCIDENCE AND PREVALENCE
A. The incidence of viral hepatitis in the United States is as follows:
  1. HBV = 19,200 cases.
  2. HCV = 30,500 cases.
  3. HDV = unknown.
B. Up to 1.4 million Americans are infected with HBV. ▶

TABLE 11.3 LIVER TRANSPLANT GUIDELINES

INDICATIONS FOR LIVER TRANSPLANT	CONTRAINDICATIONS FOR LIVER TRANSPLANT
1. Complications of acute liver failure, such as ascites, gastric bleeding, hepatic encephalopathy, bleeding esophageal varices 2. Liver-based metabolic conditions with systemic manifestations such as α_1-antitrypsin deficiency, familial amyloidosis, glycogen storage disease, hemochromatosis, primary oxaluria, Wilson disease 3. Systemic complications of liver disease such as hepatopulmonary syndrome and portopulmonary hypertension	• MELD score <15 (to calculate, see https://optn.transplant.hrsa.gov/data/allocation-calculators/meld-calculator/) • Severe cardio or pulmonary disease • AIDS • Continuing alcohol or drug abuse • Uncontrolled sepsis • Anatomic abnormality preventing transplant • Intrahepatic cholangiocarcinoma • Fulminant liver failure with ICP >50 mmHg or CPP <40 mmHg • Hemangiosarcoma • Inability or lack of desire to comply with medical treatment plan • Inadequate support system

CPP, cerebral perfusion pressure; ICP, intracranial pressure; MELD, Model for End-Stage Liver Disease.

Source: American Association for the Study of Liver Diseases. (2013). *Evaluation of liver transplantation in adults: 2013 practice guidelines by the AASLD and the American Society of Transplantation.* https://www.aasld.org/sites/default/files/2019-06/141020_Guideline_Evaluation_Adult_LT_4UFb_2015.pdf

C. Up to 2.4 million Americans are infected with HCV.

D. HCV occurs most frequently in those 40 to 59 years old.

E. HBV and HCV are the most common causes of chronic hepatitis.

F. Up to 80% of those infected with HCV will develop chronic hepatitis (Hinkle & Cheever, 2019; Huether, 2018; U.S. Department of Health & Human Services, 2016).

ETIOLOGY

A. Causative agents include HBV, HCV, and HDV.

B. HBV is transmitted parenterally and sexually.

C. HCV is primarily transmitted parenterally (rarely sexually transmitted).

D. HDV is transmitted parenterally, sexually, and through the fecal–oral route (see Table 11.4).

E. Hepatitis D is a hybrid virus that uses the HBV surface antigen to form its viral envelope. Therefore, only those who are infected with HBV can develop HDV (Hinkle & Cheever, 2019; Huether, 2018).

PATHOPHYSIOLOGY

A. The phases of viral hepatitis are prodromal, icteric, and posticteric (see Figure 11.4).

B. Chronic viral hepatitis follows the posticteric phase.

C. When chronic hepatitis develops, hepatic cell injury results from cell-mediated immune responses.

D. Chronic hepatitis is diagnosed if symptoms persist for more than 6 months after the acute phase.

E. Hepatic cell damage is most pronounced with HBV and HCV infections because these strains cause cell apoptosis (Huether, 2018).

PREDISPOSING FACTORS

A. Intravenous drug use.

B. Unprotected sexual activity.

C. Blood or blood products transfusion.

D. HDV can be transmitted through the fecal–oral route (Hinkle & Cheever, 2019; Huether, 2018; Sommers, 2019).

SUBJECTIVE DATA

A. May be asymptomatic.

B. Nausea.

C. Malaise.

D. Abdominal pain.

E. Confusion.

F. Fatigue (Hinkle & Cheever, 2019; Huether, 2018; Sommers, 2019).

OBJECTIVE DATA

A. Jaundice.

B. Weight loss.

C. Fever.

D. Vomiting.

E. Bleeding.

F. Bruising.

G. Pruritis.

H. Pale, clay-colored stools (Hinkle & Cheever, 2019; Huether, 2018; Sommers, 2019).

DIAGNOSTIC TESTS

A. See Appendix Table 11A.1 and Figure 11.5 for listing of common diagnostic tests.

DIFFERENTIAL DIAGNOSES

A. Autoimmune hepatitis.

B. Hemochromatosis.

C. Cirrhosis.

D. Drug-induced hepatopathies (Pyrsopoulos, 2021).

POTENTIAL COMPLICATIONS

A. Cirrhosis (see Table 11.1).

B. Primary hepatocellular carcinoma.

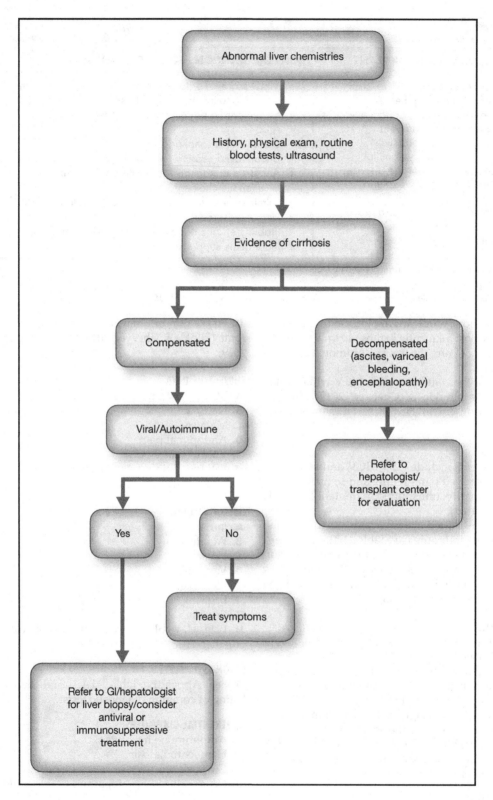

FIGURE 11.2 Management of cirrhosis.

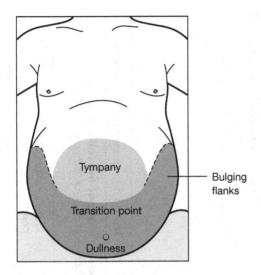

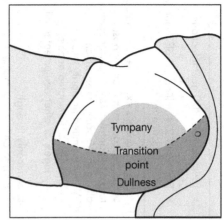

FIGURE 11.3 Ascites assessment.

C. Cryoglobulinemia.
D. Vasculitis.
E. Lymphoproliferative disease.
F. Esophageal varices.
G. Fulminant hepatitis (Huether, 2018; Sommers, 2019).

DISEASE-MODIFYING TREATMENTS
A. Lifestyle changes (alcohol and drug abstinence, weight loss; see Appendix B-6).
B. Paracentesis.
C. Postexposure prophylaxis.
D. Restriction of activities and bed rest are recommended with enlarged liver.
E. Medical management is based on etiology but may include:
   1. Antiviral medications.
   2. Interferons.
   3. Immune suppressant agents.
F. Liver transplantation (see Table 11.3; Hinkle & Cheever, 2019; Huether, 2018; Sommers, 2019).

PALLIATIVE INTERVENTIONS/SYMPTOM MANAGEMENT
A. See Appendix Table 11A.2 for listing of palliative interventions and symptom management.
B. See Appendix D-3 for overview of common symptoms.

PROGNOSIS
A. Those who have chronic, active hepatitis are carriers and can transmit the virus.
B. Roughly 15% of those who develop chronic HBV during adulthood die of cirrhosis or liver cancer.
C. Roughly 70% of those who are infected with HCV will develop chronic hepatitis (Hinkle & Cheever, 2019; Huether, 2018; World Health Organization, 2022a).

NURSING INTERVENTIONS
A. Provide education on disease process and signs of progression.

B. Teach patient to take all medications as prescribed.
C. Teach patient to reduce transmission to others by preventing contact with blood and body fluids.
D. Educate patient regarding low-fat, high-carbohydrate diet.
E. Manage pain and other symptoms.
F. Provide spiritual support.
G. Educate patient and family regarding availability of palliative care as needed.
H. Provide referral to community support groups, as needed.

NONALCOHOLIC FATTY LIVER DISEASE

DEFINITION/CHARACTERISTICS
A. Infiltration of fat cells into hepatic tissue.
B. Occurs in the absence of alcohol intake.
C. Considered the hepatic component of metabolic syndrome (Huether, 2018; Manka et al., 2021).

INCIDENCE AND PREVALENCE
A. Nonalcoholic fatty liver disease (NAFLD) is the most common liver disease in the world (see Figure 11.6).
B. Roughly a quarter of the world's population has been diagnosed with NAFLD.
C. About 24% of Americans have been diagnosed with NAFLD (Huether, 2018; Manka et al., 2021; see Figure 11.7).

ETIOLOGY
A. The exact etiology is unknown, but several risk factors have been identified (National Institute of Diabetes and Digestive and Kidney Diseases, 2022).

PATHOPHYSIOLOGY
A. The pathophysiology of NAFLD is not wholly understood.

▶

TABLE 11.4 ABCs OF HEPATITIS

THE ABCs OF HEPATITIS—FOR HEALTH PROFESSIONALS

	HEPATITIS A is caused by the HAV	**HEPATITIS B** is caused by the HBV	**HEPATITIS C** is caused by the HCV
US Statistics	• Estimated 24,900 new infections in 2018	• Estimated 21,600 new infections in 2018 • Estimated 862,000 people living with chronic HBV infection in 2016	• Estimated 50,300 new infections in 2018 • Estimated 2.4 million people living with HCV infection in 2016
Routes of transmission	Fecal–oral route. HAV is transmitted through: • Close person-to-person contact with an infected person • Sexual contact with an infected person • Ingestion of contaminated food or water Although viremia occurs early in infection, blood-borne transmission of HAV is uncommon	Percutaneous, mucosal, or nonintact skin exposure to infectious blood, semen, and other body fluids. HBV is concentrated most highly in blood, and percutaneous exposure is an efficient mode of transmission. HBV is transmitted primarily through: • Birth to an infected mother • Sexual contact with an infected person • Sharing contaminated needles, syringes, or other injection drug equipment Less commonly through: • Needlesticks or other sharp instrument injuries • Organ transplantation and dialysis • Interpersonal contact through sharing items such as razors or toothbrushes or contact with open sores of an infected person	Direct percutaneous exposure to infectious blood. Mucous membrane exposures to blood can also result in transmission, although this route is less efficient. HCV is transmitted primarily through: • Sharing contaminated needles, syringes, or other equipment to inject drugs Less commonly through: • Birth to an infected mother • Sexual contact with an infected person • Unregulated tattooing • Needlesticks or other sharp instrument injuries
Incubation period	15–50 days (average: 28 days)	60–150 days (average: 90 days)	14–182 days (average range: 14–84 days)
Symptoms of acute infection	**Symptoms of all types of viral hepatitis are similar and can include one or more of the following:** • Jaundice • Fever • Fatigue • Loss of appetite • Nausea • Vomiting • Abdominal pain • Joint pain • Dark urine • Clay-colored stool • Diarrhea (HAV only)		
Likelihood of symptomatic acute infection	• <30% of children <6 years of age have symptoms (which typically do not include jaundice) • >70% of older children and adults have jaundice	• Most children <5 years of age do not have symptoms • 30%–50% of people >5 years of age develop symptoms • Newly infected immunosuppressed adults generally do not have symptoms	• Jaundice might occur in 20%–30% of people • Nonspecific symptoms (e.g., anorexia, malaise, or abdominal pain) might be present in 10%–20% of people

THE ABCs OF HEPATITIS—FOR HEALTH PROFESSIONALS

	Hepatitis A	Hepatitis B	Hepatitis C
Potential for chronic infection after acute infection	None	Chronic infection develops in: • 90% of infants after acute infection at birth • 25%–50% of children newly infected at ages 1–5 years • 5% of people newly infected as adults	Chronic infection develops in over 50% of newly infected people
Severity	• Most people with acute disease recover with no lasting liver damage; death is uncommon but occurs more often among older people and/or those with underlying liver disease	• Most people with acute disease recover with no lasting liver damage; acute illness is rarely fatal • 15%–25% of people with chronic infection develop chronic liver disease, including cirrhosis, liver failure, or liver cancer	• Approximately 5%–25% of persons with chronic hepatitis C will develop cirrhosis over 10–20 years • People with hepatitis C and cirrhosis have a 1%–4% annual risk for hepatocellular carcinoma
Serologic tests for acute infection	• IgM anti-HAV	• HBsAg • IgM anti-HBc	• No serologic marker for acute infection
Serologic tests for chronic infection	• Not applicable—no chronic infection	Tests for chronic infection should include three HBV seromarkers: • HBsAg • anti-HBs • Total anti-HBc	• Assay for anti-HCV • Qualitative and quantitative nucleic acid tests (NAT) to detect and quantify presence of virus (HCV RNA)
Testing recommendations for chronic infection	• Not applicable—no chronic infection Note: testing for past acute infection is generally not recommended	• All pregnant women should be tested for HBsAg during an early prenatal visit in each pregnancy • Infants born to HBsAg-positive mothers (HBsAg and anti-HBs are only recommended) • People born in regions with intermediate and high HBV endemicity (HBsAg prevalence >2%) • People born in United States not vaccinated as infants whose parents were born in regions with high HBV endemicity (>8%) • Household or sexual contacts of people who are HBsAg-positive	• All adults aged 18 years and older, at least once • All pregnant women during each pregnancy • People who currently inject drugs and share needles, syringes, or other drug preparation equipment (routine periodic testing) • People who ever injected drugs • People with HIV • People who receive maintenance hemodialysis (routine periodic testing) • People who ever received maintenance hemodialysis • People with persistently abnormal ALT levels

(continued)

TABLE 11.4 ABCs OF HEPATITIS (CONTINUED)

THE ABCs OF HEPATITIS—FOR HEALTH PROFESSIONALS

	Hepatitis A	Hepatitis B	Hepatitis C

		• Men who have sex with men
		• People who inject, or have injected, drugs
		• Patients with alanine aminotransferase levels (>19 IU/L for women and >30 IU/L for men) of unknown etiology
		• People with end-stage renal disease including hemodialysis patients
		• People receiving immunosuppressive therapy
		• People with HIV
		• Donors of blood, plasma, organs, tissues, or semen
			• Prior recipients of transfusions or organ transplants, including:
			  ■ People who received clotting factor concentrates produced before 1987
			  ■ People who received a transfusion of blood or blood components before July 1992
			  ■ People who received an organ transplant before July 1992
			  ■ People who were notified that they received blood from a donor who later tested positive for HCV infection
			• Healthcare, emergency medical, and public safety personnel after needle sticks, sharps, or mucosal exposures to HCV-positive blood
			• Children born to mothers with HCV infection
			• Any person who requests hepatitis C testing should receive it

Treatment	• No medication available • Best addressed through supportive treatment	• Acute: no medication available; best addressed through supportive treatment • Chronic: regular monitoring for signs of liver disease progression; antiviral drugs are available	• Acute: AASLD/IDSA recommend treatment of acute HCV without a waiting period • Chronic: over 90% of people with hepatitis C can be cured regardless of HCV genotype with 8–12 weeks of oral therapy
Vaccination recommendations	**Children** • All children aged 12–23 months • Unvaccinated children and adolescents aged 2–18 years **People at increased risk for HAV infection** • International travelers • Men who have sex with men • People who use injection or noninjection drugs • People with occupational risk for exposure	• All infants • All unvaccinated children and adolescents aged <19 years • Sex partners of HBsAg-positive people • Sexually active people who are not in a mutually monogamous relationship • Anyone seeking evaluation or treatment for a sexually transmitted infection • Men who have sex with men • Anyone with a history of current or recent injection drug use	• There is no hepatitis C vaccine

THE ABCs OF HEPATITIS—FOR HEALTH PROFESSIONALS

• People who anticipate close personal contact with an international adoptee • People experiencing homelessness **People at increased risk for severe disease from HAV infection** • People with chronic liver disease • People with HIV infection **Other people recommended for vaccination** • Pregnant women at risk for HAV infection or severe outcome from HAV infection • Any person who requests vaccination **Vaccination during outbreaks** • Unvaccinated people in outbreak settings who are at risk for HAV infection or at risk for severe disease from HAV **Implementation strategies for settings providing services to adults** • People in settings that provide services to adults in which a high proportion of those people have risk factors for HAV infection	• Household contacts of people who are HBsAg-positive • Residents and staff of facilities for developmentally disabled people • Healthcare and public safety personnel with reasonably anticipated risk for exposure to blood or blood-contaminated body fluids • Hemodialysis, predialysis peritoneal dialysis, and home dialysis patients • People with diabetes mellitus aged <60 years and people with diabetes mellitus aged >60 years at the discretion of the treating clinician • International travelers to countries with high or intermediate levels of endemic HBV infection (HBsAg prevalence of >2%) • People living with hepatitis C • People with chronic liver disease (including cirrhosis, fatty liver disease, alcoholic liver disease, autoimmune hepatitis, and an ALT or AST level greater than twice the upper limit of normal) • People living with HIV infection • People who are incarcerated • Pregnant women who are identified as being at risk for HBV infection during pregnancy • Anyone else seeking long-term protection	• No vaccine available
Vaccination schedule		
• Single-antigen hepatitis A vaccine: two doses given 6–18 months apart depending on manufacturer • Combination hep A–hep B vaccine: typically three doses given over a 6-month period	• Infants and children: 3–4 doses given over a 6- to 18-month period depending on vaccine type and schedule • Adults: two doses, 1 month apart or three doses over a 6-month period (depending on manufacturer)	• No vaccine available

ALT, alanine transaminase; AASLD, American Association for the Study of Liver Diseases; AST, aspartate aminotransferase; HAV, hepatitis A virus; HBsAg, hepatitis B surface antigen; HBV, hepatitis B virus; HCV, hepatitis C virus; IDSA, The Infectious Diseases Society of America; TURP, transurethral prostatectomy.

Source: Adapted from Centers for Disease Control and Prevention. (2020). *The ABCs of hepatitis: For health professionals.*https://www.cdc.gov/hepatitis/resources/professionals/pdfs/abctable.pdf

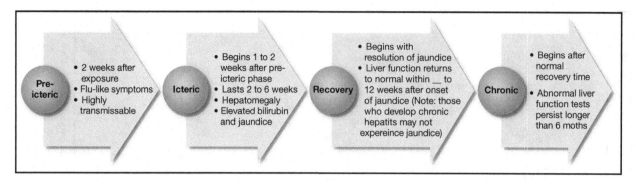

FIGURE 11.4 Phases of hepatitis.

Source: Adapted from Huether, S. E. (2018). Alternations in digestive function. In K. L. McCance & S. E. Huether (Eds.), *Pathophysiology: The biologic basis for disease in adults and children* (8th ed., pp. 1321–1372). Elsevier.

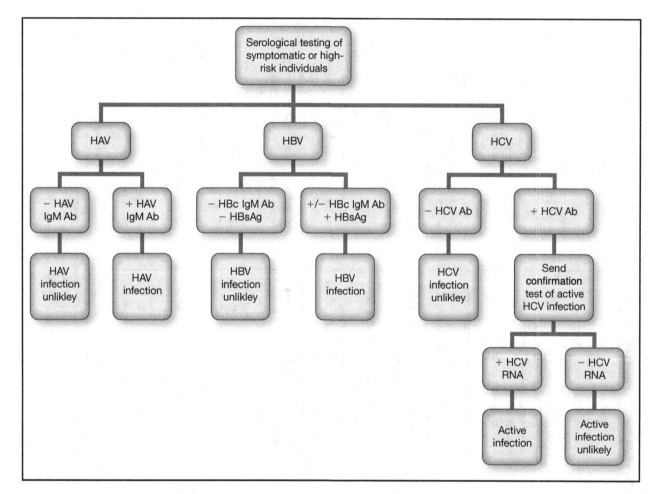

FIGURE 11.5 Testing for chronic hepatitis.

B. Fat deposition into hepatic tissues increases insulin resistance.

C. Insulin resistance can stimulate de novo lipogenesis, further exacerbating infiltration of fat cells into the liver.

D. Cellular and molecular changes can lead to impaired renal function (Jang et al., 2018; Manka et al., 2021).

PREDISPOSING FACTORS

A. Obesity.

B. Hypercholesteremia, particularly elevated triglycerides.

C. Metabolic syndrome.

D. Alterations in gut microbiome.

E. Protein malnutrition.

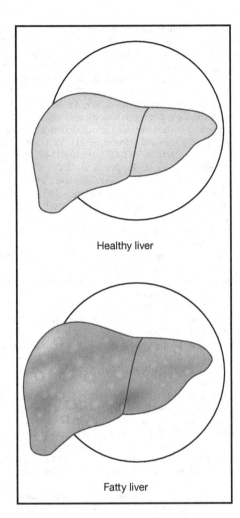

Healthy liver

Fatty liver

FIGURE 11.6 Healthy liver versus fatty liver.

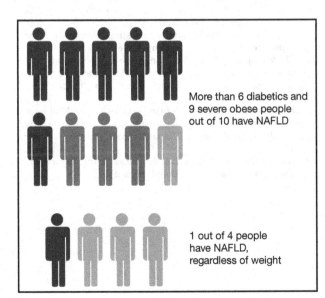

More than 6 diabetics and 9 severe obese people out of 10 have NAFLD

1 out of 4 people have NAFLD, regardless of weight

FIGURE 11.7 Prevalence of nonalcoholic fatty liver disease.

F. Coronary artery disease (CAD).
G. Long-term use of corticosteroids.
H. Sleep apnea.
I. Hypothyroidism.
J. Hypopituitarism.
K. Type 2 diabetes (Huether, 2018; Jang et al., 2018; Manka et al., 2021).

SUBJECTIVE DATA
A. Often symptomatic.
B. Fatigue.
C. Abdominal pain (Huether, 2018; Manka et al., 2021).

OBJECTIVE DATA
A. Weight loss.
B. Liver enlargement.
C. Signs of insulin resistance.
D. Splenomegaly.
E. Ascites (Huether, 2018; Manka et al., 2021).

DIAGNOSTIC TESTS
A. See Appendix Table 11A.2 for listing of common diagnostic tests.

DIFFERENTIAL DIAGNOSES
A. Alcoholic liver disease.
B. Hepatitis C.
C. Wilson disease.
D. Chemical hepatitis (Kudaravalli & John, 2022).

POTENTIAL COMPLICATIONS
A. Nonalcoholic steatohepatitis (NASH).
B. Cirrhosis.
C. End-stage liver disease.
D. Hepatocellular carcinoma.
E. Those with NAFLD are twice as likely to develop type 2 diabetes (Huether, 2018; Manka et al., 2021).

DISEASE-MODIFYING TREATMENTS
A. Lifestyle changes (alcohol and drug abstinence, weight loss; see Appendix B-6).
B. Medical management may include:
  1. Insulin sensitizers.
  2. Vitamin E.
  3. Lipid-lowering medications.
C. Liver transplantation if liver failure occurs (see Table 11.3; Huether, 2018; National Institute of Diabetes and Digestive and Kidney Diseases, 2022).

PALLIATIVE INTERVENTIONS/SYMPTOM MANAGEMENT
A. See Appendix Table 11A.2 for listing of palliative interventions and symptom management.
B. See Appendix D-3 for overview of common symptoms.

PROGNOSIS
A. Median survival is approximately 24 years.
B. The most common cause of death among those with NAFLD is cardiovascular disease (Haflidadottir et al., 2014).

NURSING INTERVENTIONS

A. Provide education on disease process and symptom management.

B. Teach patient to take all medications as prescribed.

C. Administer vitamin K injections as prescribed.

D. Monitor intake and output.

E. Measure and record abdominal girth.

F. Assess ascites (see Figure 11.3).

G. Assess bowel sounds.

H. Provide spiritual support.

I. Assess caregiver fatigue/burnout.

J. Encourage completion of advance directives.

K. Provide referral to community support groups, as needed.

REFERENCES

Abt, D., Bywater, M., Engeler, D. S., & Schmid, H. P. (2013). Therapeutic options for intractable hematuria in advanced bladder cancer. *International Journal of Urology*, 20(7), 651–660. https://doi.org/10.1111/iju.12113

American Association for the Study of Liver Diseases. (2013). Evaluation of liver transplantation in adults: 2013 practice guidelines by the AASLD and the American Society of Transplantation. https://www.aasld.org/sites/default/files/2019-06/141020_Guideline_Evaluation_Adult_LT_4UFb_2015.pdf

Aqel, B. A. (2010). *Vascular diseases of the liver.* https://doi.org/10.1002/9781444325249.ch26

Frothingham, S. (2022). *What is the Child-Pugh score?* https://www.healthline.com/health/child-Pugh-classification#:~:text=The%20Child%2DPugh%20score%20is%20determined%20by%20scoring%20five%20clinical,3%20being%20the%20most%20severe

Guyer, D. L., Almhanna, K., & McKee, K. Y. (2020). Palliative care for patients with esophageal cancer: A narrative review. *Annals of Translational Medicine*, 8(17). https://doi.org/10.21037/atm-20-3676

Haflidadottir, S., Jonasson, J. G., Norland, H., Einarsdottir, S. O., Kleiner, D. E., Lund, S. H., & Björnson, E. S. (2014). Long term follow-up and liver-related death rate in patients with non-alcoholic and alcoholic related fatty liver disease. *BMC Gastroenterology*, 14(1), 1–10. http://www.biomedcentral.com/1471-230X/14/166

Hinkle, J. L., & Cheever, K. H. (2018). *Brunner & Siddarth's textbook of medical-surgical nursing* (14th ed., pp. 1377–1427). Wolters Kluwer.

Huether, S. E. (2018). Alternations in digestive function. In K. L. McCance & S. E. Huether (Eds.), *Pathophysiology: The biologic basis for disease in adults and children* (8th ed., pp. 1321–1372). Elsevier.

Jang, H. R., Kang, D., Sinn, D. H., Gu, S., Cho, S. J., Lee, J. E., Huh, W., Paik, S. E., Ryu, S., Chang, Y., Shafi, T., Lazo, M., Guallar, E., & Gwak, G. Y. (2018). Nonalcoholic fatty liver disease accelerates kidney function decline in patients with chronic kidney disease: A cohort study. *Scientific Reports*, 8(1), 1–9. https://www.nature.com/articles/s41598-018-23014-0

Kudaravalli, P., & John, S. (2022). *Nonalcoholic fatty liver.* https://www.ncbi.nlm.nih.gov/books/NBK541033/#:~:text=The%20differential%20diagnosis%20of%20non,Wilson%20disease

Le Garf, S., Nègre, V., Anty, R., & Gual, P. (2021). Metabolic fatty liver disease in children: A growing public health problem. *Biomedicines*, 9(12), 1915 https://www.mdpi.com/2227-9059/9/12/1915/htm

Manka, P. P., Kaya, E., Canbay, A., & Syn, W. K. (2021). A review of the epidemiology, pathophysiology, and efficacy of anti-diabetic drugs used in the treatment of nonalcoholic fatty liver disease. *Digestive Diseases and Sciences*, 66(11), 3676–3688. https://link.springer.com/article/10.1007/s10620-021-07206-9

Moon, A. M., Singal, A. G., & Tapper, E. B. (2020). Contemporary epidemiology of chronic liver disease and cirrhosis. *Clinical Gastroenterology and Hepatology*, 18(12), 2650–2666. https://www.cghjournal.org/action/showPdf?pii=S1542-3565%2819%2930849-3

National Health Service. (2021). *Overview: Cirrhosis.* https://www.nhs.uk/conditions/cirrhosis/

National Institute of Diabetes and Digestive and Kidney Diseases. (2018). *Symptoms & causes of autoimmune hepatitis.* https://www.niddk.nih.gov/health-information/liver-disease/autoimmune-hepatitis/symptoms-causes

National Institute of Diabetes and Digestive and Kidney Diseases. (2019). *Cholestatic hepatitis.* https://www.ncbi.nlm.nih.gov/books/NBK548914/?report=reader

National Institute of Diabetes and Digestive and Kidney Diseases. (2022). *Symptoms & causes of NAFLD and NASH.* https://www.niddk.nih.gov/health-information/liver-disease/nafld-nash/symptoms-causes

National Organization for Rare Diseases. (2015). *Hepatorenal syndrome.* https://rarediseases.org/rare-diseases/hepatorenal-syndrome/#:~:text=Hepatorenal%20syndrome%20(HRS)%20is%20a,themselves%20are%20not%20structural%20damaged

Pugh, R. N. H., Murray-Lyon, I. M., Dawson, J. L., Pietroni, M. C., & Williams, R. (1973). Transection of the oesophagus for bleeding oesophageal varices. *British Journal of Surgery*, 60(8), 646–649.

Pyrsopoulos, N. T. (2021). *Hepatitis B differential diagnoses.* https://emedicine.medscape.com/article/177632-differential

Sharma, B., & John, S. (2021). *Hepatic cirrhosis.* https://www.ncbi.nlm.nih.gov/books/NBK482419/

Sommers, M. S. (2019). *Davis's diseases and disorders: A nursing therapeutics manual.* F.A. Davis. https://www.fadavis.com/product/nursing-fundamentals-med-surg-diseases-disorders-nursing-therapeutics-manual-sommers-6

Tariq, R., & Singal, A. K. (2020). Management of hepatorenal syndrome: A review. *Journal of Clinical and Translational Hepatology*, 8(2), 192. https://www.ncbi.nlm.nih.gov/pmc/articles/PMC7438356/

U.S. Department of Health & Human Services. (2016). *Viral hepatitis in the United States: Data and trends.* https://www.hhs.gov/hepatitis/learn-about-viral-hepatitis/data-and-trends/index.html

World Health Organization. (2022a). *Hepatitis C.* https://www.who.int/news-room/fact-sheets/detail/hepatitis-c

APPENDIX

TABLE 11A.1   DIAGNOSTIC TESTS FOR HEPATIC DISORDERS

TYPE	NOTES
Physical examination	• Thorough physical examination with detailed medical history and neurological examination
Imaging	• Abdominal ultrasound (cirrhosis) • CT scan (cirrhosis, NAFLD) • MRI (NAFLD, cirrhosis) • Liver ultrasound (chronic viral hepatitis, NAFLD) • Elastography (NAFLD)
Laboratory tests	• Percutaneous or laparoscopic liver needle biopsy (cirrhosis) • Liver enzyme tests (cirrhosis, NAFLD) • Antimitochondrial antibodies (cirrhosis) • Serum alkaline phosphate (cirrhosis) • Total serum (cirrhosis) • Serum bilirubin (cirrhosis, NAFLD) • Indirect bilirubin (cirrhosis, NAFLD) • Urine bilirubin (cirrhosis) • Serum ammonia (cirrhosis, NAFLD) • Serum albumin (cirrhosis, NAFLD) • Serum total protein (cirrhosis, NAFLD) • Prothrombin time (cirrhosis, NAFLD) • Antibody testing (chronic viral hepatitis) • Liver enzyme tests (chronic viral hepatitis, cirrhosis, NAFLD) • Serum aminotransferase (chronic viral hepatitis) • Viral hepatitis serologies (chronic viral hepatitis) • Bilirubin (chronic viral hepatitis) • Prothrombin time (chronic viral hepatitis, NAFLD) • Complete blood count (chronic viral hepatitis) • Albumin (chronic viral hepatitis) • FIB-4 score to determine need for biopsy (online calculator available: https://www.mdcalc.com/calc/2200/fibrosis-4-fib-4-index-liver-fibrosis; NAFLD)
Pathology	• Peritoneal fluid analysis (cirrhosis) • Progression of liver disease is evaluated using the Child–Pugh classification grading scale (see Table 11.2; Sommers, 2019; cirrhosis) • Liver biopsy (chronic viral hepatitis, NAFLD) • Progression of fibrosis is measured using the APRI score (online calculator available: https://www.mdcalc.com/calc/3094/ast-platelet-ratio-index-apri; NAFLD)

FIB-4, Fibrosis-4; NAFLD, nonalcoholic fatty liver disease; APRI, aspartate aminotransferase-to-platelet ratio index.

Sources: Huether, S. E. (2018). Alternations in digestive function. In K. L. McCance & S. E. Huether (Eds.), *Pathophysiology: The biologic basis for disease in adults and children* (8th ed., pp. 1321–1372). Elsevier; Manka, P. P., Kaya, E., Canbay, A., & Syn, W. K. (2021). A review of the epidemiology, pathophysiology, and efficacy of anti-diabetic drugs used in the treatment of nonalcoholic fatty liver disease. *Digestive Diseases and Sciences, 66*(11), 3676–3688. https://link.springer.com/article/10.1007/s10620-021-07206-9; Sommers, M. S. (2019). *Davis's diseases and disorders: A nursing therapeutics manual.* F.A. Davis. https://www.fadavis.com/product/nursing-fundamentals-med-surg-diseases-disorders-nursing-therapeutics-manual-sommers-6

TABLE 11A.2 PALLIATIVE INTERVENTIONS/SYMPTOM MANAGEMENT FOR HEPATIC DISORDERS

SYMPTOM	INTERVENTION
Anorexia	• Use of appetite stimulants (see Appendix D-1) • Offer small, frequent meals and snacks • Offer nutritional supplements
Anxiety and depression	• Antidepressants, anxiolytics, or benzodiazepines as indicated by patient's condition, age, and life expectancy (see Appendix D) • Non-pharmacological interventions (see Appendix D-2)
Ascites (see Figure 6.7)	• Abdominal ultrasound • Paracentesis with peritoneal fluid analysis • PleurX drain for ascites if patient is homebound • Albumin infusion if indicated • Diuretics (see Appendix D-1)
Bleeding (including epistaxis, hematemesis, melena, anemia)	• Stent placement • Cauterization • QuikClot combat gauze
Caregiver burden	• Support of interdisciplinary hospice or palliative team • Non-pharmacological interventions for caregivers (see Appendix D-2)
Fatigue and somnolence	• Alternate periods of rest with periods of activity • Utilize energy conversation techniques • Psychostimulants (see Appendix D-1)
Hepatic encephalopathy (see Figure 6.8)	• Pharmacological treatment (i.e., lactulose, diuretics; see Appendix D-1) • Antibiotic therapy • Polyethylene glycol
Hepatorenal syndrome	• Liver transplant (curative; see Table 11.3) • Dialysis • Paracentesis • Maintenance of electrolyte balance • Prompt treatment of infection • Use of vasoconstrictors • Transjugular intrahepatic portosystemic shunt (TIPS) • Address dehydration • Discontinue hepatotoxic medications • Address gastrointestinal bleeding
Pain management	• See Appendix E
Pruritis	• Thorough dermatological exam to establish cause • Depending on cause, topical agents such as ointments, barrier creams, or soaks can be trialed (e.g., calamine, menthol, oatmeal bath, antihistamine cream) • Systemic antihistamines may be used but are not recommended for older adults (see Appendix D-1) • Maintain short fingernails

Sources: Abt, D., Bywater, M., Engeler, D. S., & Schmid, H. P. (2013). Therapeutic options for intractable hematuria in advanced bladder cancer. *International Journal of Urology, 20*(7), 651–660. https://doi.org/10.1111/iju.12113; Düll, M. M., & Kremer, A. E. (2019). Treatment of pruritus secondary to liver disease. *Current Gastroenterology Reports, 21*(9), 1–9. https://link.springer.com/article/10.1007/s11894-019-0713-6#Sec9; Guyer, D. L., Almhanna, K., & McKee, K. Y. (2020). Palliative care for patients with esophageal cancer: A narrative review. *Annals of Translational Medicine, 8*(17). https://doi.org/10.21037/atm-20-3676; National Organization for Rare Diseases. (2015). *Hepatorenal syndrome.* https://rarediseases.org/rare-diseases/hepatorenal-syndrome/; Sinibaldi, V. J., Pratz, C. F., & Yankulina, O. (2018). Kidney cancer: Toxicity management, symptom control, and palliative care. *Journal of Clinical Oncology, 36*(36), 3632–3638.doi: https://doi.org/10.1200/JCO.2018.79.0188; Sommers, M. S. (2019). *Davis's diseases and disorders: A nursing therapeutics manual.* F.A. Davis. https://www.fadavis.com/product/nursing-fundamentals-med-surg-diseases-disorders-nursing-therapeutics-manual-sommers-6; Tariq, R., & Singal, A. K. (2020). Management of hepatorenal syndrome: A review. *Journal of Clinical and Translational Hepatology, 8*(2), 192. https://www.ncbi.nlm.nih.gov/pmc/articles/PMC7438356/

CHAPTER 12

IMMUNOLOGIC DISORDERS

SYSTEMIC LUPUS ERYTHEMATOSUS

DEFINITION/CHARACTERISTICS
A. There are several forms of lupus; systemic lupus erythematosus (SLE) is the most common.
B. SLE is a systemic, autoimmune disorder with inflammatory features.
C. SLE is one of the most common and complex autoimmune disorders.
D. Insidious onset characterized by periods of exacerbation and remission.
E. Characterized by an exaggerated activity of the immune system (Centers for Disease Control and Prevention, 2022; Iftimie et al., 2018; McCance & Huether, 2019; Rote & McCance, 2019).

INCIDENCE AND PREVALENCE
A. Most commonly diagnosed in women ages 20 to 40 years.
B. There are about 161,000 Americans living with SLE.
C. More than 14,000 new cases are diagnosed annually (Centers for Disease Control & Prevention, 2022; Rote & McCance, 2019).

ETIOLOGY
A. Exact cause is unknown (McCance & Huether, 2019).

PATHOPHYSIOLOGY
A. Autoimmune activation occurs in response to a trigger (often unknown).
B. Autoantibodies and immune complexes are responsible for inflammatory responses.
C. Prolonged inflammation is responsible for tissue damage to the integument and organs, especially the kidneys (Centers for Disease Control & Prevention, 2022; McCance & Huether, 2019).

PREDISPOSING FACTORS
A. Genetic predisposition.
B. Environmental factors.
C. Exposure to ultraviolet light.
D. Female sex.
E. Race (2–3 times more common among Blacks).
F. Hormonal factors, such as increased levels of estrogen and prolactin.

G. Immune factors (increased production of antibodies; Iftimie et al., 2018; McCance & Huether, 2019; Rote & McCance, 2019).

SUBJECTIVE DATA
A. Arthralgias.
B. Photosensitivity.
C. Marked fatigue (Centers for Disease Control and Prevention, 2022; McCance & Huether, 2019; Rote & McCance, 2019).

OBJECTIVE DATA
A. Butterfly shaped rash over bridge of nose and malar areas of the face (known as malar rash; see Figure 12.1).
B. Transient, diffuse rash over face, trunk, and extremities (lasting hours to days).
C. Erythematous macules and papules that develop after exposure to sun.
D. Red to purple macules or papules that appear over brown scales.
E. Raynaud's phenomenon.
F. Arthritis.
G. Vasculitis.
H. Renal disease.
I. Hematologic abnormalities, particularly anemia.
J. Cardiovascular disease.
K. Alopecia.
L. Oral ulcers.
M. Lupus anticoagulant.
N. Serositis with pleurisy (McCance & Huether, 2019; Rote & McCance, 2019).

DIAGNOSTIC TESTS
A. See Appendix Table 12A.1 for listing of common diagnostic tests.
B. See Table 12.1 for class criteria.
C. See Table 12.2 for classification criteria.

DIFFERENTIAL DIAGNOSES
A. B-cell lymphoma.
B. Fibromyalgia.
C. Epstein–Barr virus (EBV) infectious mononucleosis (mono).
D. Lyme disease.
E. Mixed connective tissue disease (MCTD)

▶

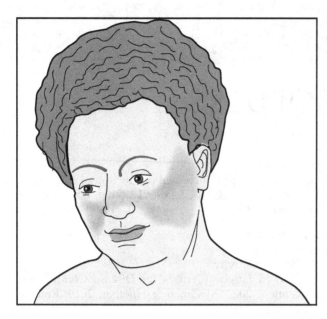

FIGURE 12.1   Malar rash.

Source: Adapted from National Institute of Arthritis and Musculoskeletal and Skin Diseases.

F. Polymyositis.
G. Rheumatoid arthritis (RA).
H. Scleroderma.
I. Sjogren syndrome (Bartles, 2022).

POTENTIAL COMPLICATIONS

A. Progressive disability.
B. Muscular pain.
C. Osteoarticular complications.
D. Cardiopulmonary involvement.
E. Gastrointestinal complications such as peritonitis, pancreatitis, or inflammatory bowel syndrome.
F. Hepatomegaly.
G. Neurological and psychiatric disturbance, including seizures, myasthenia gravis (MG), anxiety, and/or psychosis.
H. Renal damage.
I. Antiphospholipidic syndrome (Iftimie et al., 2018).

DISEASE-MODIFYING TREATMENTS

A. There is no cure for SLE.
B. Medical management may include:
   1. Anti-inflammatory medications.
   2. Antimalarial medications.
   3. Immunosuppressive medications.
   4. B-lymphocyte stimulator (BLyS)-specific inhibitors.
C. Goals of disease management:
   1. Prevent/reduce flares.
   2. Reduce/manage end-organ damage.

3. Palliative symptoms as they arise (Centers for Disease Control & Prevention, 2022; Rote & McCance, 2019).

PALLIATIVE INTERVENTIONS/SYMPTOM MANAGEMENT

A. See Appendix Table 12A.2 for listing of palliative interventions and symptom management.
B. See Appendix D-3 for overview of common symptoms.

PROGNOSIS

A. The 20-year survival rate from the time of diagnosis is about 78%.
B. Death is usually related to cardiac disease or organ failure (Rote & McCance, 2019).

NURSING INTERVENTIONS

A. Provide education on disease process and symptom management.
B. Teach patient to take all medications as prescribed.
C. Teach patient to avoid ultraviolet light.
D. Teach signs of renal involvement.
E. Encourage ambulation and activity to prevent muscle wasting and promote mobility.
F. Provide spiritual support.
G. Assess caregiver fatigue/burnout.
H. Encourage completion of advance directives.
I. Discuss wishes regarding withholding or withdrawing of life-sustaining interventions in late stage of disease with patient (if possible) and/or primary caregiver (see Appendices C-2, C-3, and C-4).
J. Educate patient and family regarding availability of palliative care.
K. Educate patient and family regarding availability of hospice services (when appropriate).
L. Provide referral to community support groups, as needed.

MULTIPLE SCLEROSIS

DEFINITION/CHARACTERISTICS

A. A chronic, progressive, autoimmune disease.
B. Characterized by demyelination of the neural sheath that surrounds nerve fibers in the central nervous system (CNS; see Figure 12.2).
C. Symptom onset can be categorized as either relapsing or progressive.
   1. Relapsing–remitting: characterized by acute episodes lasting hours to days.
   2. Non-relapsing progressive: insidious onset, occurring over months to years (Boss & Huether, 2019; Dobson & Giovannoni, 2018; Wright, 2019).

INCIDENCE AND PREVALENCE

A. Most commonly diagnosed in middle-aged women who have a first-degree relative with multiple sclerosis (MS).
B. There are roughly 2.8 million cases of MS worldwide. ▶

TABLE 12.1   DEFINITIONS OF SYSTEMIC LUPUS ERYTHEMATOSUS CLASS CRITERIA

CRITERIA	DEFINITION
ANA	ANA at a titer of ≥1:80 on HEp-2 cells or an equivalent positive test at least once. Testing by immunofluorescence on HEp-2 cells or a solid-phase ANA screening immunoassay with at least equivalent performance is highly recommended
Fever	Temperature >38.3°C
Leukopenia	White blood cell count <4,000/mm^3
Thrombocytopenia	Platelet count <100,000/mm^3
Autoimmune hemolysis	Evidence of hemolysis, such as reticulocytosis, low haptoglobin, elevated indirect bilirubin, elevated LDH, AND positive Coombs (direct antiglobulin) test
Delirium	Characterized by (a) change in consciousness or level of arousal with reduced ability to focus, (b) symptom development over hours to <2 days, (c) symptom fluctuation throughout the day, (d) either (i) acute/subacute change in cognition (e.g., memory deficit or disorientation) or (ii) change in behavior, mood, or affect (e.g., restlessness, reversal of sleep/wake cycle)
Psychosis	Characterized by (a) delusions and/or hallucinations without insight and (b) absence of delirium
Seizure	Primary generalized seizure or partial/focal seizure
Non-scarring alopecia	Non-scarring alopecia observed by a clinician[a]
Oral ulcers	Oral ulcers observed by a clinician[a]
Subacute cutaneous OR discoid lupus	Subacute cutaneous lupus erythematosus observed by a clinician[a]: Annular or papulosquamous (psoriasiform) cutaneous eruption, usually photodistributed If skin biopsy is performed, typical changes must be present (interface vacuolar dermatitis consisting of a perivascular lymphohistiocytic infiltrate, often with dermal mucin noted) OR Discoid lupus erythematosus observed by a clinician[a]: Erythematous–violaceous cutaneous lesions with secondary changes of atrophic scarring, dyspigmentation, often follicular hyperkeratosis/plugging (scalp), leading to scarring alopecia on the scalp If skin biopsy is performed, typical changes must be present (interface vacuolar dermatitis consisting of a perivascular and/or periappendageal lymphohistiocytic infiltrate. In the scalp, follicular keratin plugs may be seen. In long-standing lesions, mucin deposition may be noted)
Acute cutaneous lupus	Malar rash or generalized maculopapular rash observed by a clinician[a] If skin biopsy is performed, typical changes must be present (interface vacuolar dermatitis consisting of a perivascular lymphohistiocytic infiltrate, often with dermal mucin noted. Perivascular neutrophilic infiltrate may be present early in the course)
Pleural or pericardial effusion	Imaging evidence (such as ultrasound, x-ray, CT scan, MRI) of pleural or pericardial effusion, or both
Acute pericarditis	≥2 of (a) pericardial chest pain (typically sharp, worse with inspiration, improved by leaning forward), (b) pericardial rub, (c) EKG with new widespread ST elevation or PR depression, (d) new or worsened pericardial effusion on imaging (such as ultrasound, x-ray, CT scan, MRI)
Joint involvement	EITHER (a) synovitis involving two or more joints characterized by swelling or effusion OR (b) tenderness in two or more joints and at least 30 minutes of morning stiffness

(continued)

TABLE 12.1   DEFINITIONS OF SYSTEMIC LUPUS ERYTHEMATOSUS CLASS CRITERIA *(CONTINUED)*

CRITERIA	DEFINITION
Proteinuria >0.5 g/24 hours	Proteinuria >0.5 g/24 hours by 24-hour urine or equivalent spot urine protein-to-creatinine ratio
Class II or V lupus nephritis on renal biopsy according to ISN/RPS 2003 classification	**Class II:** Mesangial proliferative lupus nephritis: purely mesangial hypercellularity of any degree or mesangial matrix expansion by light microscopy, with mesangial immune deposit. A few isolated subepithelial or subendothelial deposits may be visible by immunofluorescence or electron microscopy, but not by light microscopy **Class V:** Membranous lupus nephritis: global or segmental subepithelial immune deposits or their morphologic sequelae by light microscopy and by immunofluorescence or electron microscopy, with or without mesangial alterations
Class III or IV lupus nephritis on renal biopsy according to ISN/RPS 2003 classification	**Class III:** Focal lupus nephritis: active or inactive focal, segmental, or global endocapillary or extracapillary glomerulonephritis involving <50% of all glomeruli, typically with focal subendothelial immune deposits, with or without mesangial alterations **Class IV:** Diffuse lupus nephritis: active or inactive diffuse, segmental, or global endocapillary or extracapillary glomerulonephritis involving ≥50% of all glomeruli, typically with diffuse subendothelial immune deposits, with or without mesangial alterations. This class includes cases with diffuse wire loop deposits but with little or no glomerular proliferation
Positive antiphospholipid antibodies	Anticardiolipin antibodies (IgA, IgG, or IgM) at medium or high titer (>40 APL, GPL, or MPL, or >the 99th percentile) or positive anti-β_2GPI antibodies (IgA, IgG, or IgM) or positive lupus anticoagulant
Low C3 OR low C4	C3 OR C4 below the lower limit of normal
Low C3 AND low C4	Both C3 AND C4 below their lower limits of normal
Anti-dsDNA antibodies OR anti-Smith antibodies	Anti-dsDNA antibodies in an immunoassay with demonstrated ≥90% specificity for SLE against relevant disease controls OR anti-Smith antibodies

[a]This may include physical examination or review of a photograph.

ANA, antinuclear antibodies; anti-β_2GPI, anti-β_2-glycoprotein I; anti-dsDNA, anti-double-stranded DNA; APL, immunoglobulin A (IgA) phospholipids units; GPL, immunoglobulin G (IgG) phospholipids units; ISN, International Society of Nephrology; LDH, lactate dehydrogenase; MPL, immunoglobulin M (IgM) phospholipids units; RPS, Renal Pathology Society; SLE, systemic lupus erythematosus.

Source: Aringer, M., Costenbader, K., Daikh, D., Brinks, R., Mosca, M., Ramsey-Goldman, R., Smolen, J. S., Wofsy, D., Boumpas, D. T., Kamen, D. L., Jayne, D., Cervera, R., Costedoat-Chalumeau, N., Diamond, B., Gladman, D. D., Hahn, B., Hiepe, F., Jacobsen, S., Khanna, D., . . . Johnson, S. R. (2019). 2019 European league against rheumatism/American College of Rheumatology classification criteria for systemic lupus erythematosus. *Arthritis & Rheumatology, 71*(9), 1400–1412. https://doi.org/10.1002/art.40930. Used with permission.

C. The 2020 global prevalence is 35.9 per 100,000 people.
D. Prevalence has been increasing in both developed and developing countries (Boss & Huether, 2019; Dobson & Giovannoni, 2018; Walton et al., 2020).

ETIOLOGY

A. Caused by an autoimmune response to a trigger (often unknown; Boss & Huether, 2019; Dobson & Giovannoni, 2018).

PATHOPHYSIOLOGY

A. There is usually a precipitating factor such as infection, trauma, or pregnancy prior to the onset of initial symptoms.
B. Demyelination of nerve fibers interrupts transmission of signals between nerves and muscles.
C. Plaque formation in the periventricular white matter, optic nerves, and spinal cord leads to degeneration of axons, which impairs the transmission of signals between neurons.

▶

TABLE 12.2   CLASSIFICATION CRITERIA FOR SYSTEMIC LUPUS ERYTHEMATOSUS

Entry criterion
ANA at a titer of ≥1:80 on HEp-2 cells or an equivalent positive test (ever)

↓

If absent, do not classify as SLE
If present, apply additive criteria

↓

Additive criteria
Do not count a criterion if there is a more likely explanation than SLE.
Occurrence of a criterion on at least one occasion is sufficient.
SLE classification requires at least one clinical criterion and ≥ 10 points.
Criteria need not occur simultaneously.
Within each domain, only the highest weighted criterion is counted toward the total score.

Clinical Domains and Criteria	Weight	Immunology Domains and Criteria	Weight
Constitutional		**Antiphospholipid antibodies**	
Fever	2	Anticardiolipin antibodies OR	
Hematologic		Anti-β_2GP1 antibodies OR	
Leukopenia	3	Lupus anticoagulant	2
Thrombocytopenia	4	**Complement proteins**	
Autoimmune hemolysis	4	Low C3 OR low C4	3
Neuropsychiatric		Low C3 AND low C4	4
Delirium	2	**SLE-specific antibodies**	
Psychosis	3	Anti-dsDNA antibody OR	
Seizure	5	Anti-Smith antibody	6
Mucocutaneous			
Non-scarring alopecia	2		
Oral ulcers	2		
Subacute cutaneous OR discoid lupus	4		
Acute cutaneous lupus	6		
Serosal			
Pleural or pericardial effusion	5		
Acute pericarditis	6		

(continued)

TABLE 12.2   CLASSIFICATION CRITERIA FOR SYSTEMIC LUPUS ERYTHEMATOSUS *(CONTINUED)*

Musculoskeletal			
Joint involvement	6		
Renal			
Proteinuria >0.5g/24 h	4		
Renal biopsy Class II or V lupus nephritis	8		
Renal biopsy Class III or IV lupus nephritis	10		
Total score:			
↓			
Classify as SLE with a score of 10 or more if entry criterion fulfilled.			

ANA, antinuclear antibodies; anti-dsDNA, anti-double-stranded DNA; SLE, systemic lupus erythematosus; anti-β_2GPI, anti-β_2-glycoprotein I.

Source: Aringer, M., Costenbader, K., Daikh, D., Brinks, R., Mosca, M., Ramsey-Goldman, R., Smolen, J. S., Wofsy, D., Boumpas, D. T., Kamen, D. L., Jayne, D., Cervera, R., Costedoat-Chalumeau, N., Diamond, B., Gladman, D. D., Hahn, B., Hiepe, F., Jacobsen, S., Khanna, D., . . . Johnson, S. R. (2019). 2019 European league against rheumatism/American College of Rheumatology classification criteria for systemic lupus erythematosus. *Arthritis & Rheumatology*, *71*(9), 1400–1412. https://doi.org/10.1002/art.40930

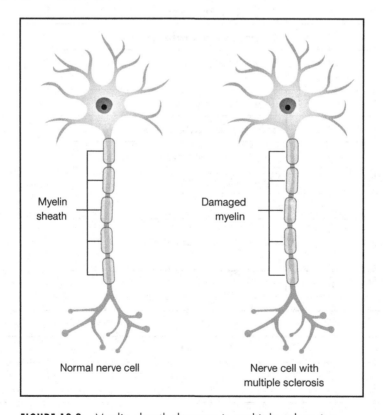

FIGURE 12.2   Myelin sheath damage in multiple sclerosis.

Source: Adapted from Stephanie021299. (n.d.). *Myelin sheath.*

D. Symptoms are related to the particular nerves that are damaged and the location of the lesions.

E. Symptoms often occur in clusters (Boss & Huether, 2019).

PREDISPOSING FACTORS

A. Vitamin D deficiency.

B. Cigarette smoking.

C. Epstein–Barr virus (EBV) infection.

D. Obesity.

E. Ultraviolet B light exposure (Boss & Huether, 2019; Dobson & Giovannoni, 2018).

SUBJECTIVE DATA

A. Overwhelming fatigue.

B. Visual disturbances (blurred or double vision).

C. Dizziness.

D. Vertigo.

E. Pain.

F. Depression.

G. Heat intolerance (Boss & Huether, 2019; Dobson & Giovannoni, 2018).

OBJECTIVE DATA

A. Visual deficits related to optic neuritis (ON).

B. Motor deficits.

C. Bowel and bladder incontinence.

D. Cognitive changes.

E. Muscle spasticity.

F. Sexual dysfunction.

G. Asymmetric paraparesis.

H. Progressive hemiparesis.

I. Cerebellar ataxia.

J. Paresthesia of the face and trunk (Boss & Huether, 2019; Dobson & Giovannoni, 2018).

DIAGNOSTIC TESTS

A. See Appendix Table 12A.1 for listing of common diagnostic tests.

B. See Table 12.3 for criteria.

DIFFERENTIAL DIAGNOSES

A. Monosymptomatic acute ON.

B. Transverse myelitis/spinal cord syndrome.

C. Vitamin deficiency.

D. Brain tumor.

E. Ischemic stroke.

TABLE 12.3 MCDONALD CRITERIA FOR MULTIPLE SCLEROSIS IN PATIENTS WITH AN ATTACK AT ONSET

NUMBER OF LESIONS WITH OBJECTIVE CLINICAL EVIDENCE		ADDITIONAL DATA NEEDED FOR A DIAGNOSIS OF MULTIPLE SCLEROSIS
≥2 clinical attacks	≥2	None[a]
≥2 clinical attacks	1 (as well as clear-cut historical evidence of a previous attack involving a lesion in a distinct anatomic location[b])	None[a]
≥2 clinical attacks	1	Dissemination in space demonstrated by an additional clinical attack implicating a different CNS site or by MRI
1 clinical attack	≥2	Dissemination in time demonstrated by an additional clinical attack or by MRI OR demonstration of CSF-specific oligoclonal bands
1 clinical attack	1	Dissemination in space demonstrated by an additional clinical attack implicating a different CNS site or by MRI AND

(continued)

TABLE 12.3 MCDONALD CRITERIA FOR MULTIPLE SCLEROSIS (CONTINUED)

NUMBER OF LESIONS WITH OBJECTIVE CLINICAL EVIDENCE		ADDITIONAL DATA NEEDED FOR A DIAGNOSIS OF MULTIPLE SCLEROSIS
		Dissemination in time demonstrated by an additional clinical attack or by MRI[d] OR demonstration of CSF-specific oligoclonal bands[c]

Note: If the 2017 McDonald criteria are fulfilled and there is no better explanation for the clinical presentation, the diagnosis is multiple sclerosis. If multiple sclerosis is suspected by virtue of a clinically isolated syndrome but the 2017 McDonald criteria are not completely met, the diagnosis is possible multiple sclerosis. If another diagnosis arises during the evaluation that better explains the clinical presentation, the diagnosis is not multiple sclerosis.

[a]No additional tests are required to demonstrate dissemination in space and time. However, unless MRI is not possible, brain MRI should be obtained in all patients in whom the diagnosis of multiple sclerosis is being considered. In addition, spinal cord MRI or CSF examination should be considered in patients with insufficient clinical and MRI evidence supporting multiple sclerosis, with a presentation other than a typical clinically isolated syndrome, or with atypical features. If imaging or other tests (e.g., CSF) are undertaken and are negative, caution needs to be taken before making a diagnosis of multiple sclerosis, and alternative diagnoses should be considered.

[b]Clinical diagnosis based on objective clinical findings for two attacks is most secure. Reasonable historical evidence for one past attack, in the absence of documented objective neurological findings, can include historical events with symptoms and evolution characteristic for a previous inflammatory demyelinating attack; at least one attack, however, must be supported by objective findings. In the absence of residual objective evidence, caution is needed.

[c]The presence of CSF-specific oligoclonal bands does not demonstrate dissemination in time per se but can substitute for the requirement for demonstration of this measure.

CNS, central nervous system; CSF, cerebral spinal fluid.

Source: Thompson, A. J., Banwell, B. L., Barkhof, F., Carroll, W. M., Coetzee, T., Comi, G., Correale, J., Fazekas, F., Filippi, M., Freedman, M. S., Fujihara, K., Galetta, S. L., Hartung, H. P., Kappos, L., Lublin, F. D., Marrie, R. A., Miller, A. E., Miller, D. H., Montalban, X., Mowry, E. M., . . . Cohen, J. A. (2018). Diagnosis of multiple sclerosis: 2017 revisions of the McDonald criteria. *The Lancet Neurology, 17*(2), 162–173. https://www.sciencedirect.com/sceience/article/abs/pii/S1474442217304702

F. Migraine.

G. Cerebral vasculitis.

H. Spinal cord compression (Dobson & Giovannoni, 2018).

POTENTIAL COMPLICATIONS

A. Loss of ambulatory ability.

B. Recurrent infections.

C. Blindness (rare).

D. Dementia (rare; Boss & Huether, 2019; Dobson & Giovannoni, 2018).

DISEASE-MODIFYING TREATMENTS

A. There is no cure for MS.

B. The goal of treatment is no evidence of disease activity (NEDA; see Figure 12.3).

C. Medical management may involve (see Table 12.4):

  1. Subcutaneous, oral, or intravenous medications.

D. Physical and occupational therapy (Boss & Huether, 2019; Dobson & Giovannoni, 2018).

PALLIATIVE INTERVENTIONS/SYMPTOM MANAGEMENT

A. See Appendix Table 12A.2 for listing of palliative interventions and symptom management.

B. See Appendix D-3 for overview of common symptoms.

PROGNOSIS

A. Women are at higher risk for MS, but men have a poorer prognosis and more severe clinical progression.

B. Life expectancy is not altered; disease progression often extends more than 30 years.

C. Death is usually related to interminable MS or complications such as aspiration pneumonia or sepsis (Boss & Huether, 2019).

NURSING INTERVENTIONS

A. Provide education on disease process and symptom management.

B. Teach patient to take all medications as prescribed.

C. Provide smoking cessation education (see Appendices B-10 and C-9).

D. Teach patient to alternate activity and rest.

E. Encourage ambulation and activity to prevent muscle wasting and promote mobility.

F. Teach patient to avoid excessive heat exposure.

G. Teach seizure precautions.

H. Educate patient on safety with ambulation.

I. Provide spiritual support.

J. Assess caregiver fatigue/burnout.

K. Encourage completion of advance directives.

▶

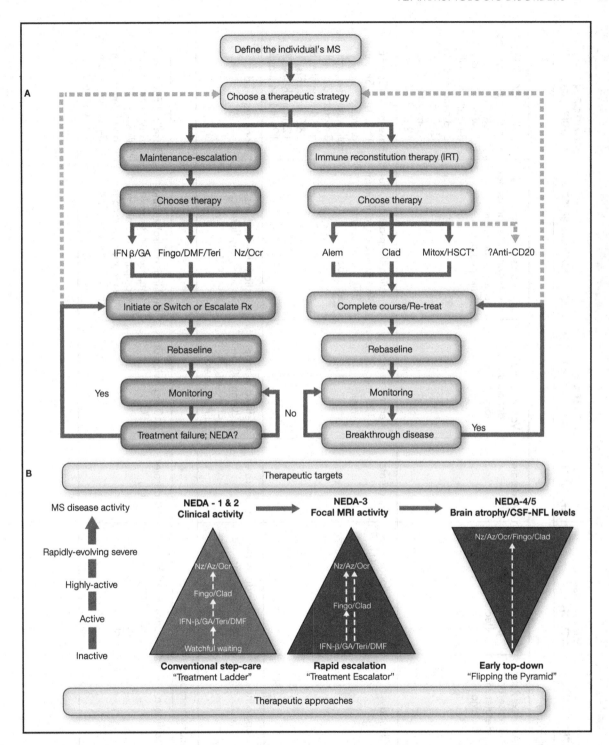

FIGURE 12.3 Therapeutic approaches to multiple sclerosis. **(A)** Treat-to-target algorithm of NEDA in relapsing forms of MS; **(B)** different therapeutic approaches to the treat-to-target algorithm.

ªMitox/HSCT, mitoxantrone/hematopoietic stem cell transplantation (not licensed in the UK for MS).

Az, alemtuzumab; Clad, oral cladribine; DMF, dimethyl fumarate; Fingo, fingolimod; GA, glatiramer acetate; IFN-β, interferon beta; NABs, neutralizing antibodies; MS, multiple sclerosis; NEDA, no evident disease activity; NEDA-2, clinical only (relapse-free and progression-free); NEDA-3, clinical and focal MRI activity; NEDA-4/5, clinical and focal MRI activity-free and normalizing brain atrophy loss and normalization of CSF neurofilament levels; Nz, natalizumab; Oer, ocrelizumab; Rx, treatment; T2T, treat-to-target; Teri, teriflunomide.

Source: Adapted from Dobson, R., & Giovannoni, G. (2019). Multiple sclerosis—a review. *European Journal of Neurology, 26*(1), 27–40. https://doi.org/10.1111/ene.13819

TABLE 12.4   DISEASE-MODIFYING THERAPIES CURRENTLY LICENSED FOR THE TREATMENT OF MULTIPLE SCLEROSIS

	TRADE NAME	MECHANISM OF ACTION	EFFICACY	ROUTE OF ADMINISTRATION	MAIN ADVERSE EFFECTS	MONITORING REQUIREMENTS
First-line injectable therapies						
IFN beta-1a and -1b	Avonex, Rebif, Betaseron, Betaferon, Extavia	Immunomodulatory, pleiotropic immune effects	Moderate	Variable and depends on formulation	Injection site reactions, flu-like symptoms, abnormal LFTs, lymphopenia, leukopenia	Baseline: FBC, U&E, LFTs, TFTs, SPE, urine protein. Follow-up: 1-month, 3-month, 6-month, and 6-monthly FBC, U&E, and LFTs. TFTs 12-monthly. NABs 12 and 24 months
Peg-IFN-beta-1a	Plegridy	Pegylated (long-circulating half-life). Immunomodulatory, pleiotropic immune effects	Moderate	Prefilled syringe 125 mcg SC 2 weekly	Injection site reactions, flu-like symptoms, abnormal LFTs, lymphopenia, leukopenia	Baseline: FBC, U&E, LFTs, TFTs, SPE, urine protein. Follow-up: 1-month, 3-month, 6-month, and 6-monthly FBC, U&E, and LFTs. TFTs 12-monthly. NABs 12 and 24 months
Glatiramer acetate	Copaxone	Immunomodulatory, pleiotropic immune effects	Moderate	Prefilled syringe 20 mg SC daily or 40 mg SC 3 times weekly	Injection site reactions, lipoatrophy, flushing reactions	None required
Oral immunomodulatory therapies						
Dimethyl fumarate	Tecfidera	Pleotropic, NRF2 activation, downregulation of nfκb	Moderate/high	240 mg twice daily PO	Flushing, gastrointestinal symptoms (dyspepsia, cramps, and diarrhea], lymphopenia, abnormal LFTs, proteinuria, PML	Baseline: FBC, U&E, LFTs, urine protein. Follow-up: FBC and urine protein 3-monthly for a year, then 6-monthly

	TRADE NAME	MECHANISM OF ACTION	EFFICACY	ROUTE OF ADMINISTRATION	MAIN ADVERSE EFFECTS	MONITORING REQUIREMENTS
Teriflunomide	Aubagio	Dihydro-orotate dehydrogenase inhibitor (reduced de novo pyrimidine synthesis), antiproliferative	Moderate	7 or 14 mg daily PO (7 mg dose only licensed in the United States)	Hair thinning, gastrointestinal symptoms (nausea, diarrhea), abnormal LFTs, leukopenia	Baseline: BP, FBC, U&E, LFTs, urine protein Follow-up: fortnightly LFTs for 6 months then every 8 weeks. Weekly LFT if ALT 2–3 × ULN. Three-monthly FBC for 1 year then 6-monthly
Oral immunosuppressive therapy						
Fingolimod	Gilenya	Selective sphingosine 1- phosphate modulator, prevents egress of lymphocytes from lymph nodes	High	0.5 mg daily PO	Bradycardia (first dose), hypertension, bronchospasm, lymphopenia, abnormal LFTs, infections, basal cell carcinoma, macular edema, opportunistic infections (PML, cryptococcosis, etc.)	Baseline: BP, FBC, U&E, LFTs, TFTs, serum immunoglobulin levels, serology (VZV, HIV 1 and 2, hepatitis B and C, syphilis), interferon gamma assay for tuberculosis (or similar), electrocardiogram Follow-up: 3-monthly FBC, U&E, and LFTs. TFTs 12-monthly. Optical coherence tomography at 3 months for macular edema

(continued)

TABLE 12.4 DISEASE-MODIFYING THERAPIES CURRENTLY LICENSED FOR THE TREATMENT OF MULTIPLE SCLEROSIS (CONTINUED)

	TRADE NAME	MECHANISM OF ACTION	EFFICACY	ROUTE OF ADMINISTRATION	MAIN ADVERSE EFFECTS	MONITORING REQUIREMENTS
Intravenous immunosuppressive therapies						
Natalizumab	Tysabri	Anti-VLA4, selective adhesion molecule inhibitor	Very high	300 mg IV 4 weekly	Infusion reactions, PML	Baseline: FBC, U&E, LFTs, JCV serology Follow-up: LFTs 3-monthly for a year. NABs at 12 months. JCV serology 6-monthly
Ocrelizumab	Ocrevus	Anti-CD20, B-cell depleter	Very high	Initially 300 mg IV, followed 2 weeks later by second dose of 300 mg IV. Subsequent dosing 600 mg IV 6-monthly	Infusion reactions, infections, possible hypogammaglobulinemia with prolonged use	Baseline: FBC, U&E, LFTs, TFTs, serum immunoglobulin levels, serology (VZV, HIV 1 and 2, hepatitis B and C, syphilis), TB elispot, cervical smear Follow-up: annual serum immunoglobulin levels
Induction/immune reconstitution therapies						
Alemtuzumab	Lemtrada	Anti-CD52, nonselective immune depleter	Very high	12 mg IVI × 5 days year 1, 12 mg IVI × 3 days year 2	Infusion reactions, infections, opportunistic infections, leukopenia, secondary autoimmunity (thyroid, immune thrombocytopenic purpura, renal, etc.)	Baseline: FBC, U&E, LFTs, TFTs, serum immunoglobulin levels, serology (VZV, HIV 1 and 2, hepatitis B and C, syphilis), TB elispot, cervical smear Follow-up (for 48 months after last course): monthly FBC, U&E, and urine analysis and 3-monthly TFTs

	TRADE NAME	MECHANISM OF ACTION	EFFICACY	ROUTE OF ADMINISTRATION	MAIN ADVERSE EFFECTS	MONITORING REQUIREMENTS
Cladribine	Mavenclad	Deoxyadenosine (purine) analogue, adenosine deaminase inhibitor, selective T- and B-cell depletion	High	10 mg tablets: cumulative dose of 3.5 mg/kg over 2 years. Tablets given for 4–5 days in months 1 and 2 in year 1 and the cycle is repeated in year 2 (8–10 days of treatment per year)	Lymphopenia, infections (in particular herpes zoster)	Baseline: FBC, U&E, LFTs, TFTs, serum immunoglobulin levels, serology (VZV, HIV 1 and 2, hepatitis B and C, syphilis), TB elispot, pregnancy test, and cervical smear. Follow-up: FBC 2 and 6 months after start of treatment in each treatment year
Mitoxantrone	Novantrone	Immune depleter (topoisomerase inhibitor)	Very high	12 mg/m² IVI 3-monthly for 2 years; maximum dose of 140 mg/m²	Leukopenia, hair loss, nausea, vomiting, infections, cardiomyopathy, amenorrhea	Baseline: FBC, U&E, LFTs, TFTs, SPE, serum immunoglobulin levels, serology (VZV, HIV 1 and 2, hepatitis B and C, syphilis), TB elispot Follow-up: 3-monthly (predosing) FBC, U&E, and LFTs. TFTs 12-monthly
Autologous hematopoietic stem cell transplantation		Autologous stem cell transplantation using standard hematology protocols	Very high	According to local protocols	Adverse events related to induction chemotherapy	Dictated by hematology protocols

ALT, alanine aminotransferase; BP, blood pressure; FBC, full blood count; IFN, interferon; IV, intravenous; IVI, intravenous infusion; JCV, John Cunningham virus; LFT, liver function test; MS, multiple sclerosis; NABs, neutralizing antibodies; nfkb, nuclear factor kappa-light-chain-enhancer of activated B cells; PML, progressive multifocal leukoencephalopathy; SQ, subcutaneous; SPE, serum protein electrophoresis; TFT, thyroid function test; U&E, urea and electrolytes; ULN, upper limit of normal; VZV, varicella zoster virus.

Source: Dobson, R., & Giovannoni, G. (2019). Multiple sclerosis–a review. European Journal of Neurology, 26(1), 27–40. https://doi.org/10.1111/ene.13819. Used with permission.

L. Discuss wishes regarding withholding or withdrawing of life-sustaining interventions in late stage of disease with patient (if possible) and/or primary caregiver (see Appendices C-2, C-3, and C-4).

M. Educate patient and family regarding availability of palliative care.

N. Educate patient and family regarding availability of hospice services (when appropriate).

O. Provide referral to community support groups, as needed.

MYASTHENIA GRAVIS

DEFINITION/CHARACTERISTICS

A. Chronic, autoimmune disease that primarily affects the neurological system.

B. Characterized by intermittent muscle weakness following activity, which is often alleviated by rest.

C. Ocular, bulbar, respiratory, and limb muscles are commonly affected (Dresser, 2011; National Institute of Neurological Disorders and Stroke [NINDS], 2022).

INCIDENCE AND PREVALENCE

A. The incidence of the disease is 4.1 to 30 cases per million person-years.

B. The prevalence rate ranges from 150 to 200 cases per million.

C. Most commonly diagnosed in women at ages 30 and 50.

D. In men, incidence increases with age, with most men being diagnosed between ages 60 and 89 (Dresser et al., 2021).

ETIOLOGY

A. MG results from immune response abnormalities.

B. Symptoms of MG results from interrupted transmission of neurotransmitters (NINDS, 2022).

PATHOPHYSIOLOGY

A. Through a cascade of intracellular processes, AChR antibodies are developed (see Figure 12.4).

B. Autoantibodies against the acetylcholine receptors (AChRs) interfere with cholinergic transmission between neurons.

C. The interrupted transmission of neurotransmitters leads to muscle weakness (see Figure 12.5; Dresser, 2021).

PREDISPOSING FACTORS

A. Age (women <40 years; men >60 years).

B. Race (more common among Blacks).

C. Environment (Whites and Asians living near the equator).

D. Female sex.

E. Genetic predisposition (Dresser, 2021; National Institute of Neurological Disorders & Stroke, 2022).

SUBJECTIVE DATA

A. Diplopia.

B. Weakness.

C. Dyspnea (Dresser, 2021; NINDS, 2022).

OBJECTIVE DATA

A. Fatigable muscle weakness worsened by activity and improved by rest (Hallmark sign).

B. Ptosis.

C. Dysarthria.

D. Dysphagia.

E. Facial and jaw weakness.

F. Head drop.

G. Limb weakness.

H. Foot drop.

I. Bulbar weakness.

J. Tongue atrophy (Dresser, 2021; NINDS, 2022).

DIAGNOSTIC TESTS

A. See Appendix Table 12A.1 for listing of common diagnostic tests.

B. See Table 12.5 for classification.

DIFFERENTIAL DIAGNOSES

A. Congenital myasthenic syndromes.

B. Lambert–Eaton syndrome.

C. Botulism.

D. Organophosphate intoxication.

E. Mitochondrial disorders involving progressive external ophthalmoplegia.

F. Acute inflammatory demyelinating polyradiculoneuropathy (AIDP).

G. Motor neuron disease.

H. Brainstem ischemia (Juel & Massey, 2007).

POTENTIAL COMPLICATIONS

A. Respiratory muscle failure requiring mechanical ventilation (myasthenia gravis [MG] crisis).

B. Treatment for MG may involve chronic suppression of the immune system (Dresser, 2021; NINDS, 2022).

DISEASE-MODIFYING TREATMENTS

A. Thymectomy.

B. Monoclonal antibodies.

C. Immunosuppressive medications.

D. Plasmapheresis.

E. Intravenous immunoglobulin (NINDS, 2022).

PALLIATIVE INTERVENTIONS/SYMPTOM MANAGEMENT

A. See Appendix Table 12A.2 for listing of palliative interventions and symptom management.

B. See Appendix D-3 for overview of common symptoms.

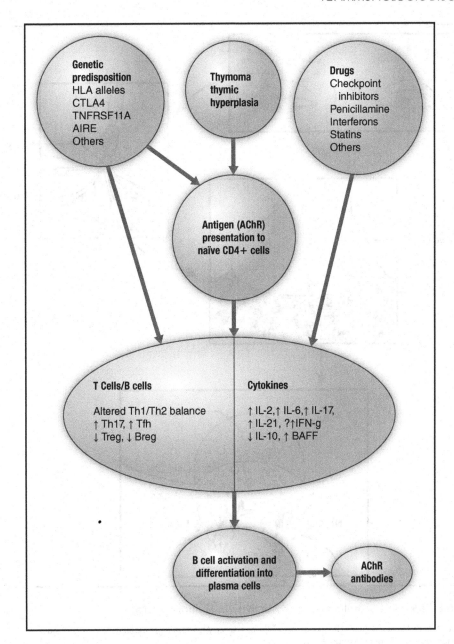

FIGURE 12.4 Pathogenesis of myasthenia gravis.

AChR, acetylcholine receptor; AIRE, autoimmune regulator; Breg, regulatory B cell; CTLA4, cytotoxic T-lymphocyte-associated protein 4; HLA, human leukocyte antigen; IL, interleukin; Tfh, T follicular helper; Th1, helper 1; Th2, helper 2; TNFRSF11A, tumor necrosis factor receptor 4 superfamily, member 11a; Treg, regulatory T cell.

Source: Adapted from Dresser, L., Wlodarski, R., Rezania, K., & Soliven, B. (2021). Myasthenia gravis: Epidemiology, pathophysiology and clinical manifestations. *Journal of Clinical Medicine, 10*(11), 2235. https://doi.org/10.3390/jcm10112235

PROGNOSIS

A. Remission is possible in about half of cases.

B. Those with refractory MG have ongoing symptom burden including:

    1. Extreme fatigue.

    2. Marked disability.

    3. Uncontrolled symptoms.

    4. Frequent myasthenic crises.

    5. Frequent hospitalizations.

    6. Reduced quality of life (NINDS, 2022; Schneider-Gold et al., 2019).

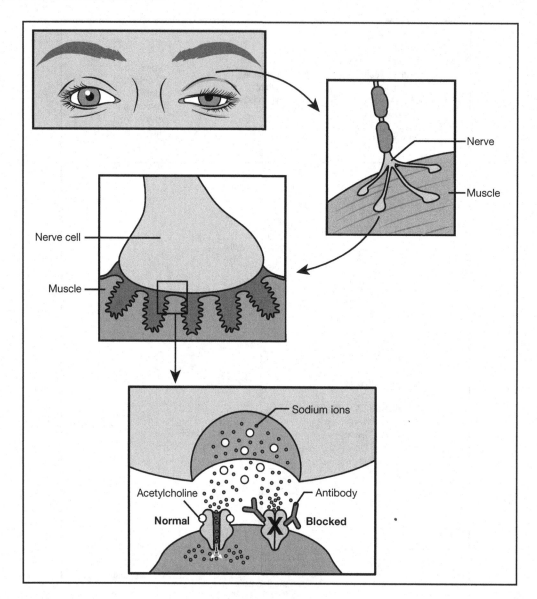

FIGURE 12.5   Acetylcholine antibody activity in multiple sclerosis.

Source: Adapted from Children's Hospital of Philadelphia. (2022). *Myasthenia gravis.* https://www.chop.edu/
conditions-diseases/myasthenia-gravis#

TABLE 12.5	CLASSIFICATION OF MYASTHENIA GRAVIS
Class I	Any ocular muscle weakness May have weakness of eye closure All other muscle strength is normal
Class II	Mild weakness affecting other than ocular muscles May also have ocular muscle weakness of any severity
IIa	Predominantly affecting limb, axial muscles, or both May also have lesser involvement of oropharyngeal muscles

(continued)

TABLE 12.5 CLASSIFICATION OF MYASTHENIA GRAVIS *(CONTINUED)*

IIb	Predominantly affecting oropharyngeal, respiratory muscles, or both May also have lesser or equal involvement of limb, axial muscles, or both
Class III	Moderate weakness affecting other than ocular muscles May also have ocular muscle weakness of any severity
IIIa	Predominantly affecting limb, axial muscles, or both May also have lesser involvement of oropharyngeal muscles
IIIb	Predominantly affecting oropharyngeal, respiratory muscles, or both May also have lesser or equal involvement of limb, axial muscles, or both
Class IV	Severe weakness affecting other than ocular muscles May also have ocular muscle weakness of any severity
IVa	Predominantly affecting limb and/or axial muscles May also have lesser involvement of oropharyngeal muscles
IVb	Predominantly affecting oropharyngeal, respiratory muscles, or both May also have lesser or equal involvement of limb, axial muscles, or both
Class V	Defined by intubation, with or without mechanical ventilation, except when employed during routine postoperative management. The use of a feeding tube without intubation places the patient in Class IVb.

Source: Jaretzki, A. I. I. I., Barohn, R. J., Ernstoff, R. M., Kaminski, H. J., Keesey, J. C., Penn, A. S., & Sanders, D. B. (2000). Myasthenia gravis: Recommendations for clinical research standards. *Neurology, 55*(1), 16–23. https://doi.org/10.1212/WNL.55.1.16. Used with permission.

NURSING INTERVENTIONS

A. Provide education on disease process and symptom management.

B. Teach patient to take all medications as prescribed.

C. Educate patient on emergency management of myasthenic crisis.

D. Teach patient to alternate activity and rest.

E. Educate patient on safety with ambulation.

F. Provide spiritual support.

G. Assess caregiver fatigue/burnout.

H. Encourage completion of advance directives.

I. Discuss wishes regarding withholding or withdrawing of life-sustaining interventions in late stage of disease with patient (if possible) and/or primary caregiver (see Appendices C-2, C-3, and C-4).

J. Educate patient and family regarding availability of palliative care.

K. Educate patient and family regarding availability of hospice services (when appropriate).

L. Provide referral to community support groups, as needed.

REFERENCES

Bartles, C. M. (2022). *Systemic lupus erythematosus (SLE) differential diagnoses.* https://emedicine.medscape.com/article/332244-differential

Boss, J. B. & Huether, S. E. (2019). Disorders of the central and peripheral nervous systems and the neuromuscular junction. In K. L. McCance & S. E. Huether (Eds.), *Pathophysiology: The biologic basis for disease in adults and children* (8th ed., pp. 550–599). Elsevier.

Centers for Disease Control and Prevention. (2022). *Systemic lupus erythematosus (SLE).* https://www.cdc.gov/lupus/facts/detailed.html#causes

Dobson, R., & Giovannoni, G. (2019). Multiple sclerosis–a review. *European Journal of Neurology, 26*(1), 27–40. https://doi.org/10.1111/ene.13819

Dresser, L., Wlodarski, R., Rezania, K., & Soliven, B. (2021). Myasthenia gravis: Epidemiology, pathophysiology and clinical manifestations. *Journal of Clinical Medicine, 10*(11), 2235. https://doi.org/10.3390/jcm10112235

Guyer, D. L., Almhanna, K., & McKee, K. Y. (2020). Palliative care for patients with esophageal cancer: A narrative review. *Annals of Translational Medicine, 8*(17). https://doi.org/10.21037/atm-20-3676

Haflidadottir, S., Jonasson, J. G., Norland, H., Einarsdottir, S. O., Kleiner, D. E., Lund, S. H., & Björnsson, E. S. (2014). Long term follow-up and liver-related death rate in patients with non-alcoholic and alcoholic related fatty liver disease. *BMC Gastroenterology, 14*(1), 1–10. http://www.biomedcentral.com/1471-230X/14/166

Huether, S. E. (2019). Alternations of renal and urinary tract function. In K. L. McCance & S. E. Huether (Eds.), *Pathophysiology: The biologic basis for disease in adults and children* (8th ed., pp. 1246–1277). Elsevier.

Iftimie, G., Pantea Stoian, A., Socea, B., Motofei, I., Marcu, D., Costache, R. S., & Diaconu, C. (2018). Complications of systemic lupus erythematosus: A review. *Romanian Journal of Military Medicine, 121*(3), 9–15. https://www.researchgate.net/profile/Raluca-Costache/publication/343166869_Complications_of_systemic_lupus_erythematosus_A_review/links/5f19e0ba299bf1720d5fb959/Complications-of-systemic-lupus-erythematosus-A-review.pdf

Juel, V. C. & Massey, J. M. (2007). Myasthenia gravis. *Orphanet Journal of Rare Diseases*, 2(44). https://ojrd.biomedcentral.com/articles/10.1186/1750-1172-2-44

National Institute of Neurological Disorders and Stroke. (2022). *Myasthenia gravis fact sheet*. https://www.ninds.nih.gov/myasthenia-gravis-fact-sheet#1

Rote, N. S. & McCance, K. L. (2019). Alterations in immunity and inflammation. In K. L. McCance & S. E. Huether (Eds.), *Pathophysiology: The biologic basis for disease in adults and children* (8th ed., pp. 255–288). Elsevier.

Schneider-Gold, C., Hagenacker, T., Melzer, N., & Ruck, T. (2019). Understanding the burden of refractory myasthenia gravis. *Therapeutic Advances in Neurological Disorders*, 12, 1756286419832242. https://doi.org/10.1177/1756286419832242

Walton, C., King, R., Rechtman, L., Kaye, W., Leray, E., Marrie, R. A., ... & Baneke, P. (2020). Rising prevalence of multiple sclerosis worldwide: Insights from the Atlas of MS. *Multiple Sclerosis Journal*, 26(14), 1816–1821. https://doi.org/10.1177%2F1352458520970841

Wright, P. M. (2019). *Certified hospice and palliative nurse (CHPN) exam review*. Springer Publishing Company.

APPENDIX

TABLE 12A.1 DIAGNOSTIC TESTS FOR IMMUNOLOGIC DISORDERS

TYPE	NOTES
Physical examination	• Thorough physical examination with detailed medical history and neurological examination
Imaging	• X-rays (SLE) • MRI (MS, MG) • Edrophonium test (MG) • Electrodiagnostics (MG) • Pulmonary function test (MG) • CT scan (MG)
Laboratory tests	• Positive ANA screening test (SLE) • Evoked potential test (MS) • Vitamin B levels (MS) • Thyroid function panel (MS) • Syphilis and human immunodeficiency virus testing (MS) • Acetylcholine receptor antibody level (MG) • MuSK antibody (MG)
Pathology	• Skin biopsy with immunofluorescent examination • Kidney biopsy • Classification of systemic lupus erythema according to severity of symptoms (see Tables 12.1 and 12.2) • Lumbar puncture with CSF analysis (MS) • Categorized according to the McDonald criteria (see Table 12.3; MS) • Progression of MG is classified according to the criteria set forth by MSAB of the MGFA (see Table 12.5; MG)

Sources: Boss, J. B. & Huether, S. E. (2019). Disorders of the central and peripheral nervous systems and the neuromuscular junction. In K. L. McCance & S. E. Huether (Eds.), *Pathophysiology: The biologic basis for disease in adults and children* (8th ed., pp. 550–599). Elsevier; Centers for Disease Control and Prevention. (2022). *Systemic lupus erythematosus (SLE).* https://www.cdc.gov/lupus/facts/detailed.html#causes; Dobson, R., & Giovannoni, G. (2019). Multiple sclerosis–a review. *European Journal of Neurology, 26*(1), 27–40. https://doi.org/10.1111/ene.13819; Dresser, L., Wlodarski, R., Rezania, K., & Soliven, B. (2021). Myasthenia gravis: Epidemiology, pathophysiology and clinical manifestations. *Journal of Clinical Medicine, 10*(11), 2235. https://doi.org/10.3390/jcm10112235; McCann and Huether (2019); National Institute of Neurological Disorders and Stroke. (2022). *Myasthenia gravis fact sheet.* https://www.ninds.nih.gov/myasthenia-gravis-fact-sheet#1; Rote, N. S. & McCance, K. L. (2019). Alterations in immunity and inflammation. In K. L. McCance & S. E. Huether (Eds.), *Pathophysiology: The biologic basis for disease in adults and children* (8th ed., pp. 255–288). Elsevier.

ANA, antinuclear antibody; CSF, cerebral spinal fluid; MG, myasthenia gravis; MGFA, Myasthenia Gravis Foundation of America; MS, multiple sclerosis; MSAB, Medical Scientific Advisory Board; SLE, systemic lupus erythematosus.

TABLE 12A.2 PALLIATIVE INTERVENTIONS/SYMPTOM MANAGEMENT FOR IMMUNOLOGIC DISORDERS

Symptom	Intervention
Anorexia	• Use of appetite stimulants (see Appendix D-1) • Offer small, frequent meals and snacks • Offer nutritional supplements
Anxiety and depression	• Antidepressants, anxiolytics, or benzodiazepines as indicated by patient's condition, age, and life expectancy (see Appendix D-1) • Non-pharmacological interventions (see Appendix D-2)

(continued)

TABLE 12A.2   PALLIATIVE INTERVENTIONS/SYMPTOM MANAGEMENT FOR IMMUNOLOGIC DISORDERS *(CONTINUED)*

Caregiver burden	• Support of interdisciplinary hospice or palliative team • Non-pharmacological interventions for caregivers (see Appendix D-2)
Communication barriers	• Use nonthreatening body language (place yourself at eye level, use therapeutic touch; MS) • Use a soft tone of voice and use short phrases (MS) • Avoid use of hand gestures when speaking as this may seem threatening to the person (MS) • Reduce distractions (MS) • Offer a limited number of choices (MS) • Use a picture board, if needed (MS)
Fatigue and somnolence	• Alternate periods of rest with periods of activity • Utilize energy conversation techniques • Psychostimulants (see Appendix D-1)
Frequent infection	• Avoid crowds or large gatherings • Wear mask when in the company of others • Wash hands frequently • Use of antibiotics or anti-infectives as indicated • Avoid animals and live plants • Avoid dental work • Avoid vaccines unless otherwise directed • Avoid raw foods
Gastrointestinal symptoms (see Appendix D-1)	• Antacids (SLE) • Antiemetics (SLE) • Promotility agents (SLE) • Laxatives (SLE) • Antidiarrheals (SLE)
Immobility	• Encourage active participation in repositioning, when possible (MS, MG) • Implement use of bed mobility devices such as a bed hoist, bed ladder, grab rail, or trapeze bar (MS, MG) • Frequently reposition patient to relieve pressure on bony surfaces (MS, MG) • Use pillows, cushions, anti-pressure mattresses to alleviate pressure wound risk (MS, MG) • If patient is at risk for falls, safety measures such as nonskid slippers, shoes, or socks, bed or chair alarms, floor sensor, or fall mat (MS, MG)
Incontinence	• Identify and correct causes of incontinence, if possible (i.e., urinary tract infection, *Clostridium difficile*, etc.; MS) • Use protective pads/undergarments (MS) • Utilize urinary diversion devices (indwelling catheter, condom catheter, etc.), as appropriate (MS) • Provide meticulous skin care and reposition patient at least every 2 hours (MS) • Utilize fecal collection devices as indicated (i.e., external pouch, rectal tubes; MS)

(continued)

TABLE 12A.2   PALLIATIVE INTERVENTIONS/SYMPTOM MANAGEMENT FOR IMMUNOLOGIC DISORDERS *(CONTINUED)*

Inflammation	• NSAIDS • Corticosteroids (see Appendix D-1; SLE, MS)
Insomnia	• Use of benzodiazepines, antidepressants, or antihistaminic agents, as indicated by patient's condition, age, and life expectancy (MS, MG) • Provide proper sleep hygiene (MS, MG) • Use non-pharmacological interventions for relaxation (MS, MG) • Address underlying anxiety and depression (MS, MG)

Neuropathy	• Pharmacological interventions (see Appendix D-1)
	  ▪ Antidepressants
	  ▪ Anticonvulsants (i.e., gabapentin)
	  ▪ Anesthetics (i.e., ketamine)
	  ▪ Opioids

Pain management	• See Appendix E
Psychosocial distress and body image changes	• Antidepressants (see Appendix D-1) • Non-pharmacological interventions (see Appendix D-2; Guyer et al., 2020)
Renal/cancer-induced anemia	• Iron supplementation (SLE) • ESA (SLE) • Red blood cell transfusions (in refractory cases when patient is symptomatic; SLE)

Seizures	• Antiepileptic medications (see Appendix D-1; SLE, MS)
	  ▪ Most commonly used is levetiracetam
	  ▪ If patient is unable to swallow, intranasal midazolam, rectal diazepam, or buccal clonazepam may be used

Sources: Abt, D., Bywater, M., Engeler, D. S., & Schmid, H. P. (2013). Therapeutic options for intractable hematuria in advanced bladder cancer. *International Journal of Urology, 20*(7), 651-660. https://doi.org/10.1111/iju.12113; Guyer, D. L., Almhanna, K., & McKee, K. Y. (2020). Palliative care for patients with esophageal cancer: A narrative review. *Annals of Translational Medicine, 8*(17). https://doi.org/10.21037/atm-20-3676; Kluger, B. M., Ney, D. E., Bagley, S. J., Mohile, N., Taylor, L. P., Walbert, T., & Jones, C. A. (2020). Top ten tips palliative care clinicians should know when caring for patients with brain cancer. *Journal of Palliative Medicine, 23*(3), 415–421. doi.10.1089/jpm.2019.0507; Sommers, M. S. (2019). *Davis's diseases and disorders: A nursing therapeutics manual.* F.A. Davis. https://www.fadavis.com/product/nursing-fundamentals-med-surg-diseases-disorders-nursing-therapeutics-manual-sommers-6; Tariq, R., & Singal, A. K. (2020). Management of hepatorenal syndrome: A review. *Journal of Clinical and Translational Hepatology, 8*(2), 192. https://www.ncbi.nlm.nih.gov/pmc/articles/PMC7438356/

ESA, erythropoiesis-stimulating agents; MG, myasthenia gravis; MS, multiple sclerosis; NSAIDS, nonsteroidal anti-inflammatory drugs; SLE, systemic lupus erythematosus.

CHAPTER 13

INFECTIOUS DISEASES

HIV/AIDS

DEFINITION/CHARACTERISTICS
A. HIV is a blood-borne retrovirus that targets CD4 cells, also known as T cells.
B. CD4 cells play an integral role in mounting immune responses.
C. If left untreated, HIV infection leads to AIDS.
D. AIDS is characterized by a decrease in the total CD4 lymphocyte count below 500 per µL.
E. HIV is transmitted through blood and other body fluids.
F. HIV infection is spread primarily through sexual contact and intravenous drug use (Centers for Disease Control and Prevention [CDC], 2022b; Klatt, 2022; Rote, 2019).

INCIDENCE AND PREVALENCE
A. Approximately 18 million people worldwide are infected with HIV.
B. Approximately 1.2 million Americans are infected with HIV.
C. About 13% of individuals who are infected with HIV are unaware of their infection.
D. About 35,000 new cases of HIV are diagnosed annually in the United States.
E. The number of newly diagnosed HIV infections has decreased by 9% since 2015.
F. About 15,800 HIV-related deaths occur in the United States annually (HIV.gov, 2022; Rote, 2019).

ETIOLOGY
A. Exposure to and subsequent infection with HIV (Rote, 2019).

PATHOPHYSIOLOGY
A. Retroviruses do not have deoxyribonucleic acid DNA and cannot replicate outside of a living host cell.
B. After entering the host, the viral particle attaches by fusion to a susceptible cell membrane and then enters the cell.
C. Once the virus is inside of the host cell, it replicates by shedding its viral capsule to release the capsid.
D. The capsid stores the two strands of viral RNA, copies of reverse transcriptase, and integrase enzymes.
E. The capsid enters via the nuclear pore complex where viral RNA integrates into the host's DNA using reverse transcription (Klatt, 2022; Figure 13.1).

PREDISPOSING FACTORS
A. Unprotected sexual activity, especially with multiple partners.
B. Needle sharing (e.g., drug use, tattoos, piercing, etc.).
C. Presence of sexually transmitted infections such as syphilis, gonorrhea, chlamydia, or herpes.
D. Accidental needlestick injury (Rote, 2019; World Health Organization [WHO], 2022d).

SUBJECTIVE DATA
A. Fever.
B. Fatigue.
C. Myalgia.
D. Arthralgia.
E. Sore throat.
F. Chills (CDC, 2022b; Rote, 2019).

OBJECTIVE DATA
A. Lymphadenopathy.
B. Chronic systemic inflammation.
C. Dyslipidemia.
D. Decreased bone density.
E. Genital inflammation.
F. Oral ulcers.
G. Recurrent opportunistic infections (see Table 13.1; CDC, 2022b; Klatt, 2022; Rote, 2019).

DIAGNOSTIC TESTS
A. See Appendix Table 13A.1 for listing of common diagnostic tests.
B. See Figure 13.2 for staging.

DIFFERENTIAL DIAGNOSES
A. Burkitt lymphoma.
B. Candidiasis.
C. Cryptococcosis.
D. Cryptosporidiosis.
E. Cytomegalovirus (CMV).
F. Herpes simplex.
G. Lymphoma.
H. Mycobacterium avium complex (MAC; mycobacterium avium-intracellulare [MAI]).
I. Toxoplasmosis (Gilroy, 2021).

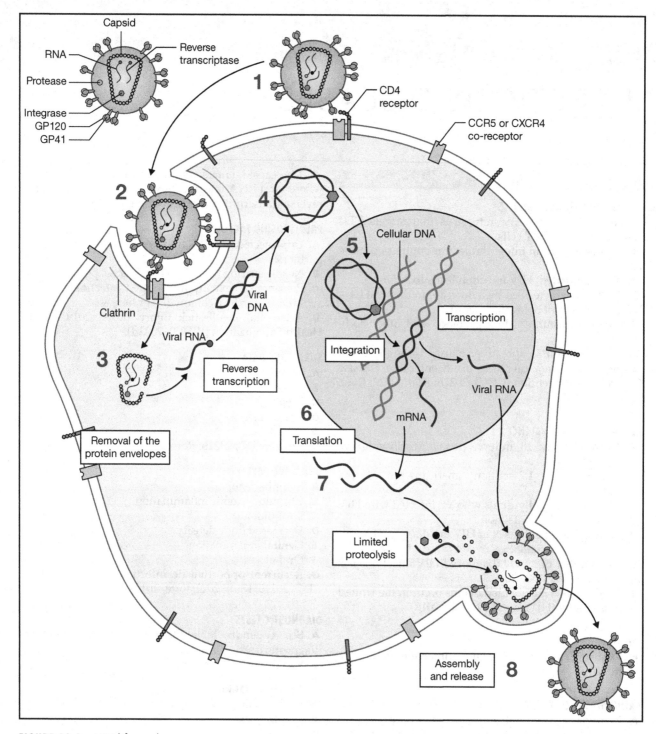

FIGURE 13.1   HIV life cycle.

POTENTIAL COMPLICATIONS

A. Opportunistic infections (see Table 13.1).
B. Heart disease.
C. Liver disease.
D. Kidney disease.

E. Encephalopathy.
F. Wasting syndrome.
G. Invasive cervical cancer.
H. Kaposi sarcoma.
I. Lymphoma.

TABLE 13.1 OPPORTUNISTIC INFECTIONS ASSOCIATED WITH HIV

Bacterial infections	*Mycobacterium avium, Mycobacterium tuberculosis,* recurrent pneumonia, Salmonella septicemia
Fungal infections	Candidiasis, coccidioidomycosis, cryptococcosis, histoplasmosis, *Pneumocystis jirovecii*
Protozoal and helminthic infections	Cryptosporidiosis, isosporiasis, toxoplasmosis
Viral infections	Cytomegalovirus, chronic herpes simplex, progressive multifocal leukoencephalopathy, varicella zoster

Source: Adapted from Rote, N. S. (2019). *Infection.* In K. L. McCance & S. E. Huether (Eds.), *Pathophysiology: The biologic basis for disease in adults and children* (8th ed., pp. 289–322). Elsevier.

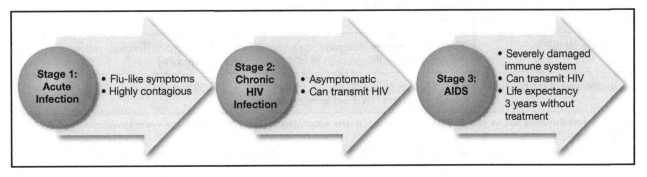

FIGURE 13.2 Staging of HIV infection.

Sources: Adpated from Centers for Disease Control and Prevention. (2022b). *About HIV.* https://www.cdc.gov/hiv/basics/whatishiv.html

J. Increased risk for:
1. Bone fractures.
2. Heart failure.
3. Renal disease.
4. Liver disease.
5. Diabetes (National Institute of Health, 2021; Rote, 2019).

DISEASE-MODIFYING TREATMENTS
A. There is no cure for HIV infection.
B. Highly active antiretroviral therapies are used to control viral replication (HAART; see Table 13.2).
C. Goals of disease management:
1. Reduce viral load.
2. Reduce HIV-associated morbidity.
3. Prolong survival.
4. Prevent HIV transmission (see Appendix B-7; CDC, 2022a; Rote & McCance, 2019).

PALLIATIVE INTERVENTIONS/SYMPTOM MANAGEMENT
A. See Appendix Table 13A.2 for listing of palliative interventions and symptom management.
B. See Appendix D-3 for overview of common symptoms.

PROGNOSIS
A. When first identified in the 1980s, mortality related to HIV was nearly 100%.
B. Today, HIV is considered a chronic illness.
C. Without interventions, progression to acute HIV takes roughly 9 to 10 years.
D. Without treatment, survival rate for AIDS is about 3 years (Rote, 2019).

NURSING INTERVENTIONS
A. Provide education on disease process and symptom management.
B. Teach patient transmission prevention strategies (see Appendix B-8).
C. Encourage smoking cessation (see Appendices B-10 and C-9).
D. Teach patient to take all medications as prescribed.
E. Teach importance of routine bloodwork.
F. Educate patient and caregiver(s) on signs of complications.
G. Provide spiritual support.
H. Assess caregiver fatigue/burnout.
I. Encourage completion of advance directives.
J. Discuss wishes regarding withholding or withdrawing of life-sustaining interventions in late stage of ▶

TABLE 13.2   ANTIRETROVIRAL THERAPY

Category	Action	Examples
NRTIs	Block the action of reverse transcriptase, which prevents replication of the virus	Zidovudine (Retrovir), tenofovir (Viread), lamivudine (Epivir), emtricitabine (Emtriva), abacavir (Ziagen)
NNRTIs	Bind to reverse transcriptase and alter it, which prevents replication of the virus	Efavirenz (Sustiva), etravirine (Intelence), nevirapine (Viramune/Viramune XR, rilpivirine (Edurant)
Fusion inhibitors	Block HIV from entering the host's CD4 cells	Enfuvirtide (Fuzeon)
CCR5 antagonists	Block CCR5 co-receptors on immune cells, which prevents the virus from entering the cell	Maraviroc (Selzentry)
Integrase inhibitors	Blocks the action of integrase, an enzyme that is important in the process of HIV replication	Dolutegravir (Tivicay), raltegravir (Isentress)
Post-attachment inhibitors	Block CD4 receptors on certain immune cells, which prevents HIV from entering the cell	Ibalizumab (Trogarzo)

CCR5, C-C motif chemokine receptor type 5; NNRTIs, non-nucleoside reverse transcriptase inhibitors; NRTIs, nucleoside reverse transcriptase inhibitors; XR, extended release.

Source: Wright, P. M. (2019). *Certified hospice and palliative nurse (CHPN) exam review: A study guide with review questions.* Springer Publishing Company.

disease with patient (if possible) and/or primary caregiver (see Appendices C-2, C-3, and C-4).

K. Educate patient and family regarding availability of palliative care.

L. Educate patient and family regarding availability of hospice services (when appropriate).

M. Provide referral to community support groups, as needed.

CORONAVIRUS DISEASE 2019

DEFINITION/CHARACTERISTICS

A. Systemic, infectious disease fist discovered in December of 2019.

B. Originally identified following an outbreak of "viral pneumonia" in Wuhan, People's Republic of China.

C. Coronavirus disease 2019 (COVID-19) has an incubation period of 2 to 14 days.

D. The acute phase of infection typically lasts 7 to 14 days.

E. Post-acute sequelae of SARS-CoV-19 (PASC) occurs when symptoms persist longer than 4 weeks. Also called:

1. Long-haul COVID.
2. Post-acute COVID-19.
3. Long-term effects of COVID.
4. Chronic COVID.
5. Post-acute COVID complications (CDC, 2022c; Chippa et al., 2021; WHO, 2022a).

INCIDENCE AND PREVALENCE

A. As of this writing, there have been 579,092,623 confirmed cases of COVID-19 (see Figure 13.3).

B. There have been 6,407,556 deaths associated with COVID-19 worldwide (WHO, 2022a).

ETIOLOGY

A. COVID-19 is caused by infection with SARS-CoV-2 virus (CDC, 2022c; Chippa et al., 2021; WHO, 2022a).

PATHOPHYSIOLOGY

A. Coronaviruses are enveloped, positive-sense, single-stranded RNA viruses.

B. COVID-19 is highly infectious and contracted through droplet and aerosol spread.

C. Once coronavirus enters a human host, it undergoes a five-step life cycle, consisting of:

1. Attachment.
2. Penetration.
3. Biosynthesis.
4. Maturation.
5. Release (see Figure 13.4).

D. Individuals have the highest viral load and are most contagious in the incubation/presymptomatic phase of the illness.

E. The virus binds to the cell-surface protein angiotensin converting enzyme-2 (ACE-2) through the receptor-binding domain (RBD) of its spike protein. ▶

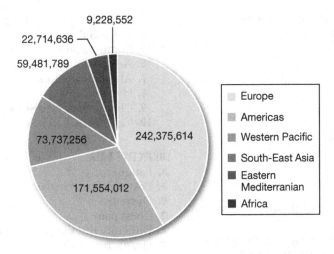

FIGURE 13.3 Confirmed cases of COVID-19.

Sources: Adapted from Centers for Disease Control and Prevention. (2022b). *About HIV.* https://www.cdc.gov/hiv/basics/whatishiv.html; National Institute of Health. (2021). *The stages of HIV infection.* https://hivinfo.nih.gov/understanding-hiv/fact-sheets/stages-hiv-infection

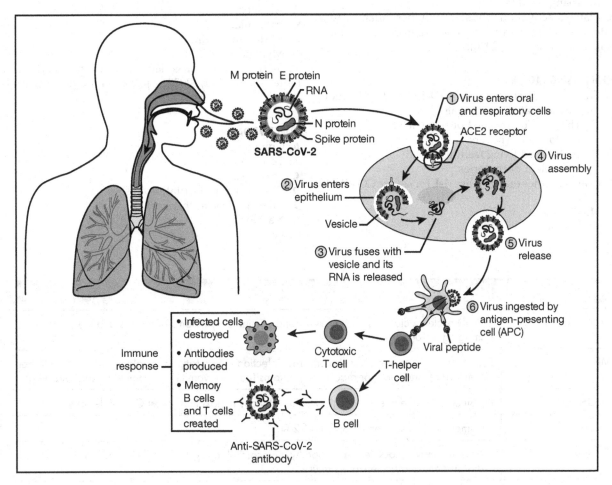

FIGURE 13.4 Transmission and life cycle of SARS-CoV-2 causing COVID-19.

Source: Adapted from Funk, C. D., Laferrière, C., & Ardakani, A. (2020). A snapshot of the global race for vaccines targeting SARS-CoV-2 and the COVID-19 pandemic. *Pharmacology, 11,* 937. https://doi.org/10.3389/fphar.2020.00937

F. ACE-2 is most commonly expressed on the:
   1. Epithelium of the nasopharynx.
   2. Upper respiratory tract.
   3. Bronchi.
   4. Type II pneumocytes.
   5. Macrophages.
   6. Monocytes.
   7. Mast cells.
   8. Vascular epithelial cells.
   9. Fat cells.
   10. Brain cells.
   11. Liver.
   12. Kidneys.
   13. Heart, which makes all of these sites potential site of viral attachment.
G. Three interconnected pathological processes take place, leading to manifestation of symptoms:
   1. Pulmonary macrophage activation syndrome with uncontrolled inflammation.
   2. Mediated endotheliosis.
   3. Procoagulant state with thrombotic microangiopathy.
H. Platelet activation leads to a hyper-inflammatory state, which increases risk for end-organ damage (Marik et al., 2021; Yuki et al., 2020).

PREDISPOSING FACTORS

A. Those at highest risk for COVID-19 infection include:
   1. Unvaccinated individuals.
   2. Those in congregate housing such as:
      a. Homeless shelters.
      b. Assisted living facilities.
      c. Student dormitories.
B. Comorbidities that increase risk for severe COVID-19 sequelae:
   1. Diabetes.
   2. Obesity.
   3. Asthma or chronic lung disease.
   4. Sickle cell anemia.
   5. Immunocompromised status.
   6. Advanced age.
   7. Atrial fibrillation.
   8. Hypertension.
   9. Chronic kidney disease.
   10. Cancer (CDC, 2022c; Yuki et al., 2020).

SUBJECTIVE DATA

A. Fatigue.
B. Post-exertional malaise.
C. Dyspnea.
D. Chest pain.
E. Difficulty thinking or concentrating ("brain fog").
F. Headache.
G. Insomnia.
H. Dizziness.
 I. Light-headedness.
 J. Neuralgias.
K. Depression.
L. Anxiety.
M. Anosmia.
N. Abdominal pain.
O. Myalgias.
P. Symptoms are classified according to severity (see Table 13.3; CDC, 2022c; Johns Hopkins Medicine, 2022).

OBJECTIVE DATA

A. Cough.
B. Tachycardia.
C. Diarrhea.
D. Dermatological irritation/rashes.
E. Menstrual cycle changes.
F. Hair loss.
G. Fever.

TABLE 13.3	CLASSIFICATION OF COVID-19 SYMPTOMS
Asymptomatic	COVID nucleic acid test positive. Without any clinical symptoms and signs and the chest imaging is normal
Mild	Symptoms of acute upper respiratory tract infection (fever, fatigue, myalgia, cough, sore throat, runny nose, sneezing) or digestive symptoms (nausea, vomiting, abdominal pain, diarrhea)
Moderate	Pneumonia (frequent fever, cough) with no obvious hypoxemia; chest CT with lesions
Severe	Pneumonia with hypoxemia (SpO2 <92%)
Critical	ARDS; may have shock, encephalopathy, myocardial injury, heart failure, coagulation dysfunction, and acute kidney injury

ARDS, acute respiratory distress syndrome.

Source: Yuki, K., Fujiogi, M., & Koutsogiannaki, S. (2020). COVID-19 pathophysiology: A review. *Clinical Immunology, 215,* 108427. https://doi.org/10.1016/j.clim.2020.108427.

H. Multi-organ effects to:
1. Kidneys.
2. Lungs.
3. Heart.
4. Skin.
5. Brain
6. Neurological system.

I. Symptoms are classified according to severity (see Figure 13.4; CDC, 2022c; Johns Hopkins Medicine, 2022).

DIAGNOSTIC TESTS
A. See Appendix Table 13A.1 for listing of common diagnostic tests.

DIFFERENTIAL DIAGNOSES
A. Community acquired pneumonia (CAP).
B. Common cold.
C. Atypical pneumonia.
D. Aspiration pneumonia.
E. *Pneumocystis jirovecii* pneumonia.
F. Middle East respiratory syndrome (MERS).
G. Avian influenza A (H5N1) virus infection.
H. Tuberculosis (TB).
I. Febrile neutropenia (BMJ Publishing Group, 2022).

POTENTIAL COMPLICATIONS
A. Multisystem inflammatory syndrome in children (MIS-C).
B. Post-acute care syndrome.
C. Mechanical ventilation.
D. Dehydration.
E. Hypoxia.
F. Stroke.
G. Venous thromboembolism.
H. Arrhythmias.
I. Heart failure.
J. Oliguria.
K. Acute respiratory distress syndrome (ARDS).
L. Acute kidney injury (AKI).
M. Neurological complications.
N. Gastrointestinal complications.
O. Cardiomyopathy.
P. Sepsis.
Q. Shock.
R. Multi-organ failure.
S. Secondary infections.
T. Pneumothorax.
U. Barotrauma.
V. Elevated liver enzymes.
W. Delirium.
X. Encephalopathy.
Y. Thrombosis.
Z. Risk factors for premature atrial contractions (PACS) include:
1. Severe COVID symptoms, especially those requiring intensive care.
2. Underlying chronic illness.

3. Lack of vaccination for COVID-19.
4. Multisystem inflammatory syndrome (MIS) during or after COVID-19 (Anesi et al., 2022; CDC, 2022c).

DISEASE-MODIFYING TREATMENTS
A. COVID-19 vaccination.
B. Medical management may involve:
1. Critical care for children with MIS-C.
2. Extracorporeal membrane oxygenation (ECMO).
3. Mechanical ventilation.
4. Critical care for adults with acute and/or multi-system complications.
5. Ritonavir-boosted nirmatrelvir (Paxlovid).

C. COVID-19 treatment guidelines are frequently updated as new information becomes available. For the most up-to-date guidelines, see: https://www.covid19treatmentguidelines.nih.gov/about-the-guidelines/(Anesi, et al., 2022; CDC, 2022c).

PALLIATIVE INTERVENTIONS/SYMPTOM MANAGEMENT
A. See Appendix Table 13A.2 for listing of palliative interventions and symptom management.
B. See Appendix D-3 for overview of common symptoms.
C. See Figure 13.5.

PROGNOSIS
A. Up to 20% of those infected with COVID-19 require hospitalization.
B. Of those requiring hospitalization, nearly 25% require intensive care.
C. Mortality ranges from 12% to 78% with an average of 25% to 50%.
D. Death often occurs from cardiac or pulmonary complications.
E. The highest death rates are among those >64 years (Anesi et al., 2022; CDC, 2022c).

NURSING INTERVENTIONS
A. Provide education on disease process and symptom management.
B. Teach patient transmission prevention strategies (see Appendix B-8).
C. Teach patient to take all medications as prescribed.
D. Teach importance of vaccination.
E. Educate patient and caregiver(s) on signs of complications.
F. Encourage smoking cessation (see Appendices B-10 and C-9).
G. Provide spiritual support.
H. Assess caregiver fatigue/burnout.
I. Encourage completion of advance directives.
J. Discuss wishes regarding withholding or withdrawing of life-sustaining interventions in late stage of disease with patient (if possible) and/or primary caregiver (see Appendices C-2, C-3, C-4, and Table 13.4).

Palliative Care for COVID-19

Relief of Dyspnea

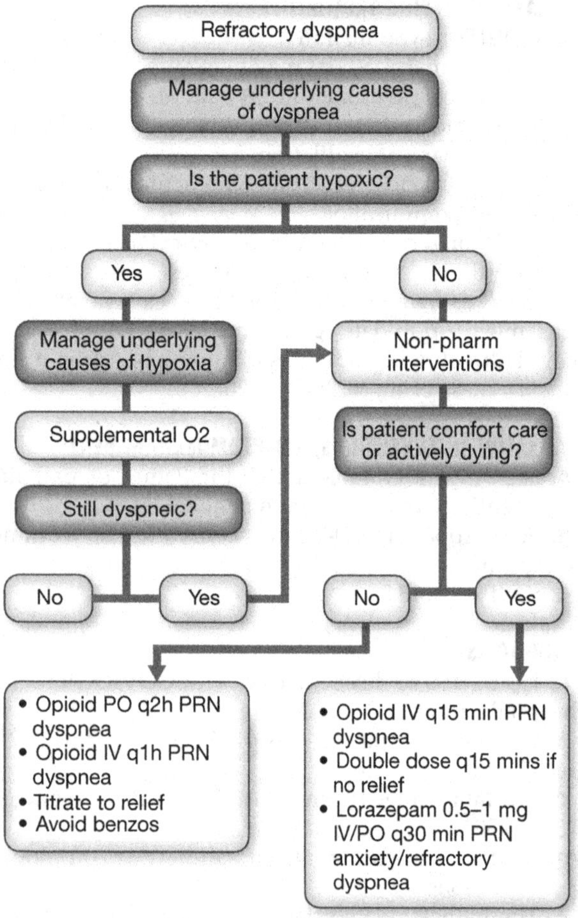

```
Refractory dyspnea
        ↓
Manage underlying causes
of dyspnea
        ↓
Is the patient hypoxic?
    ↓           ↓
   Yes          No
    ↓           ↓
Manage underlying    Non-pharm
causes of hypoxia    interventions
    ↓                   ↓
Supplemental O2    Is patient comfort care
    ↓              or actively dying?
Still dyspneic?      ↓        ↓
  ↓      ↓          No       Yes
 No     Yes
```

- Opioid PO q2h PRN dyspnea
- Opioid IV q1h PRN dyspnea
- Titrate to relief
- Avoid benzos

- Opioid IV q15 min PRN dyspnea
- Double dose q15 mins if no relief
- Lorazepam 0.5–1 mg IV/PO q30 min PRN anxiety/refractory dyspnea

Non-Pharmacologic Interventions:
- Bring patient upright or to sitting position
- Consider mindfulness, mindful breathing

Pharmacologic Interventions:
- Opioids are treatment of choice for refractory dyspnea
- For symptomatic patients, using PRN or bolus dosing titrated to relief is more effective and safe compared to starting an opioid infusion

Dosing Tips:
- For opioid-naïve patients
  - PO morphine 5–10 mg
  - PO oxycodone 2.5–5 mg
  - IV/SQ morphine 2–4 mg
  - IV/SQ hydromorphone 0.4–0.6 mg
- Consider smaller doses for older adults/frail

Opioid Quick Tips

Pharmacodynamics of Opioids:
- Time to peak effect/Duration of action
- PO opioids: 30–60 minutes/3–4 hours
- IV opioids: 5–15 minutes/3–4 hours
- Time to peak effect is the same for analgesia, relief of dyspnea, and sedation

Other Opioid Principles:
- If initial dose of IV opioid is ineffective after 2 doses at least 15 minutes apart, double the dose
- Typically need 6–8 hours of controlled symptoms to calculate a continuous opioid infusion
- If starting a continuous infusion, do not change more often than every 6 hours. Adjust infusion dose based on the 24-hour sum of PRNs

Relative Strengths and Conversion

Opioid Agent	Oral Dose	IV Dose
Morphine	30	10
Oxycodone	20	–
Hydromorphone	7.5	1.5

*Avoid fentanyl due to shortage

If Using Opioids, Start a Bowel Regimen:
- Goal is 1 BM QD or QOD, no straining
- Senna 2 tabs q HS, can increase to 4 tabs BID
- Add Miralax 17 gm daily, can increase to BID
- Bisacodyl 10 mg suppository if no BM in 72 hrs

FIGURE 13.5 COVID-19 symptom management.

BID, two times per day; BM, bowel movement; PO, by mouth; PRN, as needed, QD, every day; QOD, every other day, SQ, subcutaneous.

Source: Adapted from Center to Advance Palliative Care. (2020). *Pocket card: COVID symptom management and key communication phrases.* https://www.capc.org/documents/784/.

TABLE 13.4   COVID-19 COMMUNICATION GUIDE

Communication skills	
What they say	**What you say**
How bad is this?	From the information I have now, your loved one's situation is serious enough that your loved one should be in the hospital. **We will know more over the next day**, and we will update you.
Is my mother going to make it?	**I imagine you are scared**. Here's what I can say: Because she is 70 and is already dealing with other medical problems, **it is possible that she will not make it out of the hospital. Honestly, it is too soon to say for certain**.
Shouldn't she be in an ICU?	You/your loved one's situation does not meet criteria for the ICU right now. We are supporting her with treatments (oxygen) to relieve her shortness of breath and we are closely monitoring her condition. **We will provide all the available treatment we have that will help her and we'll keep in touch with you by phone**.
What happens if she gets sicker?	If she gets sicker, we will continue to do our best to support her with oxygen and medicines for her breathing. If she gets worse despite those best treatments, she will be evaluating for her likelihood of benefiting from treatment with a ventilator. I can see that you really care about her.
How can you just take her off a ventilator when her life depends on it?	Unfortunately, her condition has gotten worse, even though we are doing everything. She is dying now and the ventilator is not helping her to improve as we had hoped. This means that we need to take her off the ventilator to make sure she has a peaceful death and does not suffer. I wish things were different.
Resuscitation status COVID-19	**Example language**
Approach to when your clinical judgment is that a patient would not benefit from resuscitation	Given your overall condition, **I worry that if your heart or lungs stopped working, a breathing machine or CPR won't be able to help you live longer or improve your quality of life.** My recommendation is that if we get to that point, we use medications to focus on your comfort and allow you to die peacefully. This means we would not have you go to the ICU, be on a breathing machine, or use CPR. I imagine this may be hard to hear.
If in agreement:	These are really hard conversations. I think this plan makes the most sense for you.
If not in agreement:	These are really hard conversations. **We may need to talk about this again**.

Source: Center to Advance Palliative Care. (2020). *Pocket card: COVID symptom management and key communication phrases.* https://www.capc.org/documents/784/.

K. Educate patient and family regarding availability of palliative care.
L. Educate patient and family regarding availability of hospice services (when appropriate).
M. Provide referral to community support groups, as needed.

TUBERCULOSIS

DEFINITION/CHARACTERISTICS
A. Tuberculosis (TB) is a disease that usually affects the lungs but can affect the:
1. Kidneys.
2. Spine.
3. Brain.

B. There are two forms of TB (see Table 13.5):
1. Latent TB (LTB) infection.
   a. Asymptomatic.
   b. Not transmissible.
2. TB disease (TBD).
   a. Active disease.
   b. Symptomatic.
   c. Transmittable (CDC, 2021, 2022d).

INCIDENCE AND PREVALENCE
A. Worldwide, TB is the leading cause of death from curable infection.
B. The number of TB cases has declined each year since 1992, when a resurgence was caused by the HIV epidemic.

TABLE 13.5   LATENT TUBERCULOSIS VERSUS TUBERCULOSIS DISEASE

Person With LTBI	Person With TB disease
Has a small amount of TB bacteria in his/her body that are alive but **inactive**	Has a large amount of **active** TB bacteria in his/her body
Cannot spread TB bacteria to others	May spread TB bacteria to others
Does **not** feel sick, but may become sick if the bacteria in his/her body become active	May feel sick, and may have symptoms such as a cough, fever, and/or weight loss
Usually has a **positive** TB skin test or TB blood test result indicating TB infection	Usually has a **positive** TB skin test or TB blood test result indicating TB infection
Chest radiograph is typically **normal**	Chest radiograph may be **abnormal**
Sputum smears and cultures are **negative**	Sputum smears and cultures may be **positive**
Should consider treatment for LTBI to prevent TB disease	Needs treatment for TB disease
Does **not** require respiratory isolation	May require respiratory isolation
Is not a TB case	Is a TB case

LTBI, latent tuberculosis infection; TB, tuberculosis.

Source: Centers for Disease Control and Prevention. (2021). *Core curriculum on tuberculosis: What the clinician should know.* https://www.cdc.gov/tb/education/corecurr/pdf/CoreCurriculumTB-508.pdf

C. If left untreated, 1 in 10 people with LTB will develop TBD.

D. There were 7,860 cases of TB reported in the United States in 2021.

E. Up to 13 million people are living with TB worldwide.

F. Worldwide, there has been an upsurge in:
1. Multidrug-resistant TB (MDR-TB).
2. Extensively drug-resistant TB (XTR-TB; Brashers & Huether, 2019; CDC, 2022d).

ETIOLOGY

A. TB is caused by *Mycobacterium tuberculosis.*

B. *M. tuberculosis* is an acid-fast bacillus (Brashers & Huether, 2019; CDC, 2022d).

PATHOPHYSIOLOGY

A. TB is contracted through exposure to infected airborne droplets of 1 to 5 microns in diameter (see Table 13.6).

B. *M. tuberculosis* bacilli primarily invade the lungs of the host.

C. The host's immune response involves macrophage release.

D. Macrophages surround and trap the bacilli in the lungs.

E. Most bacilli are destroyed.

F. Some bacilli resist lysosomal destruction and multiply within the macrophages.

G. When the macrophages die, the bacilli are released.

H. Bacilli travel via the lymphatic system to the:
1. Lungs.
2. Lymph nodes.
3. Kidneys.
4. Brain.
5. Bone.

I. *M. tuberculosis* bacilli are present in the oropharynx and upper respiratory system of the host.

J. The bacilli are spread when the infected host coughs, sneezes, shouts, or sings.

K. TB is not transmitted on the surfaces of objects (Brashers & Huether, 2019; CDC, 2021, 2022d).

PREDISPOSING FACTORS

A. Institutional living.

B. Homelessness.

C. Substance abuse.

D. Lack of access to medical care/screening.

E. Immunocompromised status secondary to:
1. HIV.
2. Diabetes mellitus.
3. Severe kidney disease.
4. Low body mass index (BMI).
5. Medical treatments that suppress the immune response.

F. Those at risk for progression of LTB to TBD include (see Figure 13.6):
1. Immunocompromised patients.
2. Children younger than 5 years.

TABLE 13.6   FACTORS THAT INCREASE TRANSMISSION OF TB

Factor	Description
Concentration of infectious droplet nuclei	The more droplet nuclei in the air, the more probable that *M. tuberculosis* will be transmitted
Space	Exposure in small, enclosed spaces
Ventilation	Inadequate local or general ventilation that results in insufficient dilution or removal of infectious droplet nuclei
Air circulation	Recirculation of air containing infectious droplet nuclei
Specimen handling	Improper specimen-handling procedures that generate infectious droplet nuclei
Air pressure	Lack of negative air pressure in infectious patient's room that causes *M. tuberculosis* organisms to flow to other areas

TB, tuberculosis.

Source: Centers for Disease Control and Prevention. (2021). *Core curriculum on tuberculosis: What the clinician should know.* https://www.cdc.gov/tb/education/corecurr/pdf/CoreCurriculumTB-508.pdf

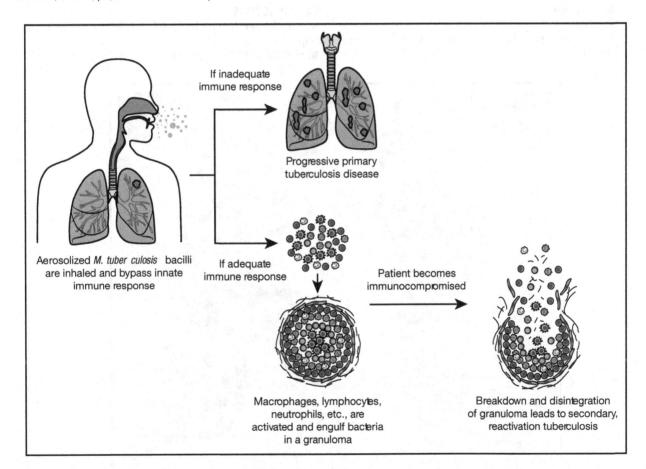

FIGURE 13.6.   Activation or reactivation of tuberculosis disease.

3. Medically underserved groups.
4. History of:
   a. Gastric bypass surgery.
   b. Untreated or inadequately treated TBD.
   c. Diabetes mellitus.
   d. Silicosis.
   e. Chronic renal failure.
   f. Acute Renal Failure.
   g. Cancer.
   h. Low BMI.
   i. Cigarette smoking.
   j. Alcohol or drug abuse (Brashers & Huether, 2019; CDC, 2021, 2022d).

SUBJECTIVE DATA

A. LTB is asymptomatic with no radiologic evidence of disease.
B. TBD involves:
   1. Fatigue.
   2. Lethargy.
   3. Dyspnea.
   4. Chest pain.
   5. Bone pain (Brashers & Huether, 2019; CDC, 2021, 2022d).

OBJECTIVE DATA

A. LTB is asymptomatic with no radiologic evidence of disease.
B. TBD involves:
   1. Weight loss.
   2. Anorexia.
   3. Low-grade fever that usually occurs in the afternoon.
   4. Night sweats.
   5. Productive cough.
   6. Hemoptysis.
   7. Neurological deficits.
   8. Meningitis.
   9. Dysuria.
   10. Chest x-ray reveals (see Figure 13.7):
      a. Nodules.
      b. Calcifications.
      c. Cavities.
      d. Hilar enlargement (Brashers & Huether, 2019; CDC, 2021, 2022d).

DIAGNOSTIC TESTS

A. See Appendix Table 13A.1 for listing of common diagnostic tests.
B. See Table 13.7 for classification.

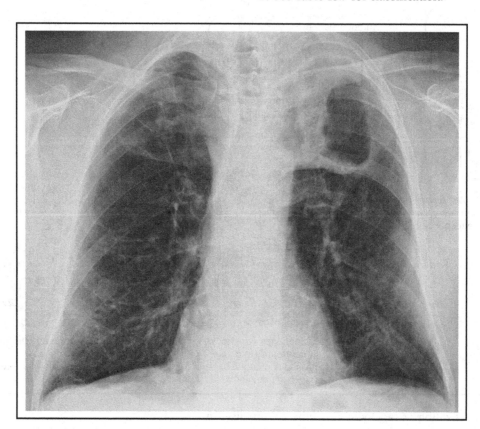

FIGURE 13.7   X-ray image of tuberculosis disease.

Source: Epontzer. (2020). *Chest x-ray of severe tuberculosis of the lungs.*

TABLE 13.7   CLASSIFICATION OF TUBERCULOSIS

Class	Type	Description
0	No TB exposure—**not** infected	• No history of TB exposure and no evidence of *M. tuberculosis* infection or disease • Negative reaction to TST or IGRA
1	TB exposure—no evidence of infection	• History of exposure to *M. tuberculosis* • Negative reaction to TST or IGRA (test given at least 8 to 10 weeks after exposure)
2	TB infection—no TB disease	• Positive reaction to TST or IGRA • Negative bacteriological studies (smear and cultures) • No clinical or radiographic evidence of active TB disease
3	TB disease clinically active	• Positive culture for *M. tuberculosis* **OR** • Positive reaction to TST or IGRA, plus clinical, bacteriological, or radiographic evidence of current active TB disease
4	Previous TB disease (**not** clinically active)	• May have past medical history of TB disease • Abnormal but stable radiographic findings • Positive reaction to the TST or IGRA • Negative bacteriological studies (smear and cultures) • No clinical or radiographic evidence of current active TB disease
5	TB disease suspected	Signs and symptoms of active TB disease, but medical evaluation **not** complete

IGRA, interferon-gamma release assay; TB, tuberculosis; TST, tuberculin skin test.

Source: Centers for Disease Control and Prevention. (2021). *Core curriculum on tuberculosis: What the clinician should know.* https://www.cdc.gov/tb/education/corecurr/pdf/CoreCurriculumTB-508.pdf

DIFFERENTIAL DIAGNOSES
A. Blastomycosis.
B. Tularemia.
C. Actinomycosis.
D. Other mycobacterium infections.
E. Squamous cell carcinoma (Herchline, 2020).

POTENTIAL COMPLICATIONS
A. Back pain.
B. Arthralgia.
C. Arthritis.
D. Meningitis.
E. Liver damage.
F. Kidney damage.
G. Cardiac tamponade.
H. Adverse effects related to medication management:
   1. Paresthesias.
   2. Weakness.
   3. Fatigue.
   4. Bruising or bleeding.
   5. Vision changes.
   6. Anorexia.
   7. Nausea.
   8. Jaundice.
   9. Discolored urine (Mayo Clinic, 2023).

DISEASE-MODIFYING TREATMENTS
A. Bacille Calmette–Guérin (BCG) vaccine.
B. Antibiotics.
   1. Isoniazid.
   2. Rifampin.
   3. Pyrazinamide.
   4. Ethambutol.
C. Antibiotic therapy can last 6 to 24 months, depending on the strain of TB (Brashers & Huether, 2019; CDC, 2021, 2022d; National Health Service, 2022).

PALLIATIVE INTERVENTIONS/SYMPTOM MANAGEMENT
A. See Appendix Table 13.A2 for listing of palliative interventions and symptom management.
B. See Appendix D-3 for overview of common symptoms.

PROGNOSIS
A. The prognosis for TB, when treated, is very good.
B. If TB is left untreated, the mortality rate is 50%.
C. For those with LTB, the risk for developing TBD is:
   1. About 10% during their lifetime.
   2. About 30% during their lifetime with a concomitant diagnosis of diabetes.

▶

3. About 7% to 10% every year with a concomitant diagnosis of HIV (Adigun & Singh, 2022; CDC, 2021).

NURSING INTERVENTIONS

A. Provide education on disease process and symptom management.

B. Teach patient transmission prevention strategies.

C. Teach patient to take all medications as prescribed.

D. Teach importance of adherence to treatment plan.

E. Teach patient not to ingest alcohol during treatment.

F. Manage symptoms of comorbidities.

G. Report suspected or confirmed cases of TB to the Department of Health within 24 hours.

H. Educate patient and caregiver(s) on signs of complications.

I. Encourage smoking cessation (see Appendices B-10 and C-9).

J. Provide spiritual support.

K. Assess caregiver fatigue/burnout (Appendix B-5).

L. Encourage completion of advance directives.

M. Discuss wishes regarding withholding or withdrawing of life-sustaining interventions in late stage of disease with patient (if possible) and/or primary caregiver (see Appendices C-2, C-3, C-4, and Figure 13.5).

N. Educate patient and family regarding availability of palliative care.

O. Educate patient and family regarding availability of hospice services (when appropriate).

P. Provide referral to community support groups, as needed.

REFERENCES

Adigun, R., & Singh, R. (2022). *Tuberculosis.* https://www.ncbi.nlm.nih.gov/books/NBK441916/

Anesi, G. L., Manaker, S., & Finlay, G. (2022). *COVID-19: Epidemiology, clinical features, and prognosis of the critically ill adult.* https://www.uptodate.com/contents/covid-19-epidemiology-clinical-features-and-prognosis-of-the-critically-ill-adult

BMJ Publishing Group. (2022). *Coronavirus disease 2019 (COVID-19).* https://bestpractice.bmj.com/topics/en-us/3000168/differentials

Bramati, P., & Bruera, E. (2021). Delirium in palliative care. *Cancers, 13*(23), 5893. https://www.mdpi.com/2072-6694/13/23/5893

Brashers, V. L., & Huether, S. E. (2019). Alterations in pulmonary function. In K. L. McCance & S. E. Huether (Eds.), *Pathophysiology: The biologic basis for disease in adults and children* (8th ed., pp. 1163–1201). Elsevier.

Centers for Disease Control and Prevention. (2021). *Core curriculum on tuberculosis: What the clinician should know.* https://www.cdc.gov/tb/education/corecurr/pdf/CoreCurriculumTB-508.pdf

Centers for Disease Control and Prevention. (2022a). *Systemic lupus erythematosus (SLE).* https://www.cdc.gov/lupus/facts/detailed.html#causes

Centers for Disease Control and Prevention. (2022b). *About HIV.* https://www.cdc.gov/hiv/basics/whatishiv.html

Centers for Disease Control and Prevention. (2022c). *COVID-19.* https://www.cdc.gov/coronavirus/2019-ncov/your-health/about-covid-19.html

Centers for Disease Control and Prevention. (2022d). *Tuberculosis (TB).* https://www.cdc.gov/tb/default.htm

Chang, L., & Shukla, D. K. (2018). Imaging studies of the HIV-infected brain. *Handbook of Clinical Neurology, 152,* 229–264. https://www.sciencedirect.com/science/article/abs/pii/B9780444638496000189

Chippa, V., Aleem, A., & Anjum, F. (2021). *Post acute coronavirus (COVID-19) syndrome.* https://europepmc.org/article/NBK/nbk570608

Düll, M. M., & Kremer, A. E. (2019). Treatment of pruritus secondary to liver disease. Current gastroenterology reports, 21(9), 1–9. https://link.springer.com/article/10.1007/s11894-019-0713-6#Sec9

Fusco, F. (2021). Mouth care. In E. Bruera, I. J. Higginson, C. F. von Gunten, & T. Morita (Eds.), *Textbook of palliative medicine and supportive care.* Taylor & Francis Group.

Gilroy, S. A. (2021). *HIV infection and AIDS differential diagnoses.* https://emedicine.medscape.com/article/211316-differential

Guyer, D. L., Almhanna, K., & McKee, K. Y. (2020). Palliative care for patients with esophageal cancer: A narrative review. *Annals of Translational Medicine, 8*(17). https://doi.org/10.21037/atm-20-3676

Herchline, T. E. (2020). *Tuberculosis (TB) differential diagnoses.* https://emedicine.medscape.com/article/230802-differential

HIV.gov. (2022). *US statistics.* https://www.hiv.gov/hiv-basics/overview/data-and-trends/statistics

Johns Hopkins Medicine. (2022). *Coronavirus diagnosis: What should I expect?* https://www.hopkinsmedicine.org/health/conditions-and-diseases/coronavirus/diagnosed-with-covid-19-what-to-expect.gvfv

Klatt, E. C. (2022). *Pathology of HIV/AIDS.* (33rd ed.). Mercer University. https://webpath.med.utah.edu/AIDS2022.PDF

Kluger, B. M., Ney, D. E., Bagley, S. J., Mohile, N., Taylor, L. P., Walbert, T., & Jones, C. A. (2020). Top ten tips palliative care clinicians should know when caring for patients with brain cancer. *Journal of Palliative Medicine, 23*(3), 415–421. https://doi.org/10.1089/jpm.2019.0507

Marik, P. E., Iglesias, J., Varon, J., & Kory, P. (2021). A scoping review of the pathophysiology of COVID-19. *International Journal of Immunopathology and Pharmacology, 35.* https://doi.org/20587384211048026

Mayo Clinic. (2023). *Tuberculosis.* https://www.mayoclinic.org/diseases-conditions/tuberculosis/diagnosis-treatment/drc-20351256

McCance, A., & Huether, S. E. (2019). Structure, function, and disorders of the integument. In K. L. McCance & S. E. Huether (Eds.), *Pathophysiology: The biologic basis for disease in adults and children* (8th ed., pp. 1496–1529). Elsevier.

National Health Service. (2022). *Treatment: Tuberculosis (TB).* https://www.nhs.uk/conditions/tuberculosis-tb/treatment

National Institute of Health. (2021). *The stages of HIV infection.* https://hivinfo.nih.gov/understanding-hiv/fact-sheets/stages-hiv-infection

Rote, N. S. (2019). Infection. In K. L. McCance & S. E. Huether (Eds.), *Pathophysiology: The biologic basis for disease in adults and children* (8th ed., pp. 289–322). Elsevier.

Rote, N. S., & McCance, K. L. (2019). Alterations in immunity and inflammation. In K. L. McCance & S. E. Huether (Eds.), *Pathophysiology: The biologic basis for disease in adults and children* (8th ed., pp. 255–288). Elsevier.

Sommers, M. S. (2019). *Davis's diseases and disorders: A nursing therapeutics manual.* F.A. Davis. https://www.fadavis.com/

product/nursing-fundamentals-med-surg-diseases-disorders-nursing-therapeutics-manual-sommers-6

Tariq, R., & Singal, A. K. (2020). Management of hepatorenal syndrome: A review. *Journal of Clinical and Translational Hepatology, 8*(2), 192. https://www.ncbi.nlm.nih.gov/pmc/articles/PMC7438356/

Walker, Z., Possin, K. L., Boeve, B. F., & Aarsland, D. (2015). Lewy body dementias. *The Lancet, 386*(10004), 1683–1697. https://doi.org/10.1016/S0140-6736(15)00462-6

World Health Organization. (2022a). *HIV.* https://www.who.int/news-room/fact-sheets/detail/hiv-Aids

World Health Organization. (2022b). *Coronavirus disease pandemic (COVID-19).* https://www.who.int/emergencies/diseases/novel-coronavirus-2019

World Health Organization. (2022c). *WHO coronavirus (COVID-19) dashboard.* https://covid19.who.int/

World Health Organization. (2022d). *Hepatitis C.* https://www.who.int/news-room/fact-sheets/detail/hepatitis-c#

Yuki, K., Fujiogi, M., & Koutsogiannaki, S. (2020). COVID-19 pathophysiology: A review. *Clinical Immunology, 215,* 108427. https://doi.org/10.1016/j.clim.2020.108427

APPENDIX

TABLE 13A.1 DIAGNOSTIC TESTS FOR INFECTIOUS DISEASES

Type	Notes
Physical examination	• Thorough physical examination with detailed medical history and neurological examination
Imaging	• CT scan • MRI (HIV/AIDS) • X-ray (COVID-19, TB) • Electrocardiogram (COVID-19) • Lung ultrasound (COVID-19)
Laboratory tests	• Antibody test (HIV, AIDS) • Antigen/antibody test (HIV, AIDS) • Nucleic acid test (HIV, AIDS) • CBC (COVID-19) • Rapid antigen test (COVID-19) • PCR test (COVID-19) • COVID-19 antibody test (COVID-19) • D-dimer (COVID-19) • PT (COVID-19) • PTT (COVID-19) • TST (PPD; TB) • Immunoassays (TB): ▪ QFT-GIT ▪ T-SPOT®.TB test (T-Spot)
Pathology	• Staging aligns with disease progression (see Figure 13.2; HIV, AIDS) • Lung pathology (usually consistent with ARDS; COVID-19) • Sputum microscopy (TB) • Sputum culture (TB) • Indirect DST (TB) • Sputum staining (TB) • Tuberculosis-specific NAATs (TB) • TB severity is classified in stages 1 through 5 (See Table 13.7; TB)

CBC, complete blood count; COVID-19, coronavirus disease 2019; DST, drug susceptibility testing; NAATs, nucleic acid amplification tests; PCR, polymerase chain reaction; PPD, purified protein derivative; PT, prothrombin time; PTT, partial thromboplastin time; QFT-GIT, QuantiFERON®-TB Gold In-Tube test; TST, tuberculin skin test; TB, tuberculosis.

Sources: (Brashers, V. L., & Huether, S. E. (2019). Alterations in pulmonary function. In K. L. McCance & S. E. Huether (Eds.), *Pathophysiology: The biologic basis for disease in adults and children.* (8th ed., pp. 1163–1201). Elsevier; Centers for Disease Control & Prevention. (2021b). *Core curriculum on tuberculosis: What the clinician should know.* https://www.cdc.gov/tb/education/corecurr/pdf/CoreCurriculumTB-508.pdf; Centers for Disease Control and Prevention. (2022b). *About HIV.* https://www.cdc.gov/hiv/basics/whatishiv.html; Centers for Disease Control and Prevention. (2022c). *COVID-19.* https://www.cdc.gov/coronavirus/2019-ncov/your-health/about-covid-19.html; Centers for Disease Control and Prevention. (2022d). *Tuberculosis (TB).* https://www.cdc.gov/tb/default.htm; Chang, L., & Shukla, D. K. (2018). Imaging studies of the HIV-infected brain. *Handbook of clinical neurology, 152,* 229–264. https://www.sciencedirect.com/science/article/abs/pii/B9780444638496000189; Johns Hopkins Medicine. (2022). Coronavirus diagnosis: What should I expect? https://www.hopkinsmedicine.org/health/conditions-and-diseases/coronavirus/diagnosed-with-covid-19-what-to-expect.gvfv)

TABLE 13A.2 PALLIATIVE INTERVENTIONS/SYMPTOM MANAGEMENT FOR INFECTIOUS DISEASES

Symptom	Intervention
Anorexia	• Use of appetite stimulants (see Appendix D-1) • Offer small, frequent meals and snacks • Offer nutritional supplements
Anxiety and depression	• Antidepressants, anxiolytics, or benzodiazepines as indicated by patient's condition, age, and life expectancy (see Appendix D-1) • Non-pharmacological interventions (see Appendix D-2)
Brain fog	• Psychostimulants (see Appendix D-1), if necessary (COVID-19) • Occupational therapy (COVID-19) • Write a list of daily tasks (COVID-19) • Prepare for the next day the night before (COVID-19) • Label drawers or storage containers for easy access (COVID-19) • Designate locations of important items such as car keys and glasses (COVID-19) • Keep important phone numbers handy (COVID-19) • Keep a notepad handy to write down reminders (COVID-19) • Enlist helps from others as needed (COVID-19)
Caregiver burden	• Support of interdisciplinary hospice or palliative team • Non-pharmacological interventions for caregivers (see Appendix D-2)
Constipation	• Promotility agents (see Appendix D-1; TB) • Laxatives (see Appendix D-1; TB) • Ambulation (TB) • Increased dietary fiber (TB) • Increased fluids (as tolerated; TB)
Delirium	• Reverse the cause, if possible (HIV, TB) • Pharmacological and non-pharmacological interventions (see Appendices D-1, D-2; HIV, TB) • Frequently reorient patient if this is not distressing (HIV, TB) • Remove dangerous objects such as razors, lighters, etc. (HIV, TB) • Dim lights at night; ensure adequate lighting during the day (HIV, TB) • Provide peaceful and calming environment (HIV, TB) • Avoid immobilization (HIV, TB) • Manage pain and other symptoms (HIV, TB) • Ensure adequate nutrition and hydration within the limits of the disease process (HIV, TB)
Dyspnea (see Appendix D, Figure 13.5)	• Corticosteroids for reducing inflammation (COVID-19, TB) • Opioids to reduce inspiratory effort and tachypnea (COVID-19, TB) • Bronchodilators for opening airways (mechanism of action of relaxation of muscular bands that surround bronchi, thus widening the airway; COVID-19, TB) • Diuretics to reduce systemic congestion (COVID-19, TB) • Anticholinergics to reduce secretions, especially at the end of life (COVID-19, TB) • Use of fans (COVID-19, TB) • Lower temperature in the room (COVID-19, TB)
Fatigue and somnolence	• Alternate periods of rest with periods of activity • Utilize energy conversation techniques • Psychostimulants (see Appendix D-1)

(continued)

TABLE 13A.2 PALLIATIVE INTERVENTIONS/SYMPTOM MANAGEMENT FOR INFECTIOUS DISEASES *(CONTINUED)*

Symptom	Intervention
Fever	<ul><li>Address underlying cause, when possible</li><li>Use of antipyretics</li><li>Application of cool compresses</li><li>Increase fluids to address dehydration, if applicable</li></ul>
Frequent infection	<ul><li>Avoid crowds or large gatherings (HIV, AIDS)</li><li>Wear mask when in the company of others (HIV, AIDS)</li><li>Wash hands frequently (HIV, AIDS)</li><li>Use of antibiotics or anti-infectives as indicated (HIV, AIDS)</li><li>Avoid animals and live plants (HIV, AIDS)</li><li>Avoid dental work (HIV, AIDS)</li><li>Avoid vaccines unless otherwise directed (HIV, AIDS)</li><li>Avoid raw foods (HIV, AIDS)</li></ul>
Gastrointestinal symptoms (see Appendix D-1)	<ul><li>Antacids (TB)</li><li>Antiemetics (TB)</li><li>Promotility agents (TB)</li><li>Laxatives (TB)</li></ul>
Hypoxia	<ul><li>Elevate head of bed (COVID-19, TB)</li><li>Use deep breathing and coughing techniques (COVID-19, TB)</li><li>Provide supplemental oxygen (COVID-19, TB)</li><li>Use opioids or bronchodilators as indicated (COVID-19, TB)</li><li>Address underlying anxiety and depression (COVID-19, TB)</li></ul>
Insomnia	<ul><li>Use of benzodiazepines, antidepressants, or antihistaminic agents, as indicated by patient's condition, age, and life expectancy (see Appendix D-1)</li><li>Provide proper sleep hygiene</li><li>Use non-pharmacological interventions for relaxation</li><li>Address underlying anxiety and depression</li></ul>
Lymphedema	<ul><li>Topical application of emollients containing lactic acid, urea, ceramides, glycerin, dimethicone, olive oil, or salicylic acid (HIV, AIDS)</li><li>Frequently assess for and promptly treat secondary infection (HIV, AIDS)</li><li>Use of topical steroids if skin becomes inflamed (HIV, AIDS)</li><li>Silver-containing polymer dressing for ulcers associated with primary lymphedema (HIV, AIDS)</li><li>Frequent dressing changes if lymphorrhea (drainage of lymphatic fluid directly through the skin) occurs to prevent skin breakdown (HIV, AIDS)</li><li>Application of low-pressure (40–60 mmHg) compression therapy (HIV, AIDS)</li><li>Physical and/or occupational therapy to increase muscle mass and stimulate lymphatic flow (HIV, AIDS)</li><li>Assess and treat pain associated with limb heaviness, fluid retention, and immobility (HIV, AIDS)</li><li>Address body image issues related to lymphedema (HIV, AIDS)</li></ul>
Nausea	<ul><li>Antiemetics (see Appendix D-1; TB)</li><li>Non-pharmacological interventions (see Appendix D-2; TB)</li></ul>

(continued)

TABLE 13A.2 PALLIATIVE INTERVENTIONS/SYMPTOM MANAGEMENT FOR INFECTIOUS DISEASES *(CONTINUED)*

Symptom	Intervention

Neuropathy	• Pharmacological interventions (see Appendix D-1; HIV, TB)
	  ▪ Antidepressants
	  ▪ Anticonvulsants (i.e., gabapentin)
	  ▪ Anesthetics (i.e., ketamine)
	  ▪ Opioids

Night sweats	• Review medications and lower dosages on or discontinue medications that can cause hyperhidrosis (i.e., hormones, antidepressants, aromatase inhibitors, etc.) • Use cotton bed linens and light pajamas • Offer cool washcloths to forehead and under arms • Open window and/or use fan • Increase fluid intake as appropriate • Avoid alcohol use • Consider use of nonsteroidal anti-inflammatory medications and/or corticosteroids
Pain management	• See Appendix E
Pruritus	• Thorough dermatological exam to establish cause (TB) • Depending on cause, topical agents such as ointments, barrier creams, or soaks can be trialed (e.g., calamine, menthol, oatmeal bath, antihistamine cream; TB) • Systemic antihistamines may be used but are not recommended for older adults (see Appendix D-1; TB) • Maintain short fingernails (TB)
Psychosocial distress and body image changes	• Antidepressants • Non-pharmacological interventions (see Appendix D-2)
Stomatitis	• Treat underlying cause, if possible (e.g. candidiasis, viral infections; HIV, AIDS) • Use of amifostine, if indicated (HIV, AIDS) • Offer patient ice chips or sips of water as tolerated (HIV, AIDS) • Oral topical anesthetics (HIV, AIDS)
Xerostomia (HIV, AIDS)	• Ensure adequate fluid intake; provide sips of water or ice chips as tolerated (HIV, AIDS) • Discontinue medications that cause xerostomia, if possible (HIV, AIDS) • If supplemental oxygen is in use, add humidification (HIV, AIDS) • Use salivary supplements or stimulants (e.g., pilocarpine; HIV, AIDS) • Offer patient sugar-free gum, if able to chew without pain (HIV, AIDS) • Provide moist, soft foods at mealtimes (HIV, AIDS) • Non-pharmacological interventions (Appendix D-2; HIV, AIDS)

Sources: Bramati, P., & Bruera, E. (2021). Delirium in palliative care. *Cancers, 13*(23), 5893. https://www.mdpi.com/2072-6694/13/23/5893; Düll & Kremer, 2019; Fusco, F. (2021). Mouth care. In E. Bruera, I. J. Higginson, C. F. von Gunten, & T. Morita (Eds.), *Textbook of palliative medicine and supportive care.* Taylor & Francis Group; Guyer, D. L., Almhanna, K., & McKee, K. Y. (2020). Palliative care for patients with esophageal cancer: A narrative review. *Annals of Translational Medicine, 8*(17). https://doi.org/10.21037/atm-20-3676; Kluger, B. M., Ney, D. E., Bagley, S. J., Mohile, N., Taylor, L. P., Walbert, T., & Jones, C. A. (2020). Top ten tips palliative care clinicians should know when caring for patients with brain cancer. *Journal of Palliative Medicine, 23*(3), 415–421. https://doi.org/10.1089/jpm.2019.0507; Sommers, M. S. (2019). *Davis's diseases and disorders: A nursing therapeutics manual.* F.A. Davis. https://www.fadavis.com/product/nursing-fundamentals-med-surg-diseases-disorders-nursing-therapeutics-manual-sommers-6; Tariq, R., & Singal, A. K. (2020). Management of hepatorenal syndrome: A review. *Journal of Clinical and Translational Hepatology, 8*(2), 192. https://www.ncbi.nlm.nih.gov/pmc/articles/PMC7438356/; Walker, Z., Possin, K. L., Boeve, B. F., & Aarsland, D. (2015). Lewy body dementias. *The Lancet, 386*(10004), 1683–1697. https://doi.org/10.1016/S0140-6736(15)00462-6

CHAPTER 14

NEUROLOGICAL DISORDERS

AMYOTROPHIC LATERAL SCLEROSIS

DEFINITION/CHARACTERISTICS
A. Also called Lou Gehrig disease.
B. Progressive neurodegenerative disease.
C. Characterized by loss of motor neurons.
D. Results in progressive muscle weakness (ALS Association, 2022; Boss & Huether, 2019).

INCIDENCE AND PREVALENCE
A. Amyotrophic lateral sclerosis (ALS) is the most common motor neuron disease.
B. There are approximately 32,000 cases in the United States.
C. Each year, between 4,861 and 6,045 new cases are diagnosed.
D. Worldwide, ALS affects about 5 in 100,000 people.
E. Prevalence is higher among males (Boss & Huether, 2019; Centers for Disease Control and Prevention [CDC], 2022; Ingre et al., 2015; U.S. National Library of Medicine, 2022).

ETIOLOGY
A. Etiology is not known.
B. Genetic mutations have been found in ALS patients (Boss & Huether, 2019).

PATHOPHYSIOLOGY
A. Progressive degeneration and death of upper and lower motor neurons result in loss of muscle control and function.
B. Paresis often begins with a single muscle group.
C. Gradually, all striated muscles are affected, except for the heart and extraocular muscles.
D. It is uncommon for the urethral and anal sphincters to be affected.
E. The disease progresses to paralysis without remission (Boss & Huether, 2019).

PREDISPOSING FACTORS
A. Older age.
B. Male sex.
C. Exposure to:
  1. Heavy metals.
  2. Pesticides.
  3. Electromagnetic fields (EMFs).
D. Low body mass index (BMI).
E. Nutritional state (low-caloric intake; Ingre et al., 2015; Nowicka et al., 2019; see Figure 14.1).

SUBJECTIVE DATA
A. Sialorrhea.
B. Dyspnea.
C. Apathy.
D. Disinhibition.
E. Diminished emotional control.
F. Perseveration.
G. Depression.
H. Impaired quality of life.
I. Anxiety.
J. Fatigue.
K. Insomnia.
L. Weight loss (ALS Association, 2022; Caga et al., 2019; Mayo Clinic, 2022; U.S. National Library of Medicine, 2022).

OBJECTIVE DATA
A. Slurred speech.
B. Impaired gag reflex.
C. Uncontrolled laughing or crying.
D. Muscle weakness.
E. Incoordination.
F. Dysphagia.
G. Dysmasesis.
H. Muscle atrophy.
I. Impaired gait; tripping.
J. Spasticity.
K. Paresis.
L. Hypotonia.
M. Loss of body hair.
N. Thickening of nails.
O. Diaphoresis.
P. Clasp-knife reflex.
Q. Hyperactive deep tendon reflexes.
R. Diminished or absent cremasteric reflex or Babinski sign.
S. Coexistence of frontotemporal dementia.
T. Dystonia.
U. Poor respiratory effort (ALS Association, 2022; Caga et al., 2019; Mayo Clinic, 2022; U.S. National Library of Medicine, 2022).

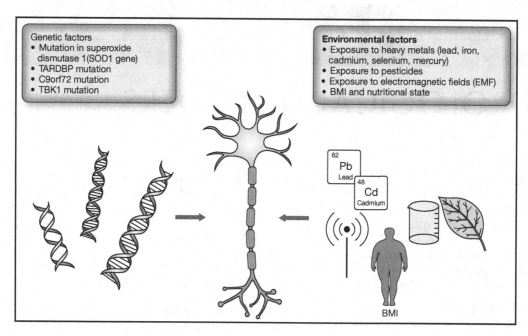

FIGURE 14.1 Risk factors for amyotrophic lateral sclerosis.

Source: Adapted from Nowicka, N., Juranek, J., Juranek, J. K., & Wojtkiewicz, J. (2019). Risk factors and emerging therapies in amyotrophic lateral sclerosis. *International Journal of Molecular Sciences, 20*(11), 2616. https://www.mdpi.com/142 2-0067/20/11/2616

DIAGNOSTIC TESTS

A. See Appendix Table 14A.1 for listing of common diagnostic tests.

B. See Figure 14.2 for staging.

DIFFERENTIAL DIAGNOSES

A. Brainstem lesion.

B. Brain mass or central nervous system (CNS) tumor.

C. Stroke.

D. Cranial nerve palsy.

E. Radiculopathy.

F. Neuropathy.

G. Polymyositis.

H. Acute viral infection.

I. Lymphoma.

J. Vasculitis.

K. Lyme disease.

L. Multiple sclerosis (Armon, 2018).

POTENTIAL COMPLICATIONS

A. Aspiration pneumonia.

B. Dependence for activities of daily living (ADLs).

C. Respiratory failure.

D. Weight loss.

E. Skin breakdown (U.S. National Library of Medicine, 2022).

DISEASE-MODIFYING TREATMENTS

A. There is no cure for ALS.

B. Treatments are directed at slowing progression and maintaining function and may include:

  1. Edaravone (Radicava).

  2. Riluzole (Rilutek).

  3. Baclofen.

  4. Diazepam.

  5. Trihexyphenidyl.

  6. Amitriptyline.

  7. Intercostal pump.

  8. Noninvasive positive pressure ventilation.

  9. Percutaneous endoscopic gastrostomy (PED).

  10. Diaphragmatic pacing (see Figure 14.3).

  11. Physical therapy.

  12. Occupational therapy.

  13. Speech therapy (ALS Association, 2022; Boss & Huether, 2019; Mayo Clinic, 2022; U.S. National Library of Medicine, 2022).

PALLIATIVE INTERVENTIONS/SYMPTOM MANAGEMENT

A. See Appendix Table 14A.2 for listing of palliative interventions and symptom management.

B. See Appendix D-3 for overview of common symptoms.

PROGNOSIS

A. Mean survival time is 2 to 5 years.

B. A small percentage of patients live up to 10 years after diagnosis (ALS Association, 2022; Boss & Huether, 2019).

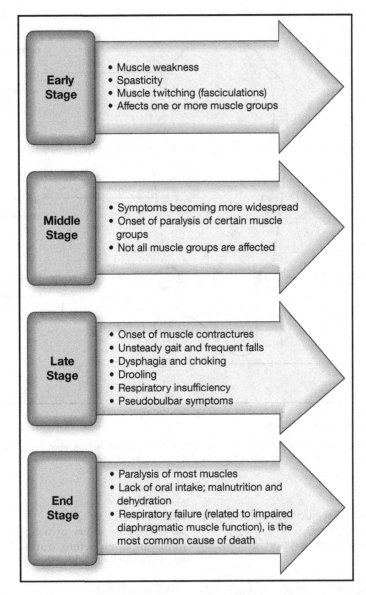

FIGURE 14.2 Stages of amyotrophic lateral sclerosis.

Source: Adapted from Muscular Dystrophy Association. (2022). *Amyotrophic lateral sclerosis (ALS).* https://www.mda.org/disease/amyotrophic-lateral-sclerosis/signs-and-symptoms/stages-of-als

NURSING INTERVENTIONS

A. Provide education on disease process and symptom management.

B. Teach patient how to use communication devices.

C. Teach patient to take all medications as prescribed.

D. Modify diet as needed to address dysphagia and dysmasesis.

E. Educate patient and caregiver(s) on disease trajectory.

F. Provide meticulous skin care.

G. Address dyspnea and respiratory distress.

H. Provide assistance with ADLs as needed.

I. Provide spiritual support.

J. Assess caregiver fatigue/burnout.

K. Encourage completion of advance directives.

L. Discuss wishes regarding withholding or withdrawing of life-sustaining interventions in late stage of disease with patient (if possible) and/or primary caregiver (see Appendices C-2, C-3, and C-4).

M. Educate patient and family regarding availability of palliative care.

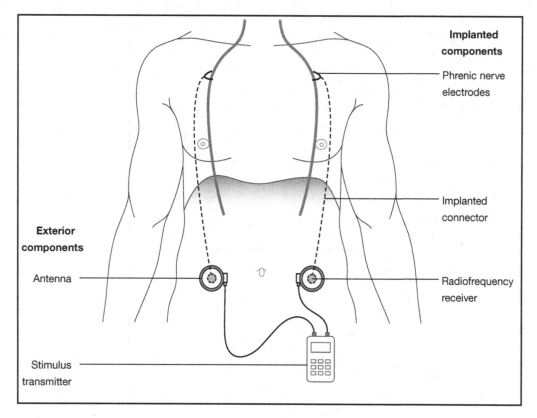

FIGURE 14.3 Diaphragmatic pacing.

Source: Adapted from Gu, X. Y., Ren, S., Shi, Y., Wang, N., Tong, Z. H., & Cai, M. L. (2020). Restoration methods of respiratory function for spinal cord injury. *Mathematical Problems in Engineering, 2020.* https://www.hindawi.com/journals/mpe/2020/7398789/

N. Educate patient and family regarding availability of hospice services (when appropriate).

O. Provide referral to community support groups, as needed.

CEREBRAL PALSY

DEFINITION/CHARACTERISTICS

A. Disorder of the cerebral cortex, which directs muscle function.

B. Results in impaired muscle tone and posture.

C. Symptoms typically appear in infancy or early childhood (Butterfield & Huether, 2019; National Institute of Neurological Disorders & Stroke [NINDS], 2022).

INCIDENCE AND PREVALENCE

A. Cerebral palsy (CP) is one of the most common diseases of childhood.

B. Affects nearly 500,000 (1 in 232) children in the United States.

C. Occurs in 2 to 3 out of 1,000 live births worldwide (Butterfield & Huether, 2019; Vitrikas et al., 2020).

ETIOLOGY

A. Caused by injury or abnormal development in the immature brain before, during, or after birth, or up to age 1 (Butterfield & Huether, 2019; Vitrikas et al., 2020).

PATHOPHYSIOLOGY

A. Thought to be related to inflammation that results in brain injury.

B. The cerebral changes caused by CP lead to:

1. Shortened muscles.
2. Contractures.
3. Muscle weakness.
4. Muscle stiffness.

C. Defects in muscle stem cells prevent regeneration of muscles and muscle growth (Morgan & McGinley, 2018).

PREDISPOSING FACTORS

A. Most cases are idiopathic.

B. Often, perinatal injury/complications are involved, such as:

1. Prenatal or perinatal hypoxia.
2. Hemorrhage.

3. Infection.

4. Genetic abnormalities.

5. Low birth weight.

6. Congenital abnormalities.

7. Mechanical or iatrogenic injuries.

8. Head trauma.

9. Metabolic disorders.

10. Electrolyte imbalances.

11. Toxicosis.

12. Maternal–fetal blood incompatibilities.

13. Premature labor.

14. Exposure to radiation.

15. Multiple gestation.

16. Complicated labor and delivery.

17. Intrauterine growth restriction.

18. Acidosis (Butterfield & Huether, 2019; Vitrikas et al., 2020).

SUBJECTIVE DATA

A. Emotional dysregulation.

B. Depression.

C. Constipation.

D. Nausea (Mayo Clinic, 2022; NINDS, 2022; Vitrikas et al., 2020).

OBJECTIVE DATA

A. Spinal deformities.

B. Hearing loss.

C. Incontinence.

D. Contractures.

E. Malnutrition.

F. Diplegia, hemiplegia, or tetraplegia.

G. Ataxia.

H. Spasticity.

I. Muscle weakness.

J. Walking on toes.

K. Crouched gait.

L. Scissor walking.

M. Drooling.

N. Dysphagia.

O. Dysarthria.

P. Tremors.

Q. Delayed muscle development.

R. Fine motor impairment.

S. Intellectual disabilities (possible).

T. Seizures.

U. Abnormal physical sensations or perceptions.

V. Impaired vision.

W. Vomiting.

X. Bowel obstruction.

Y. Osteoporosis (Mayo Clinic, 2022; NINDS, 2022; Vitrikas et al., 2020).

DIAGNOSTIC TESTS

A. See Appendix Table 14A.1 for listing of common diagnostic tests.

DIFFERENTIAL DIAGNOSES

A. Inherited metabolic disorders.

B. Intellectual disabilities.

C. Metabolic myopathies.

D. Tumors.

E. Arteriovenous malformations.

F. Fistulas of the spinal cord.

G. Metabolic neuropathies.

H. Rhett syndrome (Abdel-Hamid, 2018; Hallman-Cooper & Cabrero, 2021).

POTENTIAL COMPLICATIONS

A. Osteoarthritis.

B. Post-impairment syndrome.

C. Pressure ulcers.

D. Depression.

E. Premature aging.

F. Scoliosis.

G. Hypertension.

H. Incontinence.

I. Bladder dysfunction.

J. Dysphagia.

K. Aspiration pneumonia.

L. Bone fractures.

M. Hip displacement.

N. Epilepsy.

O. Equinus deformity (NINDS, 2022; Vitrikas et al., 2020).

DISEASE-MODIFYING TREATMENTS

A. There is no cure for CP.

B. Treatments are directed at slowing progression and maintaining function and may include:

1. Botulinum toxin A (BoNT-A).

2. Intrathecal baclofen.

3. Orthopedic surgery.

4. Neurosurgery (selective dorsal rhizotomy).

5. Assistive devices.

6. Stem cell therapy.

7. Nerve blocks.

8. Soft tissue lengthening surgery.

9. Tendon transfer (surgical).

10. Joint stabilization.

11. Physical therapy.

12. Occupational therapy.

13. Speech therapy.

14. Recreational therapy (NINDS, 2022; Sadowska et al., 2020).

PALLIATIVE INTERVENTIONS/SYMPTOM MANAGEMENT

A. See Appendix Table 14A.2 for listing of palliative interventions and symptom management.

B. See Appendix D-3 for overview of common symptoms.

PROGNOSIS

A. Related to the gestational age at the time of injury.

B. Severe disease lowers life expectancy due to respiratory complications.

C. Life expectancy is not reduced in those with mild impairment.

D. Aspiration pneumonia is the most common cause of death.

E. The 20-year survival rate is 85% to 94%.

F. In severe cases, life expectancy is 45 to 54 years (Barkoudah, 2022; Blair et al., 2019; Butterfield & Huether, 2019).

NURSING INTERVENTIONS

A. Provide education on disease process and symptom management.

B. Educate patient and caregiver(s) on disease trajectory.

C. Teach patient to take all medications as prescribed.

D. Address caregiver fatigue and emotional distress.

E. Address proper technique for lifting and transfers.

F. Monitor bone health; assess for risk of fractures.

G. Provide assistance with activities of daily living (ADLs) as needed, including application of braces, if used.

H. Implement fall precautions.

I. Provide proper incontinence care, as needed.

J. Implement pain management (pharmacological and non-pharmacological).

K. Provide spiritual support.

L. Encourage completion of advance directives.

M. Discuss wishes regarding withholding or withdrawing of life-sustaining interventions in late stage of disease with patient (if possible) and/or primary caregiver (see Appendices C-2, C-3, and C-4).

N. Educate patient and family regarding availability of palliative care.

O. Educate patient and family regarding availability of hospice services (when appropriate).

P. Provide referral to community support groups, as needed.

MUSCULAR DYSTROPHY

DEFINITION/CHARACTERISTICS

A. An umbrella term used to describe:

　　1. Neurological, genetic conditions that cause:

　　　　a. Progressive muscle weakness.

　　　　b. Muscle atrophy.

B. There are several types of muscular dystrophy (MD):

　　1. Sex-related (male) MDs.

　　　　a. Duchenne muscular dystrophy (DMD).

　　　　b. Becker muscular dystrophy (BMD).

　　　　c. Emery–Dreifuss.

　　2. Autosomal dominant MDs.

　　　　a. Distal.

　　　　b. Ocular.

　　　　c. Facioscapulohumeral dystrophy.

　　　　d. Oculopharyngeal.

　　3. Autosomal recessive MD.

　　　　a. Limb-girdle MD (CDC, 2020; Do, 2021; Sommers, 2019; Wright, 2019).

INCIDENCE AND PREVALENCE

A. DMD and BMD are the most common forms.

B. DMD and BMD primarily affects males.

C. MD has a higher prevalence among White males.

D. Worldwide, MD affects 3.6 per 100,000 people.

E. In the Americas, 5.1 per 100,000 people are affected (CDC, 2020; Do, 2021; Salari et al., 2022).

ETIOLOGY

A. MD results from a genetic mutation that affects muscle proteins (NINDS, 2020).

PATHOPHYSIOLOGY

A. Duchenne and Becker MD:

　　1. Genetic alterations reduce dystrophin levels, which causes cellular instability, leading to muscle cell degradation, and death.

B. Other forms of MD:

　　1. Genetic alterations cause altered coding of dystrophin-associated glycoproteins, which, due to their location, manifest in specific areas. Examples are:

　　　　a. Oculopharyngeal MD.

　　　　b. Limb-girdle MD (Do, 2021).

PREDISPOSING FACTORS

A. Genetic predisposition (Do, 2021).

SUBJECTIVE DATA

A. Dyspnea.

B. Extreme fatigue (Wright, 2019).

OBJECTIVE DATA

A. Impaired gait; tripping.

B. Lower extremity edema.

C. Cognitive dysfunction (possible).

D. Incontinence.

E. Muscle cramping.

F. Frequent falls.

G. Dysphagia.

H. Arrythmias.

I. Cardiomyopathies.

J. Difficulty rising from a seated or lying position.

K. Elevated serum creatine kinase.

L. Neck flexor weakness.

M. Waddling gait.

N. Respiratory insufficiency.

O. Scoliosis (Wright, 2019; Yiu & Kornberg, 2015).

DIAGNOSTIC TESTS
A. See Appendix Table 14A.1 for listing of common diagnostic tests.
B. See Table 14.1 for staging.

DIFFERENTIAL DIAGNOSES
A. Spinal muscle atrophy (Do, 2021).

POTENTIAL COMPLICATIONS
A. Left ventricular dysfunction.
B. Pulmonary failure (Mospan et al., 2016).

DISEASE-MODIFYING TREATMENTS
A. There is no cure for MD.
B. Treatments are directed at slowing progression and maintaining function and may include:
    1. Eteplirsen (Exondys 51)
    2. Steroids.
    3. Angiotensin converting enzyme (ACE) inhibitors.
    4. Beta-blockers.
    5. Physical therapy.
    6. Occupational therapy.
    7. Speech therapy.

PALLIATIVE INTERVENTIONS/SYMPTOM MANAGEMENT
A. See Appendix Table 14A.2 for listing of palliative interventions and symptom management.
B. See Appendix D-3 for overview of common symptoms.

PROGNOSIS
A. The prognosis for DMD is 20 to 30 years.
B. The average survival rate for DMD is 23 to 27.8 years.
C. The leading cause of death for those with DMD is cardiac or respiratory failure.
D. For patients who have BMD, life expectancy can be 40 years or more (Schwartz, 2019; Van Ruiten et al., 2016).

NURSING INTERVENTIONS
A. Provide education on disease process and symptom management.
B. Educate patient and caregiver(s) on disease trajectory.
C. Teach patient to take all medications as prescribed.
D. Address caregiver fatigue and emotional distress.
E. Address proper technique for lifting and transfers.
F. Promote cardiac health; monitor for symptoms of cardiac failure.
G. Address dyspnea and respiratory distress.
H. Monitor bone health; assess for risk of fractures.
I. Provide assistance with activities of daily living (ADLs) as needed, including application of braces, if used.
J. Provide spiritual support.
K. Encourage completion of advance directives.
L. Discuss wishes regarding withholding or withdrawing of life-sustaining interventions in late stage of disease with patient (if possible) and/or primary caregiver (see Appendices C-2, C-3, and C-4).

TABLE 14.1   CLINICAL STAGES OF MUSCULAR DYSTROPHY

STAGE	CLINICAL FEATURES
Stage 1: Early/Presymptomatic	Muscular dystrophy not yet diagnosed Developmental delays may be noticed during infancy
Stage 2: Early ambulatory	Begins to exhibit signs of motor dysfunction by walking on toes, using waddling gait, or using triad poses to move from floor to standing position (leaning hands on calves, then knees, then thighs to stand)
Stage 3: Late ambulatory	Difficulty noted with ambulation and with climbing stairs. Frequent falls and inability to stand after fall. Upper extremity weakness
Stage 4: Early nonambulatory	Nonambulatory. Able to propel wheelchair. Diminished trunk control and risk for scoliosis
Stage 5: Late nonambulatory	Progressive upper extremity dysfunction. Increased dependence for activities of daily living. Diminished cardiac and respiratory function
Stage 6: End-of-life care	Dependence for all activities of daily living. May require mechanical ventilation and/or tracheostomy. Severe cardiac disease that interferes with activities may be present

Source: Adapted from Sharma, A., Badhe, P., Gokulchandran, N., Chopra, G., Lohia, M., & Kulkarni, P. (2011). Stem cell therapy and other recent advances in muscular dystrophy. *Neurogen Brain and Spine Institute (EDs) publication.* https://www.stemcellsmumbai.com/book/Muscular%20 Dystrophy%20Book.pdf

M. Educate patient and family regarding availability of palliative care.

N. Educate patient and family regarding availability of hospice services (when appropriate).

O. Provide referral to community support groups, as needed.

PARKINSON DISEASE

DEFINITION/CHARACTERISTICS

A. A complex disorder involving motor and non-motor symptoms.

B. Categorized as:
  1. Primary (idiopathic).
  2. Secondary (cause can be identified; Boss & Huether, 2019).

INCIDENCE AND PREVALENCE

A. Onset of primary Parkinson disease (PD) is typically after age 40, with rising incidence after age 60.

B. There are about 60,000 new cases of PD diagnosed annually.

C. Roughly 10 million people are living with PD worldwide.

D. The incidence of PD has been rising over the past two decades (Bloem et al., 2021; Boss & Huether, 2019).

ETIOLOGY

A. Most cases of PD are idiopathic (primary).

B. About 10% of cases are familial.

C. Common causes of secondary PD are:
  1. Other neurodegenerative disorders.
  2. Acquired disorders.
  3. Drug-induced (Boss & Huether, 2019).

PATHOPHYSIOLOGY

A. The pathology of primary PD is not well understood.

B. PD is characterized by:
  1. Loss of dopamine.
  2. Basal ganglia deterioration.
  3. Lewy body formation.
  4. Decreased levels of norepinephrine.

C. Patterns of symptoms and disease progression are highly variable.

D. Often involves a lengthy prodromal period (see Figure 14.4; Bloem et al., 2021; Boss & Huether, 2019).

PREDISPOSING FACTORS

A. Genetic predisposition.

B. Exposure to certain neurotoxins.

C. Head injury (Bloem et al., 2021).

SUBJECTIVE DATA

A. Altered mentation.

B. Altered sensory status.

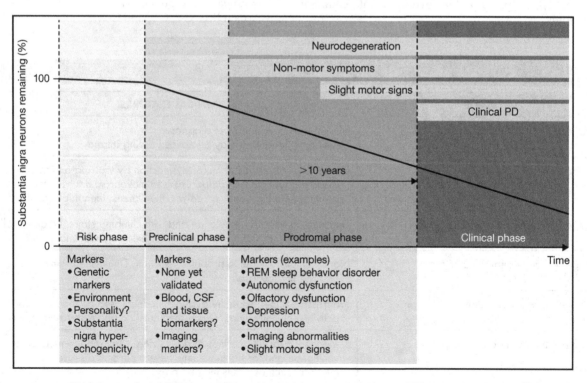

FIGURE 14.4 Parkinson disease trajectory.

Source: Adapted from Postuma, R. B., & Berg, D. (2016). Advances in markers of prodromal Parkinson disease. *Nature Reviews Neurology,* *12*(11), 622–634. https://www.nature.com/articles/nrneurol.2016.152

C. Sleep disorders.
 1. Frequent nightmares.
 2. Hyposomnia.
 3. Daytime drowsiness.
D. Pain.
E. Altered sense of smell and taste.
F. Visual changes.
G. Urinary urgency.
H. Difficulty concentrating.
I. Depression.
J. Apathy.
K. Hallucinations.
L. Alterations in executive functioning.
M. Impaired memory.
N. Visuospatial deficits.
O. Cognitive decline.
P. Pain.
Q. Postprandial fullness.
R. Asymmetric, vague shoulder pain (Bloem et al., 2021; Boss & Huether, 2019; Sveinbjornsdottir, 2016).

OBJECTIVE DATA
A. Resting tremor.
B. Rigidity.
C. Bradykinesia (or akinesia).
D. Postural disturbances.
E. Dysarthria.
F. Dysphagia.
G. Impaired ambulation.
H. Difficulty initiating movement.
I. Diaphoresis.
J. Orthostatic hypotension.
K. Drooling.
L. Constipation.
M. Dementia symptoms.
N. Masked facies.
O. Short, shuffling steps.
P. Muscle rigidity.

Q. Stooped posture.
R. Wide-based gait (Bloem et al., 2021; Boss & Huether, 2019; Sveinbjornsdottir, 2016).

DIAGNOSTIC TESTS
A. See Appendix Table 14A.1 for listing of common diagnostic tests.
B. See Table 14.2 for staging.

DIFFERENTIAL DIAGNOSES
A. Chorea in adults.
B. Dopamine-responsive dystonia.
C. Alzheimer disease.
D. Dementia with Lewy bodies.
E. Muscle system atrophy.
F. Progressive supranuclear palsy.
G. Corticobasal syndrome.
H. Drug-induced parkinsonism.
I. Vascular parkinsonism.
J. Normal pressure hydrocephalus.
K. Wilson disease.
L. Huntington disease.
M. Spinocerebellar ataxia.
N. Fragile-X dementia with parkinsonism.
O. Cardioembolic stroke.
P. Psychogenic parkinsonism.
Q. Atypical parkinsonism (Greenland & Barker; 2018; Hauser, 2020).

POTENTIAL COMPLICATIONS
A. Falls.
B. Aspiration pneumonia.
C. Pain.
D. Behavioral disturbances.
E. Psychosis.
F. Sleep attacks.
G. Dyskinesias.
H. Parkinsonism-hyperreflexia syndrome.
I. Impulse control disorders.

TABLE 14.2 STAGES OF PARKINSON DISEASE

STAGE 1	STAGE 2	STAGE 3	STAGE 4	STAGE 5
• Unilateral involvement • Limited functional impairment, if any	• Bilateral or midline involvement • Impaired balance • Risk for falls	• Impaired ability to right self when losing balance, resulting in falls • Mild to moderate disability	• Unassisted ambulation is unsteady but possible • Disease is severe and disabling	• Bedbound status • Complete dependence for activities of daily living

Source: Adapted from Hoehn, M. M., & Yahr, M. D. (2001). Parkinsonism: Onset, progression and mortality. *Neurology, 57*(10, Suppl. 3), S11–S26. https://psycnet.apa.org/record/2001-05820-00

J. Dysphagia.

K. Dysarthria.

L. Rapid eye motion (REM) sleep behavior disorder (Bloem et al., 2021; Simonet et al., 2020).

DISEASE-MODIFYING TREATMENTS

A. There is no cure for PD.

B. Pharmacological interventions include:

   1. Carbidopa–levodopa.

   2. Monoamine oxidase-B inhibitors.

   3. Dopamine agonists.

C. Deep brain stimulation.

D. Physical therapy.

E. Occupational therapy.

F. Speech therapy (Armstrong & Okun, 2020; Boss & Huether, 2019).

PALLIATIVE/SYMPTOM MANAGEMENT INTERVENTIONS

A. See Appendix Table 14A.2 for listing of palliative interventions and symptom management.

B. See Appendix D-3 for overview of common symptoms.

PROGNOSIS

A. Typical life expectancy is 6.9 to 14.3 years after diagnosis.

B. Rates of disease progression vary widely.

C. Common causes of death include complications from a fall or aspiration pneumonia (Armstrong & Okun, 2020; Bloem et al., 2021).

NURSING INTERVENTIONS

A. Provide education on disease process and symptom management.

B. Educate patient and caregiver(s) on disease trajectory (see Figure 14.4).

C. Teach patient to take all medications as prescribed.

D. Address caregiver fatigue and emotional distress.

E. Address proper technique for lifting and transfers.

F. Implement communication measures.

G. Address psychological aspects of PD.

H. Monitor risk for falls and implement appropriate interventions.

I. Provide assistance with activities of daily living (ADLs) as needed.

J. Provide spiritual support.

K. Encourage completion of advance directives.

L. Discuss wishes regarding withholding or withdrawing of life-sustaining interventions in late stage of disease with patient (if possible) and/or primary caregiver (see Appendices C-2, C-3, and C-4).

M. Educate patient and family regarding availability of palliative care.

N. Educate patient and family regarding availability of hospice services (when appropriate).

O. Provide referral to community support groups, as needed.

REFERENCES

Abdel-Hamid, H. (2018). *Cerebral palsy: Differential diagnoses.* https://emedicine.medscape.com/article/1179555-differential

ALS Association. (2022). *Understanding ALS.* https://www.als.org/understanding-als

Armon, C. A. (2018). *Amyotrophic lateral sclerosis differential diagnoses.* https://emedicine.medscape.com/article/1170097-differential

Armstrong, M. J., & Okun, M. S. (2020). Diagnosis and treatment of Parkinson disease: A review. *JAMA, 323*(6), 548–560. https://doi.org/10.1001/jama.2019.22360

Barkoudah, E. (2022). *Cerebral palsy: Overview of management and prognosis.* https://www.medilib.ir/uptodate/show/6176#rid85

Blair, E., Langdon, K., McIntyre, S., Lawrence, D., & Watson, L. (2019). Survival and mortality in cerebral palsy: Observations to the sixth decade from a data linkage study of a total population register and National Death Index. *BMC Neurology, 19*(1), 1–11. https://bmcneurol.biomedcentral.com/articles/10.1186/s12883-019-1343-1

Bloem, B. R., Okun, M. S., & Klein, C. (2021). Parkinson's disease. *The Lancet, 397*(10291), 2284–2303. https://doi.org/10.1016/S0140-6736(21)00218-X

Boss, J. B., & Huether, S. E. (2019). Alternations in cognitive systems, cerebral hemodynamics, and motor function. In K. L. McCance & S. E. Huether (Eds.), *Pathophysiology: The biologic basis for disease in adults and children* (8th ed., pp. 504–549). Elsevier.

Butterfield, R. J., & Huether, S. E. (2019). Alternations in neurological function in children. In K. L. McCance & S. E. Huether (Eds.), *Pathophysiology: The biologic basis for disease in adults and children* (8th ed., pp. 619–643). Elsevier.

Caga, J., Hsieh, S., Lillo, P., Dudley, K., & Mioshi, E. (2019). The impact of cognitive and behavioral symptoms on ALS patients and their caregivers. *Frontiers in Neurology, 10*, 192. https://www.frontiersin.org/articles/10.3389/fneur.2019.00192/full

Centers for Disease Control and Prevention. (2020). *What is muscular dystrophy?* https://www.cdc.gov/ncbddd/musculardystrophy/facts.html

Centers for Disease Control and Prevention. (2022). *National amyotrophic lateral sclerosis (ALS) registry.* https://www.cdc.gov/als/dashboard/index.html

Do, T. T. (2021). *Muscular dystrophy.* https://emedicine.medscape.com/article/1259041-overview#a8

Fusco, F. (2021). Mouth care. In E. Bruera, I. J. Higginson, C. F. von Gunten, & T. Morita (Eds.), *Textbook of palliative medicine and supportive care.* Taylor & Francis Group.

Greenland, J. C., & Barker, R. A. (2018). *The differential diagnosis of Parkinson's disease.* In T. B. Stoker & J. C. Greenland (Eds.), *Parkinson's disease: Pathogenesis and clinical aspects.* https://www.ncbi.nlm.nih.gov/books/NBK536715/ https://doi.org/10.15586/codonpublications.parkinsonsdisease.2018.ch6

Gu, X. Y., Ren, S., Shi, Y., Wang, N., Tong, Z. H., & Cai, M. L. (2020). Restoration methods of respiratory function for spinal cord injury. *Mathematical Problems in Engineering, 2020.* https://www.hindawi.com/journals/mpe/2020/7398789/

Guyer, D. L., Almhanna, K., & McKee, K. Y. (2020). Palliative care for patients with esophageal cancer: A narrative review. *Annals of Translational Medicine, 8*(17). https://doi.org/10.21037/atm-20-3676

Hallman-Cooper, J. L., & Cabrero, F. R. (2021). *Cerebral palsy.* https://www.ncbi.nlm.nih.gov/books/NBK538147/

Hauser, R. A. (2020). *Parkinson's disease: Differential diagnoses.* https://emedicine.medscape.com/article/1831191-differential

Hoehn, M. M., & Yahr, M. D. (2001). Parkinsonism: Onset, progression and mortality. *Neurology, 57*(10, Suppl 3), S11–S26. https://psycnet.apa.org/record/2001-05820-002

Ingre, C., Roos, P. M., Piehl, F., Kamel, F., & Fang, F. (2015). Risk factors for amyotrophic lateral sclerosis. *Clinical Epidemiology*, 7, 181. https://www.ncbi.nlm.nih.gov/pmc/articles/PMC4334292/

Khan, F., Amatya, B., Bensmail, D., & Yelnik, A. (2019). Non-pharmacological interventions for spasticity in adults: An overview of systematic reviews. *Annals of Physical and Rehabilitation Medicine*, 62(4), 265–273. https://pubmed.ncbi.nlm.nih.gov/29042299/

Kluger, B. M., Ney, D. E., Bagley, S. J., Mohile, N., Taylor, L. P., Walbert, T., & Jones, C. A. (2020). Top ten tips palliative care clinicians should know when caring for patients with brain cancer. *Journal of Palliative Medicine*, 23(3), 415–421. https://doi.org/10.1089/jpm.2019.0507

Kondziella, D., Amiri, M., Othman, M. H., Beghi, E., Bodien, Y. G., Citerio, G., Giacino, J. T., Mayer, S. A., Lawson, T. N., Menon, D. K., Rass, V., Sharshar, T., Stevens, R. D., Tinti, L., Vespa, P., McNett, M., Rao, C. P., V., Helbok, R., & Curing Coma Campaign Collaborators. (2022). Incidence and prevalence of coma in the UK and the USA. *Brain Communications*, 4(5), fcac188. https://doi.org/10.1093/braincomms/fcac188

Mayo Clinic. (2022). *Amyotrophic lateral sclerosis (ALS)*. https://www.mayoclinic.org/diseases-conditions/amyotrophic-lateral-sclerosis/diagnosis-treatment/drc-20354027

McGeachan, A. J., & Mcdermott, C. J. (2017). Management of oral secretions in neurological disease. *Practical Neurology*, 17(2), 96–103. https://doi.org/10.1136/practneurol-2016-001515

Morgan, P., & McGinley, J. L. (2018). Cerebral palsy. In B. L. Day & S. R. Lord (Eds.), *Handbook of clinical neurology: Balance, gait & falls* (Vol. 159., pp. 323–336). Elsevier.

Mospan, G. A., Vickery, P. B., & Riley, T. T. (2016). Muscular dystrophy: Options for complication management. *U.S. Pharmacist*, 41(1), HS2–6. https://www.uspharmacist.com/article/muscular-dystrophy-options-for-complication-management

Muscular Dystrophy Association. (2022). *Amyotrophic lateral sclerosis (ALS)*. https://www.mda.org/disease/amyotrophic-lateral-sclerosis/signs-and-symptoms/stages-of-als

National Heart, Lung, and Blood Institute. (2022). *Stroke diagnosis*. https://www.nhlbi.nih.gov/health/stroke/diagnosis

National Institute of Child Health and Human Development. (2020). *What causes muscular dystrophy (MD)?* https://www.nichd.nih.gov/health/topics/musculardys/conditioninfo/causes

National Institute of Neurological Disorders and Stroke. (2022). *Cerebral palsy: Hope through research*. https://www.ninds.nih.gov/health-information/patient-caregiver-education/hope-through-research/cerebral-palsy-hope-through-research

Nowicka, N., Juranek, J., Juranek, J. K., & Wojtkiewicz, J. (2019). Risk factors and emerging therapies in amyotrophic lateral sclerosis. *International Journal of Molecular Sciences*, 20(11), 2616. https://pubmed.ncbi.nlm.nih.gov/31141951/

Postuma, R. B., & Berg, D. (2016). Advances in markers of prodromal Parkinson disease. *Nature Reviews Neurology*, 12(11), 622–634. https://www.nature.com/articles/nrneurol.2016.152

Rabinstein, A. A. (2018). Coma and brain death. *CONTINUUM: Lifelong Learning in Neurology*, 24(6), 1708–1731. http://medcell.org/tbl/files/coma/coma_and_brain_death.pdf

Sadowska, M., Hujar, B. S., & Kopyta, I. (2020). Cerebral palsy: Current opinions on definition, epidemiology, risk factors, classification and treatment options. *Neuropsychiatric Disease & Treatment*, 16, 1505–1518. https://doi.org/10.2147/NDT.S235165

Salari, N., Fatahi, B., Valipour, E., Kazeminia, M., Fatahian, R., Kiaei, A., Shohaimi, S., & Mohammadi, M. (2022). Global prevalence of Duchenne and Becker muscular dystrophy: A systematic review and meta-analysis. *Journal of Orthopaedic Surgery and Research*, 17(1), 1–12. https://josr-online.biomedcentral.com/articles/10.1186/s13018-022-02996-8

Schwartz, M. A. (2019). Neurological disorders. In B. R. Ferrell, N. Coyle, & J. A. Paice (Eds.), *Oxford textbook of palliative nursing* (5th ed., pp. 291–318). Oxford University Press.

Sharma, A., Badhe, P., Gokulchandran, N., Chopra, G., Lohia, M., & Kulkarni, P. (2011). *Stem cell therapy & other recent advances in muscular dystrophy*. Neurogen Brain and Spine Institute (EDs) publication. https://www.stemcellsmumbai.com/book/Muscular%20Dystrophy%20Book.pdf

Simonet, C., Tolosa, E., Camara, A., & Valldeoriola, F. (2020). Emergencies and critical issues in Parkinson's disease. *Practical Neurology*, 20(1), 15–25. https://pn.bmj.com/content/practneurol/20/1/15.full.pdf

Sommers, M. S. (2019). *Davis's diseases and disorders: A nursing therapeutics manual*. F.A. Davis. https://www.fadavis.com/product/nursing-fundamentals-med-surg-diseases-disorders-nursing-therapeutics-manual-sommers-6

Sveinbjornsdottir, S. (2016). The clinical symptoms of Parkinson's disease. *Journal of Neurochemistry*, 139, 318–324. https://doi.org/10.1111/jnc.13691

Tariq, R., & Singal, A. K. (2020). Management of hepatorenal syndrome: A review. *Journal of Clinical and Translational Hepatology*, 8(2), 192. https://www.ncbi.nlm.nih.gov/pmc/articles/PMC7438356/

U.S. National Library of Medicine. (2022). *Amyotrophic lateral sclerosis (ALS)*. https://medlineplus.gov/ency/article/000688.htm

Van Ruiten, H. J. A., Bettolo, C. M., Cheetham, T., Eagle, M., Lochmuller, H., Bushby, K., & Guglieri, M. (2016). Why are some patients with Duchenne muscular dystrophy dying young: An analysis of causes of death in Northeast England? *Journal of European Paediatric Neurology*, 20, 904–909. https://doi.org/10.1016/j.ejpn.2016.07.020

Vitrikas, K., Dalton, H., & Breish, D. (2020). Cerebral palsy: An overview. *American Family Physician*, 101(4), 213–220. https://www.aafp.org/pubs/afp/issues/2020/0215/p213.html

Walker, Z., Possin, K. L., Boeve, B. F., & Aarsland, D. (2015). Lewy body dementias. *The Lancet*, 386(10004), 1683–1697. https://doi.org/10.1016/S0140-6736(15)00462-6

Wright, P. M. (2019). *Certified hospice and palliative nurse (CHPN) exam review*. Springer Publishing Company.

Yiu, E. M., & Kornberg, A. J. (2015). Duchenne muscular dystrophy. *Journal of Paediatrics and Child Health*, 51(8), 759–764 https://doi.org/10.1111/jpc.12868

APPENDIX

TABLE 14A.1   DIAGNOSTIC TESTS FOR NEUROLOGICAL DISORDERS

TYPE	NOTES
Physical examination	• Thorough physical examination with detailed medical history and neurological examination
Imaging	• CT scan • MRI • Swallowing studies (CP) • Cranial ultrasound (CP) • Perinatal ultrasound (CP)
Laboratory tests	• NCV (ALS) • EMG (ALS) • Serum protein electrophoresis (ALS) • Thyroid and parathyroid panels (ALS) • 24-hour urine analysis (ALS) • Electroencephalogram (CP) • Dual-energy x-ray absorptiometry (CP) • Metabolic panel (CP) • Genetic testing (MD) • Needle electromyography (MD) • Nerve conduction studies (MD) • Serum creatinine kinase (MD) • Serum alanine transaminase (MD) • Aspartate transaminase levels (MD) • Immunostaining and/or Western blot analysis (MD)
Pathology	• Staging aligns with disease progression (see Figure 14.2; ALS) • CSF analysis (ALS) • Muscle or nerve biopsy (ALS) • Classified according to severity and symptoms (see https://www.cpqcc.org/sites/default/files/GMFCS-ER.pdf; CP) • Staging aligns with disease progression (see Table 14.1; MD) • Muscle biopsy (if serum creatinine is inconclusive; MD)

ALS, amyotrophic lateral sclerosis; CP, cerebral palsy; CSF, cerebral spinal fluid; EMG, electromyography; MD, muscular dystrophy; NCV, nerve conduction velocity.

Sources: Boss, J. B., & Huether, S. E. (2019). Alternations in cognitive systems, cerebral hemodynamics, and motor function. In K. L. McCance & S. E. Huether (Eds.), *Pathophysiology: The biologic basis for disease in adults and children* (8th ed., pp. 504–549). Elsevier; Butterfield, R. J., & Huether, S. E. (2019). Alternations in neurological function in children. In K. L. McCance & S. E. Huether (Eds.), *Pathophysiology: The biologic basis for disease in adults and children* (8th ed., pp. 619–643). Elsevier; National Heart, Lung, and Blood Institute. (2022). *Stroke diagnosis.* https://www.nhlbi.nih.gov/health/stroke/diagnosis; National Institute of Neurological Disorders and Stroke. (2022). *Cerebral palsy: Hope through research.* https://www.ninds.nih.gov/health-information/patient-caregiver-education/hope-through-research/cerebral-palsy-hope-through-research; Rabinstein, A. A. (2018). Coma and brain death. *CONTINUUM: Lifelong Learning in Neurology, 24*(6), 1708–1731. http://medcell.org/tbl/files/coma/coma_and_brain_death.pdf; U.S. National Library of Medicine. (2022). *Amyotrophic lateral sclerosis (ALS).* https://medlineplus.gov/ency/article/000688.htm; Vitrikas, K., Dalton, H., & Breish, D. (2020). Cerebral palsy: An overview. *American Family Physician, 101*(4), 213–220. https://www.aafp.org/pubs/afp/issues/2020/0215/p213.html; Wright, P. M. (2019). *Certified hospice and palliative nurse (CHPN®) exam review.* Springer Publishing Company; Yiu, E. M., & Kornberg, A. J. (2015). Duchenne muscular dystrophy. *Journal of Paediatrics and Child Health, 51*(8), 759–764 https://doi.org/10.1111/jpc.12868.

TABLE 14A.2 PALLIATIVE INTERVENTIONS/SYMPTOM MANAGEMENT FOR NEUROLOGICAL DISORDERS

SYMPTOM	INTERVENTION
Angina (stable/typical)	• Encourage rest (MD) • Administer nitroglycerin as prescribed (MD) • Offer small, frequent meals (MD) • Reduction of emotional stress (MD)
Anorexia	• Use of appetite stimulants (see Appendix D-1; ALS, MD) • Offer small, frequent meals and snacks (ALS, MD) • Offer nutritional supplements (ALS, MD)
Anxiety and depression	• Antidepressants, anxiolytics, or benzodiazepines as indicated by patient's condition, age, and life expectancy (see Appendix D-1) • Non-pharmacological interventions (see Appendix D-2)
Bone-modifying interventions (see Appendix D-1)	• Bisphosphonates to strengthen bones and reduce bone loss (CP, MD)
Caregiver burden	• Support of interdisciplinary hospice or palliative team • Non-pharmacological interventions for caregivers (see Appendix D-2)
Communication barriers	• Use nonthreatening body language (place yourself at eye level, use therapeutic touch; ALS) • Use a soft tone of voice and use short phrases (ALS) • Avoid use of hand gestures when speaking as this may seem threatening to the person (ALS) • Reduce distractions (ALS) • Offer a limited number of choices (ALS) • Use a picture board, if needed (ALS)
Diaphoresis	• Review medications and lower dosages on or discontinue medications that can cause hyperhidrosis (i.e., hormones, antidepressants, aromatase inhibitors, etc.; ALS) • Use cotton bed linens and light pajamas (ALS) • Offer cool washcloths to forehead and underarms (ALS) • Open window and/or use fan (ALS) • Increase fluid intake as appropriate (ALS) • Avoid alcohol use (ALS) • Consider use of nonsteroidal anti-inflammatory medications and/or corticosteroids (ALS)
Drooling	• Use of anticholinergic medications (see Appendix D-1; ALS) • Injection of botulinum toxin A into salivary glands (ALS) • Skin care to prevent excoriation from saliva (ALS)
Dysphagia	• Stent placement for dilation of esophagus • Dietary modification (puree, thickened liquids, etc.) • Crush medications or use liquid formulations when possible

(continued)

TABLE 14A.2 PALLIATIVE INTERVENTIONS/SYMPTOM MANAGEMENT FOR NEUROLOGICAL DISORDERS *(CONTINUED)*

SYMPTOM	INTERVENTION
Dyspnea (see Appendix D)	• Corticosteroids for reducing inflammation (ALS, MD) • Opioids to reduce inspiratory effort and tachypnea (ALS, MD) • Bronchodilators for opening airways (mechanism of action of relaxation of muscular bands that surround bronchi, thus widening the airway; ALS, MD) • Diuretics to reduce systemic congestion (ALS, MD) • Anticholinergics to reduce secretions, especially at the end of life (ALS, MD) • Use of fans (ALS, MD) • Lower temperature in the room (ALS, MD)

Dysrhythmias	• Treatment depends on underlying cause (see section on dysrhythmias; MD)
	• Possible interventions (see Appendix D-1; MD)
	  ▪ Medications (e.g., adenosine, atropine, beta-blockers, calcium channel blockers, epinephrine, amiodarone, anticoagulants, lidocaine)
	  ▪ Pacemaker placement
	  ▪ Cardioversion (as indicated by patient preference and disease progression)
	  ▪ Cardiac ablation

Edema (see Appendix D)	• Use of diuretics as indicted (MD) • Elevation of extremity (MD) • Compression (MD)
Fatigue and somnolence	• Alternate periods of rest with periods of activity • Utilize energy conversation techniques • Psychostimulants (see Appendix D-1)
Hypoxia	• Elevate head of bed (ALS, MD) • Use deep breathing and coughing techniques (ALS, MD) • Provide supplemental oxygen (ALS, MD) • Use opioids or bronchodilators as indicated (ALS, MD) • Address underlying anxiety and depression (ALS, MD)
Immobility	• Encourage active participation in repositioning, when possible (ALS) • Implement use of bed mobility devices such as a bed hoist, bed ladder, grab rail, or trapeze bar (ALS) • Frequently reposition patient to relieve pressure on bony surfaces (ALS) • Use pillows, cushions, anti-pressure mattresses to alleviate pressure wound risk (ALS) • If patient is at risk for falls, safety measures such as nonskid slippers, shoes, or socks, bed or chair alarms, floor sensor, or fall mat (ALS)

(continued)

TABLE 14A.2   PALLIATIVE INTERVENTIONS/SYMPTOM MANAGEMENT FOR NEUROLOGICAL DISORDERS *(CONTINUED)*

SYMPTOM	INTERVENTION
Incontinence	• Identify and correct causes of incontinence, if possible (i.e., urinary tract infection, *Clostridium difficile*, etc.; CP) • Use protective pads/undergarments (CP) • Utilize urinary diversion devices (indwelling catheter, condom catheter, etc.), as appropriate (CP) • Provide meticulous skin care and reposition patient at least every 2 hours (CP) • Utilize fecal collection devices as indicated (i.e., external pouch, rectal tubes; CP)
Insomnia	• Use of benzodiazepines, antidepressants, or antihistaminic agents, as indicated by patient's condition, age, and life expectancy (see Appendix D; ALS) • Provide proper sleep hygiene (ALS) • Use non-pharmacological interventions for relaxation (ALS) • Address underlying anxiety and depression (ALS)

Muscle spasm	• Stretching (ALS, MD)
	• Exercise as tolerated (ALS, MD)
	• Alternate activity with periods of rest (ALS, MD)
	• Massage (ALS, MD)
	• Heat therapy (ALS, MD)
	• Frequent position change (ALS, MD)
	• Joint splinting (ALS, MD)
	• Pharmacological interventions (see Appendix D-1; ALS, MD)
	  ▪ Antispasmodics
	  ▪ Benzodiazepines
	  ▪ Muscle relaxants
	  ▪ Calcium channel blockers

Neuropathy	• Pharmacological interventions (see Appendix D-1; ALS)
	  ▪ Antidepressants
	  ▪ Anticonvulsants (i.e., gabapentin)
	  ▪ Anesthetics (i.e., ketamine)
	  ▪ Opioids

Pain management	See Appendix E
Pathological fractures	• Treatment of localized pain (CP, MD) • Joint stabilization (CP, MD) • For lower extremity compression fractures, surgical stabilization with or without joint replacement, if patient's condition and prognosis are favorable (CP, MD) • For vertebral compression fractures, VP or BKP may be considered, depending on patient's condition and prognosis (CP, MD)
Psychosocial distress and body image changes	• Antidepressants (see Appendix D-1) • Non-pharmacological interventions (see Appendix D-2)

(continued)

TABLE 14A.2   PALLIATIVE INTERVENTIONS/SYMPTOM MANAGEMENT FOR NEUROLOGICAL DISORDERS *(CONTINUED)*

SYMPTOM	INTERVENTION
Seizures	• Antiepileptic medications (see Appendix D-1; CP) ▪ Most commonly used is levetiracetam • If patient is unable to swallow, intranasal midazolam, rectal diazepam, or buccal clonazepam may be used (CP)
Xerostomia	• Ensure adequate fluid intake; provide sips of water or ice chips as tolerated (ALS) • Discontinue medications that cause xerostomia, if possible (ALS) • If supplemental oxygen is in use, add humidification (ALS) • Use salivary supplements or stimulants (e.g., pilocarpine; ALS) • Offer patient sugar-free gum, if able to chew without pain (ALS) • Provide moist, soft foods at mealtimes (ALS) • Non-pharmacological interventions (Appendix D-2; ALS)

ALS, amyotrophic lateral sclerosis; BKP, balloon kyphoplasty; CP, cerebral palsy; MD, muscular dystrophy; VP, vertebroplasty.

Sources: Guyer, D. L., Almhanna, K., & McKee, K. Y. (2020). Palliative care for patients with esophageal cancer: A narrative review. *Annals of Translational Medicine, 8*(17). https://doi.org/10.21037/atm-20-3676; Khan, F., Amatya, B., Bensmail, D., & Yelnik, A. (2019). Non-pharmacological interventions for spasticity in adults: An overview of systematic reviews. *Annals of Physical and Rehabilitation Medicine, 62*(4), 265–273. https://pubmed.ncbi.nlm.nih.gov/29042299/; Kluger, B. M., Ney, D. E., Bagley, S. J., Mohile, N., Taylor, L. P., Walbert, T., & Jones, C. A. (2020). Top ten tips palliative care clinicians should know when caring for patients with brain cancer. *Journal of Palliative Medicine, 23*(3), 415–421. https://doi.org/10.1089/jpm.2019.0507; McGeachan, A. J., & Mcdermott, C. J. (2017). Management of oral secretions in neurological disease. *Practical Neurology, 17*(2), 96–103. https://doi.org/10.1136/practneurol-2016-001515; Sommers, M. S. (2019). *Davis's diseases and disorders: A nursing therapeutics manual.* F.A. Davis. https://www.fadavis.com/product/nursing-fundamentals-med-surg-diseases-disorders-nursing-therapeutics-manual-sommers-6; Tariq, R., & Singal, A. K. (2020). Management of hepatorenal syndrome: A review. *Journal of Clinical and Translational Hepatology, 8*(2), 192. https://www.ncbi.nlm.nih.gov/pmc/articles/PMC7438356/; Walker, Z., Possin, K. L., Boeve, B. F., & Aarsland, D. (2015). Lewy body dementias. *The Lancet, 386*(10004), 1683–1697. https://doi.org/10.1016/S0140-6736(15)00462-6

CHAPTER 15

NEUROVASCULAR DISORDERS

CEREBROVASCULAR ACCIDENT/STROKE

DEFINITION/CHARACTERISTICS
A. Damage to the brain tissue secondary to loss of blood flow.
B. Generally, results from (see Figure 15.1):
    1. Blockage of cerebral vessel.
    2. Rupture of cerebral artery (Centers for Disease Control and Prevention [CDC], 2022; National Cancer Institute, 2022).

INCIDENCE AND PREVALENCE
A. Leading cause of disability and death in women.
B. Fifth leading cause of death in men.
C. Most (75%) occur in those older than 65 years.
D. There are about 795,000 new stroke diagnoses each year.
E. Roughly 129,000 deaths occur from stroke each year.
F. Incidence of stroke is 150% greater among Blacks than in Whites (Boss & Huether, 2019).

ETIOLOGY
A. Genetic predisposition.
B. Cardioembolism.
C. Large artery atherosclerosis (Boss & Huether, 2019; Tiedt et al., 2020).

PATHOPHYSIOLOGY
A. Ischemic stroke results from obstruction of cerebral blood flow due to:
    1. Thrombus formation.
    2. Embolus associated with atherosclerosis.
    3. Hypoperfusion.
B. Hemorrhagic stroke results from a ruptured artery in the brain (Boss & Huether, 2019; CDC, 2022).

PREDISPOSING FACTORS
A. Older age.
B. Poorly or uncontrolled hypertension.
C. Smoking (increases risk by 50%).
D. Obesity.
E. Insulin resistance.
F. Polycythemia.
G. Thrombocythemia.
H. Postmenopausal hormone therapy.
I. High sodium intake (>2,300 mg/day).
J. Low potassium intake (<4,700 mg/day).
K. Heart failure.
L. Sickle cell disease.
M. Peripheral vascular disease.
N. Hyperhomocysteinemia.
O. Atrial fibrillation.
P. Genetic predisposition.
Q. Physical inactivity.
R. Sleep apnea.
S. Depression.
T. *Chlamydia pneumoniae* infection (Boss & Huether, 2019; Tiedt et al., 2020).

SUBJECTIVE DATA
A. Symptoms depend on affected area of damage (see Figure 15.2).
B. Loss of sensation.
C. Dizziness.
D. Numbness.
E. Vertigo (Boss & Huether, 2019; National Cancer Institute, 2022; Tehrani et al., 2018).

OBJECTIVE DATA
A. Hemiparesis or hemiplegia.
B. Aphasia.
C. Dysarthria.
D. Contralateral homonymous, hemianopsia, or quadrantanopia.
E. Mirror movements.
F. Visual or sensory neglect.
G. Apraxia (Boss & Huether, 2019; National Cancer Institute, 2022; Tehrani et al., 2018).

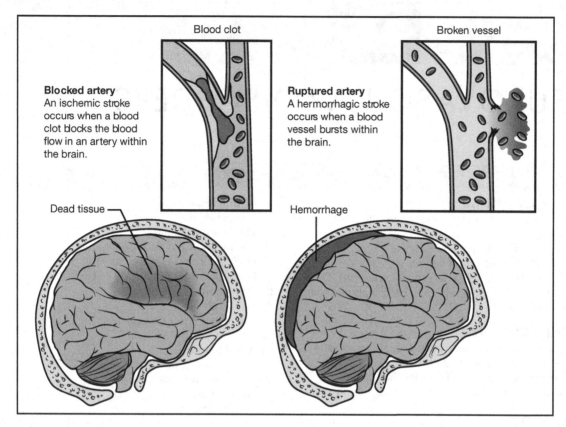

FIGURE 15.1 Causes of stroke.

Source: Adapted from Centers for Disease Control and Prevention. (2022). *About stroke.* https://www.cdc.gov/stroke/about.htm

DIAGNOSTIC TESTS
A. See Appendix Table 15A.1 for listing of common diagnostic tests.

DIFFERENTIAL DIAGNOSES
A. Seizure.
B. Syncope.
C. Sepsis.
D. Migraine.
E. Brain tumor.
F. Hypoglycemia.
G. Peripheral vestibular disease.
H. Neuropathy.
I. Dementia.
J. Extradural or subdural hemorrhage.
K. Drug or alcohol use.
L. Transient global amnesia.
M. Vestibular neuritis (Hankey et al., 2015).

POTENTIAL COMPLICATIONS
A. Seizures.
B. Incontinence.
C. Cognitive impairment.
D. Spasticity.
E. Hypertonicity.
F. Hemiplegic shoulder pain.
G. Limb contracture.
H. Depression and anxiety.
I. Emotional lability.
J. Hydrocephalus.
K. Recurrent stroke (Chonan et al., 2019; Singh et al., 2018).

DISEASE-MODIFYING TREATMENTS
A. Intravenous thrombolysis (for ischemic stroke).
B. Control bleeding (hemorrhagic stroke).
C. Management of hypertension.
D. Surgical intervention.
E. Physical therapy.
F. Occupational therapy.
G. Speech therapy (Boss & Huether, 2019; Chonan et al., 2019).

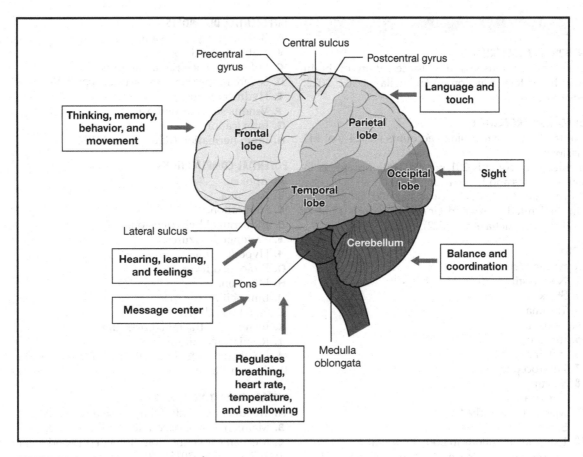

FIGURE 15.2 Brain structure and function.

PALLIATIVE INTERVENTIONS/SYMPTOM MANAGEMENT
A. See Appendix Table 15A.2 for listing of palliative interventions and symptom management.

PROGNOSIS
A. Long-term disability is common.
B. Recurrent stroke occurs in nearly half of patients within 10 years.
C. Mortality is often related to:
  1. Recurrent stroke.
  2. Cardiovascular complications.
  3. Aspiration pneumonia.
  4. Pulmonary embolism.
  5. Urosepsis or other infection (Singh et al., 2018).

NURSING INTERVENTIONS
A. Provide education on disease process, symptom management, and recurrence (see Appendix B-9).
B. Teach patient how to use communication devices.
C. Teach patient to take all medications as prescribed.
D. Modify diet as needed to address/prevent hypertension.
E. Educate patient on smoking cessation techniques (see Appendices B-10 and C-9)

F. Educate patient and caregiver(s) on disease trajectory.
G. Provide meticulous skin care.
H. Address dysphagia with dietary modifications, as needed.
I. Assess and address symptoms of depression and anxiety.
J. Provide assistance with activities of daily living (ADLs) as needed.
K. Provide spiritual support.
L. Assess caregiver fatigue/burnout (see Appendix B-5).
M. Encourage completion of advance directives.
N. Discuss wishes regarding withholding or withdrawing of life-sustaining interventions in late stage of disease with patient (if possible) and/or primary caregiver (see Appendices C-2, C-3, and C-4).
O. Educate patient and family regarding availability of palliative care.
P. Educate patient and family regarding availability of hospice services (when appropriate).
Q. Provide referral to community support groups, as needed.

COMA

DEFINITION/CHARACTERISTICS
A. Loss of consciousness due to cessation of brain and/or brainstem function (Kondziella et al., 2022; Rabinstein, 2018).

INCIDENCE AND PREVALENCE
A. Coma of unknown etiology accounts for 0.4% of ED admissions.
B. Incidence of coma is 201 per 100,000 population in the United States and United Kingdom.
C. Prevalence of coma is 20 cases per 100,000 population in the United States and United Kingdom (Huff & Tadi, 2022; Kondziella et al., 2022).

ETIOLOGY
A. Coma can result from:
   1. Neoplasms.
   2. Stroke.
   3. Trauma.
   4. Anoxia.
   5. Infection.
   6. Inflammation.
   7. Hydrocephalus.
   8. Seizures.
   9. Intoxication.
   10. Metabolic disturbances.
   11. Sepsis.
   12. Extreme alterations in body temperature.
   13. Coronavirus disease 2019 (COVID-19; Huff & Tadi, 2022; Kondziella et al., 2022; Rabinstein, 2018).

PATHOPHYSIOLOGY
A. Neuronal dysfunction and brain cell death results from:
   1. Diminished glucose to brain.
   2. Brain tissue hypoxia (Huff & Tadi, 2022).

PREDISPOSING FACTORS
A. Hypertension.
B. Stroke.
C. Diabetes.
D. Encephalopathy.
E. Meningitis.
F. Drug or alcohol overdose (Obiako et al., 2011).

OBJECTIVE DATA
A. Unresponsiveness to all stimuli (Rabinstein, 2018).

DIAGNOSTIC TESTS
A. See Appendix Table 15A.1 for listing of common diagnostic tests.
B. See Figure 15.3 for assessment.

DIFFERENTIAL DIAGNOSES
A. Basilar artery occlusion.
B. Status epilepticus.
C. Fulminant bacterial meningitis.
D. Severe herpes simplex virus encephalitis.
E. Hydrocephalus.
F. Venous sinus thrombosis.
G. Intoxication.
H. Brain herniation (Rabinstein, 2018).

POTENTIAL COMPLICATIONS
A. Anoxia.
B. Ischemia.
C. Herniation.
D. Intracranial hypertension.
E. Prolonged seizures.
F. Hypoglycemia.
G. Prolonged fever.
H. Infection.
I. Immobility.
J. Skin breakdown.
K. Increased intracranial pressure.
L. Respiratory failure.
M. Death (Huff & Tadi, 2022; Kondziella et al., 2022; Rabinstein, 2018).

DISEASE-MODIFYING TREATMENTS
A. Treatment of underlying cause (if reversible).
B. Maintenance of adequate blood pressure.
C. Mechanical ventilation, if needed (Kondziella et al., 2022; Rabinstein, 2018).

PALLIATIVE INTERVENTIONS/SYMPTOM MANAGEMENT
A. See Appendix Table 15A.2 for listing of palliative interventions and symptom management.

PROGNOSIS
A. Prognosis is dependent on cause and duration of coma.
B. Mortality rate in hospitalized patients is 26.5%.
C. When coma is associated with cancer, mortality rate is almost 90%.
D. When coma is associated with poisoning, mortality rate is <15% (Huff & Tadi, 2022; Rabinstein, 2018).

NURSING INTERVENTIONS
A. Provide education on disease process and symptom management.
B. Administer all medications as prescribed.
C. Administer nutritional supplements as prescribed.
D. Provide meticulous skin care.
E. Assess caregiver fatigue/burnout (see Appendix B-5).
F. Encourage completion of advance directives.
G. Discuss wishes regarding withholding or withdrawing of life-sustaining interventions in late stage of disease with patient (if possible) and/or primary caregiver (see Appendices C-2, C-3, and C-4).

Best eye opening
- Spontaneous (4)
- In response to speech (3)
- In response to painful stimuli (See Box A) (2)
- No response (1)
- Unable to open eyes due to swelling or trauma (C)

Best verbal response
- Alert, oriented, and verbally responsive (5)
- Disoriented, but verbal (4)
- Speech is inappropriae or disorganized (3)
- Speech is incoherent, no distinguishable words, or groaning (2)
- No audible response (1)
- Intubated (T)

Best motor response
- Obeys one-stage command (6)
- Moves arm above shoulder in response to pain (5)
- Flexes arm toward painful stimulus (4)
- Decorticate posturing in response to pain (See Box B) (3)
- Decerebrate posturing in response to pain (See Box B) (2)
- No response to pain (1)

Scoring
- 13–15 = mild brain injury
- 9–12 = moderate brain injury
- 8 or less = severe brain injury

Box A

To determine response to painful stimuli:
1. Press on fingertip
2. Press on trapezius muscle
3. Press on suborbital notch

Box B

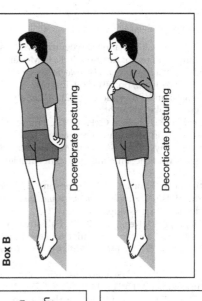

Decerebrate posturing

Decorticate posturing

FIGURE 15.3 Coma assessment.

Source: Adapted from Teasdale, G., & Jennett, B. (1974). Assessment of coma and impaired consciousness: A practical scale. *The Lancet, 304*(7872), 81–84.

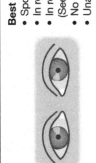
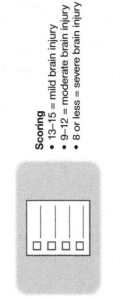

H. Educate patient and family regarding availability of palliative care.

I. Educate patient and family regarding availability of hospice services (when appropriate).

J. Provide referral to community support groups, as needed.

REFERENCES

Boss, J. B., & Huether, S. E. (2019). Alternations in cognitive systems, cerebral hemodynamics, and motor function. In K. L. McCance & S. E. Huether (Eds.), *Pathophysiology: The biologic basis for disease in adults and children* (8th ed., pp. 504–549). Elsevier.

Centers for Disease Control and Prevention. (2022). *About stroke.* https://www.cdc.gov/stroke/about.htm

Chohan, S. A., Venkatesh, P. K., & How, C. H. (2019). Long-term complications of stroke and secondary prevention: an overview for primary care physicians. *Singapore Medical Journal, 60*(12), 616. https://www.ncbi.nlm.nih.gov/pmc/articles/PMC7911065/

Fusco, F. (2021). Mouth care. In E. Bruera, I. J. Higginson, C. F. von Gunten, & T. Morita (Eds.), *Textbook of palliative medicine and supportive care.* Taylor & Francis Group.

Guyer, D. L., Almhanna, K., & McKee, K. Y. (2020). Palliative care for patients with esophageal cancer: A narrative review. *Annals of Translational Medicine, 8*(17). https://doi.org/10.21037/atm-20-3676

Hankey, G. J. (2017). Stroke. *Lancet, 389*(10069), 641–654. https://news.medlive.cn/uploadfile/20150116/14213992808171.pdf

Huff J. S., & Tadi P. (2022) *Coma.* In: StatPearls [Internet]. StatPearls Publishing. https://www.ncbi.nlm.nih.gov/books/NBK430722/#_NBK430722_pubdet_

Khan, F., Amatya, B., Bensmail, D., & Yelnik, A. (2019). Non-pharmacological interventions for spasticity in adults: An overview of systematic reviews. *Annals of Physical and Rehabilitation Medicine, 62*(4), 265–273. https://pubmed.ncbi.nlm.nih.gov/29042299/

Kluger, B. M., Ney, D. E., Bagley, S. J., Mohile, N., Taylor, L. P., Walbert, T., & Jones, C. A. (2020). Top ten tips palliative care clinicians should know when caring for patients with brain cancer. *Journal of Palliative Medicine, 23*(3), 415–421. https://doi.org/10.1089/jpm.2019.0507

Kondziella, D., Amiri, M., Othman, M. H., Beghi, E., Bodien, Y. G., Citerio, G., Giacino, J. T., Mayer, S. A., Lawson, T. N., Menon, D. K., Rass, V., Sharshar, T., Stevens, R. D., Tinti, L., Vespa, P., McNett, M., Rao, C. P., V., Helbok, R., & Curing Coma Campaign Collaborators. (2022). Incidence and prevalence of coma in the UK and the USA. *Brain Communications, 4*(5), fcac188. https://doi.org/10.1093/braincomms/fcac188

National Cancer Institute. (2022). *CVA.* https://www.cancer.gov/publications/dictionaries/cancer-terms/def/cva

Obiako, O. R., Oparah, S., & Ogunniyi, A. (2011). Causes of medical coma in adult patients at the University College Hospital, Ibadan Nigeria. *Nigerian Postgraduate Medical Journal, 18*(1), 1–7. https://www.researchgate.net/publication/50892178

Rabinstein, A. A. (2018). Coma and brain death. *CONTINUUM: Lifelong Learning in Neurology, 24*(6), 1708–1731. http://medcell.org/tbl/files/coma/coma_and_brain_death.pdf

Singh, R. J., Chen, S., Ganesh, A., & Hill, M. D. (2018). Long-term neurological, vascular, and mortality outcomes after stroke. *International Journal of Stroke, 13*(8), 787–796. https://doi.org/10.1177/174749301879852

Sommers, M. S. (2019). *Davis's diseases and disorders: A nursing therapeutics manual.* F.A. Davis. https://www.fadavis.com/product/nursing-fundamentals-med-surg-diseases-disorders-nursing-therapeutics-manual-sommers-6

Tariq, R., & Singal, A. K. (2020). Management of hepatorenal syndrome: A review. *Journal of Clinical and Translational Hepatology, 8*(2), 192. https://www.ncbi.nlm.nih.gov/pmc/articles/PMC7438356/

Tehrani, A. S., Kattah, J. C., Kerber, K. A., Gold, D. R., Zee, D. S., Urrutia, V. C., & Newman-Toker, D. E. (2018). Diagnosing stroke in acute dizziness and vertigo: Pitfalls and pearls. *Stroke, 49*(3), 788–795. https://www.ahajournals.org/doi/pdf/10.1161/STROKEAHA.117.016979

Tiedt, S., Herzberg, M., Küpper, C., Feil, K., Kellert, L., Dorn, F., … & Wollenweber, F. A. (2020). Stroke etiology modifies the effect of endovascular treatment in acute stroke. *Stroke, 51*(3), 1014-1016. https://www.ahajournals.org/doi/pdf/10.1161/STROKEAHA.119.028383

APPENDIX

TABLE 15A.1   DIAGNOSTIC TESTS FOR NEUROVASCULAR DISORDERS

TYPE	NOTES
Physical examination	• Thorough physical examination with detailed medical history and neurological examination
Imaging	• Angiography (stroke) • Carotid ultrasound (stroke) and cerebral scintigraphy (coma) • CT scan (stroke) • Echocardiogram (stroke) • Electrocardiography (stroke) • MRI • Transcranial doppler (coma)
Laboratory tests	• Arterial blood gas (coma) • Blood glucose (coma, stroke) • Blood urea nitrogen (coma) • Platelet count (stroke) • PT (stroke) • PTT (stroke) • Serum ammonia level (coma) • Toxicology screening (coma)
Pathology	• Lumbar puncture with cerebral spinal fluid analysis • Coma is staged according to the Glasgow Coma Scale (see https://www.mdcalc.com/calc/64/glasgow-coma-scale-score-gcs and Figure 15.1)

PT, prothrombin time; PTT, partial thromboplastin time.

Sources: Boss, J. B., & Huether, S. E. (2019). Alternations in cognitive systems, cerebral hemodynamics, and motor function. In K. L. McCance & S. E. Huether (Eds.), *Pathophysiology: The biologic basis for disease in adults and children* (8th ed., pp. 504–549). Elsevier; National Heart, Lung, and Blood Institute. (2022). *Stroke diagnosis.* https://www.nhlbi.nih.gov/health/stroke/diagnosis; Rabinstein, A. A. (2018). Coma and brain death. *CONTINUUM: Lifelong Learning in Neurology, 24*(6), 1708–1731. http://medcell.org/tbl/files/coma/coma_and_brain_death.pdf

TABLE 15A.2   PALLIATIVE INTERVENTIONS/SYMPTOM MANAGEMENT FOR NEUROVASCULAR DISORDERS

SYMPTOM	INTERVENTION
Anxiety and depression	• Antidepressants, anxiolytics, or benzodiazepines as indicated by patient's condition, age, and life expectancy (see Appendix D-1) • Non-pharmacological interventions (see Appendix D-2)
Caregiver burden	• Support of interdisciplinary hospice or palliative team • Non-pharmacological interventions for caregivers (see Appendix D-2)
Communication barriers	• Use nonthreatening body language (place yourself at eye level, use therapeutic touch; stroke) • Use a soft tone of voice and use short phrases (stroke) • Avoid use of hand gestures when speaking as this may seem threatening to the person (stroke) • Reduce distractions (stroke) • Offer a limited number of choices (stroke) • Use a picture board, if needed (stroke)

(continued)

TABLE 15A.2 PALLIATIVE INTERVENTIONS/SYMPTOM MANAGEMENT FOR NEUROVASCULAR DISORDERS *(CONTINUED)*

SYMPTOM	INTERVENTION
Dysphagia	• Stent placement for dilation of esophagus (stroke) • Dietary modification (puree, thickened liquids, etc.; stroke) • Crush medications or use liquid formulations when possible (stroke)
Fatigue and somnolence	• Alternate periods of rest with periods of activity (stroke) • Utilize energy conversation techniques (stroke) • Psychostimulants (see Appendix D; stroke)
Immobility	• Encourage active participation in repositioning, when possible • Implement use of bed mobility devices such as a bed hoist, bed ladder, grab rail, or trapeze bar • Frequently reposition patient to relieve pressure on bony surfaces • Use pillows, cushions, anti-pressure mattresses to alleviate pressure wound risk • If patient is at risk for falls, safety measures such as nonskid slippers, shoes, or socks, bed or chair alarms, floor sensor, or fall mat
Incontinence	• Identify and correct causes of incontinence, if possible (i.e., urinary tract infection, *Clostridium difficile*, etc.) • Use protective pads/undergarments • Utilize urinary diversion devices (indwelling catheter, condom catheter, etc.), as appropriate • Provide meticulous skin care and reposition patient at least every 2 hours • Utilize fecal collection devices as indicated (i.e., external pouch, rectal tubes)
Insomnia	• Use of benzodiazepines, antidepressants, or antihistaminic agents, as indicated by patient's condition, age, and life expectancy (see Appendix D-1; stroke) • Provide proper sleep hygiene (stroke) • Use non-pharmacological interventions for relaxation (stroke) • Address underlying anxiety and depression (stroke)

Intracranial swelling	• Corticosteroids
	  ■ Dexamethasone is most frequently used
	  ■ Lowest possible dose should be used
	  ■ Monitor for effects of long-terms steroid use
	  ■ In certain cases of steroid dependency, bevacizumab may be considered as a palliative care intervention to reduce steroid dose

Muscle spasm	• Stretching (stroke)
	• Exercise as tolerated (stroke)
	• Alternate activity with periods of rest (stroke)
	• Massage (stroke)
	• Heat therapy (stroke)
	• Frequent position change (stroke)
	• Joint splinting (stroke)
	• Pharmacological interventions (see Appendix D-1; stroke)
	  ■ Antispasmodics
	  ■ Benzodiazepines
	  ■ Muscle relaxants
	  ■ Calcium channel blockers

(continued)

TABLE 15A.2 PALLIATIVE INTERVENTIONS/SYMPTOM MANAGEMENT FOR NEUROVASCULAR DISORDERS *(CONTINUED)*

SYMPTOM	INTERVENTION
Neuropathy	• Antidepressants (see Appendix D-1; stroke) • Anticonvulsants (i.e., gabapentin; stroke) • Anesthetics (i.e., ketamine; stroke) • Opioids (stroke)
Pain management	See Appendix E
Psychosocial distress and body image changes (stroke)	• Antidepressants (see Appendix D-1) • Non-pharmacological interventions (see Appendix D-2)
Seizures	• Antiepileptic medications (see Appendix D-1) • Most commonly used is levetiracetam ▪ If patient is unable to swallow, intranasal midazolam, rectal diazepam, or buccal clonazepam may be used

Sources: Fusco, F. (2021). Mouth care. In E. Bruera, I. J. Higginson, C. F. von Gunten, & T. Morita (Eds.), *Textbook of palliative medicine and supportive care.* Taylor & Francis Group; Guyer, D. L., Almhanna, K., & McKee, K. Y. (2020). Palliative care for patients with esophageal cancer: A narrative review. *Annals of Translational Medicine, 8*(17). https://doi.org/10.21037/atm-20-3676; Khan, F., Amatya, B., Bensmail, D., & Yelnik, A. (2019). Non-pharmacological interventions for spasticity in adults: An overview of systematic reviews. *Annals of Physical and Rehabilitation Medicine, 62*(4), 265–273. https://pubmed.ncbi.nlm.nih.gov/29042299/; Kluger, B. M., Ney, D. E., Bagley, S. J., Mohile, N., Taylor, L. P., Walbert, T., & Jones, C. A. (2020). Top ten tips palliative care clinicians should know when caring for patients with brain cancer. *Journal of Palliative Medicine, 23*(3), 415–421. https://doi.org/10.1089/jpm.2019.0507; Sommers, M. S. (2019). *Davis's diseases and disorders: A nursing therapeutics manual.* F.A. Davis. https://www.fadavis.com/product/nursing-fundamentals-med-surg-diseases-disorders-nursing-therapeutics-manual-sommers-6; Tariq, R., & Singal, A. K. (2020). Management of hepatorenal syndrome: A review. *Journal of Clinical and Translational Hepatology, 8*(2), 192. https://www.ncbi.nlm.nih.gov/pmc/articles/PMC7438356/; Walker, Z., Possin, K. L., Boeve, B. F., & Aarsland, D. (2015). Lewy body dementias. *The Lancet, 386*(10004), 1683–1697. https://doi.org/10.1016/S0140-6736(15)00462-6.

CHAPTER 16

PULMONARY DISORDERS

CHRONIC OBSTRUCTIVE PULMONARY DISEASE

DEFINITION/CHARACTERISTICS
A. Chronic respiratory illness characterized by:
1. Airflow limitation.
2. Progressive nature with exacerbations.
3. Productive cough.
4. Enlargement of airways.
5. Destruction of alveolar walls.
6. Chronic inflammation (Brashers & Huether, 2019).

INCIDENCE AND PREVALENCE
A. Chronic obstructive pulmonary disease (COPD) is the third leading cause of death in the United States.
B. Nearly 15.7 million (6%) Americans have been diagnosed with COPD (Boss & Huether, 2019; Centers for Disease Control and Prevention, 2022).

ETIOLOGY
A. Respiratory toxins:
1. Tobacco or marijuana smoke.
2. Biomass fuel smoke.
3. Outdoor air pollution (vehicle or industrial).
4. Occupational exposure to:
   a. Gases.
   b. Fumes.
   c. Dust.
   d. Chemicals.
   e. Smoke (Huang et al., 2019).

PATHOPHYSIOLOGY
A. Chronic irritant exposure leads to:
1. Progressive inflammation.
2. Narrowing of airways.
3. Hypersecretion of mucus.
4. Hypertrophied bronchial smooth muscle (see Figure 16.1).

PREDISPOSING FACTORS
A. Smoking (tobacco or marijuana).
B. Inhaled chemicals.
C. Occupational hazards.
D. Air pollution.
E. Genetic predisposition.
F. History of emphysema or asthma (Brashers & Huether, 2019b).

SUBJECTIVE DATA
A. Progressively worsening dyspnea.
B. Anorexia.
C. Fatigue.
D. Anxiety.
E. Decreased physical endurance.
F. Insomnia.
G. Depression (Brashers & Huether, 2019; Vogelmeier et al., 2020).

OBJECTIVE DATA
A. Poor inspiratory effort.
B. Tripod positioning.
C. Productive cough.
D. Wheezing.
E. Barrel chest (see Figure 16.2).
F. Cyanosis.
G. Cor pulmonale.
H. Polycythemia.
I. Weight loss (Boss & Heuther, 2019; Vogelmeier et al., 2020).

DIAGNOSTIC TESTS
A. See Appendix Table 16A.1 for listing of common diagnostic tests.

DIFFERENTIAL DIAGNOSES
A. Asthma.
B. Heart failure.
C. Bronchiectasis.
D. Tuberculosis.
E. Bronchiolitis obliterans.
F. Emphysema (Leader, 2022; Mosenfar, 2022).

POTENTIAL COMPLICATIONS
A. Frequent infections and exacerbations.
B. Bronchospasm.
C. Exertional dyspnea progressing to dyspnea at rest.
D. Chronic productive cough (Brashers & Huether, 2019b).

DISEASE-MODIFYING TREATMENTS
A. COPD is not reversible.
B. Treatment is based on GOLD guidelines.
C. Smoking cessation.
D. Chest physiotherapy.

▶

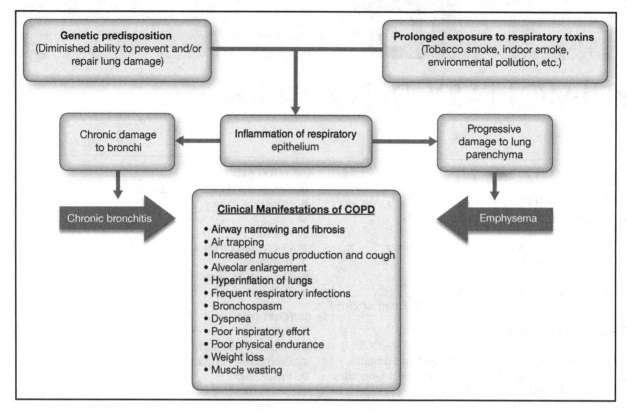

FIGURE 16.1   Pathogenesis of chronic obstructive pulmonary disease.

Sources: Adapted from Brashers, V. L., & Huether, S. E. (2019). *Alterations in pulmonary function.* In K. L. McCance & S. E. Huether (Eds.), *Pathophysiology: The biologic basis for disease in adults and children* (8th ed., pp. 1163–1201). Elsevier; The Calgary Guide to Understanding Disease. (2022). *COPD.* https://calgaryguide.ucalgary.ca/copd-pathogenesis/

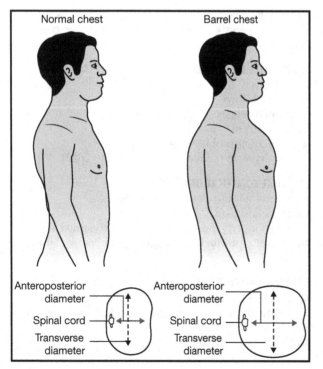

FIGURE 16.2   Barrel chest.

E. Deep breathing.
F. Oxygen therapy.
G. Mechanical ventilation.
H. Lung volume reduction surgery.
I. Lung transplantation (Boss & Huether, 2019; Vogelmeier et al., 2020).

PALLIATIVE INTERVENTIONS/SYMPTOM MANAGEMENT
A. See Appendix Table 16A.2 for listing of palliative interventions and symptom management.
B. See Appendix D-3 for overview of common symptoms.
C. See Figure 16.3 for approaches to patient with dyspnea.

PROGNOSIS
A. The course of COPD is marked with periods of stability and exacerbation (see Figure 16.4).
B. Prognosis is dependent on disease severity and comorbidities.
C. About 20% to 24% die within 5 years of diagnosis.
D. Estimated 4-year survival can be calculated here: www.mdcalc.com/calc/3916/bode-index-copd-survival (Kiddle et al., 2020)

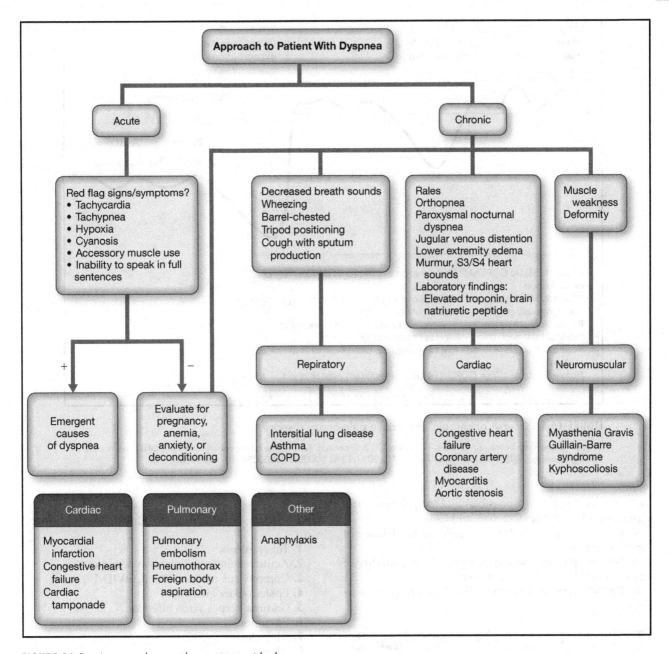

FIGURE 16.3 Approaches to the patient with dyspnea.

NURSING INTERVENTIONS
A. Provide education on disease process and symptom management.
B. Teach patient importance of smoking cessation (see Appendices B-10 and C-9).
C. Teach patient to take all medications as prescribed.
D. Modify diet as needed.
E. Educate patient and caregiver(s) on disease trajectory (Figure 16.4).
F. Teach pursed-lip breathing.
G. Teach energy conservation techniques.

H. Assess and address symptoms of depression and anxiety.
I. Provide assistance with activities of daily living (ADLs) as needed.
J. Provide education on oxygen therapy.
K. Encourage routine vaccination (influenza, pneumococcal, coronavirus disease 2019 [COVID-19]).
L. Provide spiritual support.
M. Assess caregiver fatigue/burnout (see Appendix B-5).
N. Encourage completion of advance directives.
O. Discuss wishes regarding withholding or withdrawing of life-sustaining interventions in late stage of ▶

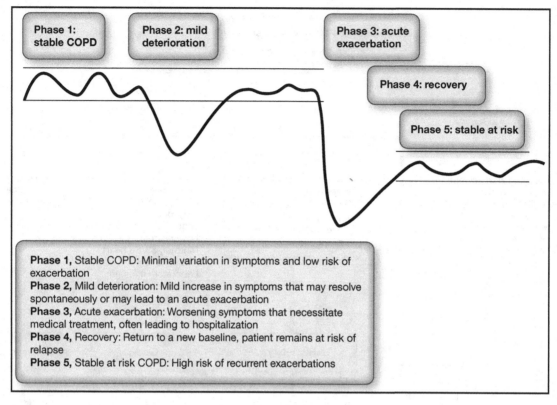

Phase 1, Stable COPD: Minimal variation in symptoms and low risk of exacerbation
Phase 2, Mild deterioration: Mild increase in symptoms that may resolve spontaneously or may lead to an acute exacerbation
Phase 3, Acute exacerbation: Worsening symptoms that necessitate medical treatment, often leading to hospitalization
Phase 4, Recovery: Return to a new baseline, patient remains at risk of relapse
Phase 5, Stable at risk COPD: High risk of recurrent exacerbations

FIGURE 16.4   Course of chronic obstructive pulmonary disease.

Source: Adapted from Baltaji, S., Cheronis, N., Bajwa, O., & Cheema, T. (2021). The role of palliative care in COPD. *Critical Care Nursing Quarterly, 44*(1), 113–120. https://doi.org/10.1097/CNQ.0000000000000344. Used with permission.

disease with patient (if possible) and/or primary caregiver (see Appendices C-2, C-3, and C-4).

P. Educate patient and family regarding availability of palliative care.

Q. Educate patient and family regarding availability of hospice services (when appropriate).

R. Provide referral to community support groups, as needed.

PULMONARY FIBROSIS

DEFINITION/CHARACTERISTICS
A. Restrictive lung disease.
B. Associated with development of excessive fibrous tissue within the lungs (see Figure 16.5; Brashers & Huether, 2019b; Sommers, 2019).

INCIDENCE AND PREVALENCE
A. Onset generally occurs over a 6-month period.
B. Most commonly diagnosed in those over 50 (Sommers, 2019).

ETIOLOGY
A. Formation of scar tissue related to pulmonary insult.
  1. Tuberculosis.
  2. Acute respiratory distress syndrome.
  3. Coronavirus disease 2019 (COVID-19).
  4. Epstein–Barr virus.
  5. Gamma herpes virus infection.
  6. Pneumonia.
  7. Atelectasis.
  8. Alveolar cell cancer.
  9. Pulmonary edema.
  10. Lung surgery or trauma.
B. Non-respiratory disorders.
  1. Rheumatoid arthritis.
  2. Progressive systemic sclerosis.
  3. Sarcoidosis.
  4. Guillain–Barré syndrome.
  5. Amyotrophic lateral sclerosis.
  6. Myasthenia gravis.
  7. Muscular dystrophy.

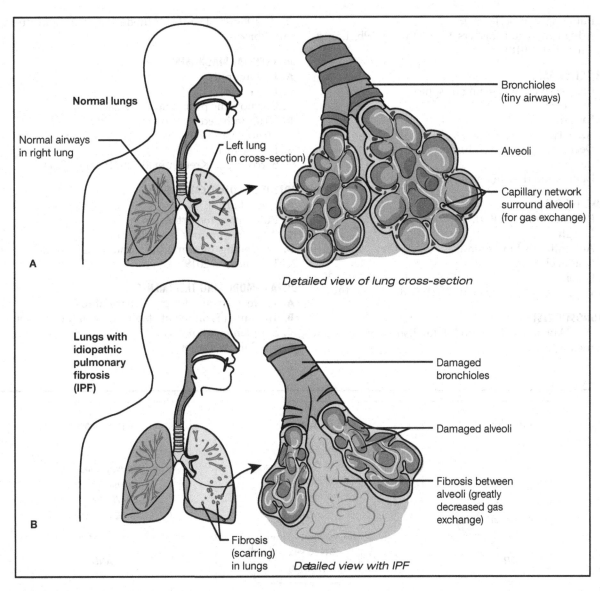

Normal lungs

Normal airways in right lung

Left lung (in cross-section)

Bronchioles (tiny airways)

Alveoli

Capillary network surround alveoli (for gas exchange)

A

Detailed view of lung cross-section

Lungs with idiopathic pulmonary fibrosis (IPF)

Damaged bronchioles

Damaged alveoli

Fibrosis between alveoli (greatly decreased gas exchange)

B

Fibrosis (scarring) in lungs

Detailed view with IPF

FIGURE 16.5 Pulmonary fibrosis.

Source: Adapted from National Heart Lung and Blood Institute. (2013). *Pulmonary fibrosis.* NIH.

C. Inhalation of toxins:
  1. Coal dust.
  2. Asbestos.
  3. Cigarette smoke.
  4. Silica.
D. May be idiopathic (Brashers & Huether, 2019b; Doane et al., 2021; López-Ramírez et al., 2018; Rai et al., 2021; Sommers, 2019).

PATHOPHYSIOLOGY
A. Chronic inflammation leads to:
  1. Fibrosis.
  2. Alveolar epithelialization.
  3. Myofibroblast proliferation

B. Scarring and distortion of lung tissue leads to:
  1. Lung tissue stiffness, causing hypoperfusion (Brashers & Huether, 2019b; Sommers, 2019).

PREDISPOSING FACTORS
A. Smoking.
B. Inhaled chemicals.
C. Occupational hazards.
D. Air pollution.
E. Genetic predisposition.
F. History of emphysema or asthma.
G. Certain viral infections.
H. Respiratory infections.
I. Gastroesophageal reflux.

▶

J. Pulmonary hypertension.

K. Advancing age (Brashers & Huether, 2019b; López-Ramírez et al., 2018).

SUBJECTIVE DATA

A. Progressively worsening dyspnea.

B. Anorexia.

C. Fatigue.

D. Anxiety.

E. Decreased physical endurance.

F. Insomnia.

G. Depression (Kreuter et al., 2021; Sommers, 2019).

OBJECTIVE DATA

A. Poor inspiratory effort.

B. Cough.

C. Adventitious lung sounds.

D. Digital clubbing.

E. Fever.

F. Weight loss (Kreuter et al., 2021; Sommers, 2019).

DIAGNOSTIC TESTS

A. See Appendix Table 16A.1 for listing of common diagnostic tests.

B. See Figure 16.6, GAP model for staging of pulmonary fibrosis.

DIFFERENTIAL DIAGNOSES

A. Pneumonitis.

B. Pneumonia.

C. Cardiogenic pulmonary edema.

D. Drug-induced pulmonary toxicity.

E. Histoplasmosis.

F. Lung cancer.

G. Sarcoidosis (Kreuter et al., 2021; Sayf, 2021).

POTENTIAL COMPLICATIONS

A. Heart failure.

B. Pulmonary hypertension.

C. Acute respiratory exacerbations.

D. Worsening of comorbid conditions (Kreuter et al., 2021; Sommers, 2019).

DISEASE-MODIFYING TREATMENTS

A. There is no cure for pulmonary fibrosis.

B. Treatment is aimed at stabilization and palliation.

C. Supplemental oxygen.

D. Smoking cessation.

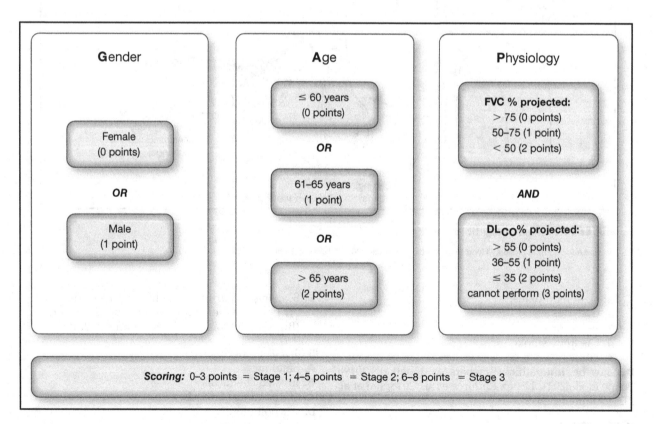

FIGURE 16.6 GAP model.

Source: Adapted from Ley, B., Ryerson, C. J., Vittinghoff, E., Ryu, J. H., Tomassetti, S., Lee, J. S., Poletti, V., Buccioli, M., Elicker, B. M., Jones, K. D., King, T. E., Jr., & Collard, H. R. (2012). A multidimensional index and staging system for idiopathic pulmonary fibrosis. *Annals of Internal Medicine, 156*(10), 684–691. https://www.acpjournals.org/doi/abs/10.7326/0003-4819-156-10-201205150-00004

E. Medication management:
1. Nintedanib
2. Pirfenidone

F. Lung transplant (American Lung Association [ALS], 2022; Sommers, 2019).

PALLIATIVE INTERVENTIONS/SYMPTOM MANAGEMENT
A. See Appendix Table 16A.2 for listing of palliative interventions and symptom management.
B. See Appendix D-3 for overview of common symptoms.

PROGNOSIS
A. Median survival time is 3 to 5 years after diagnosis.
B. Half of those hospitalized with acute exacerbation die in the hospital.
C. Median survival time after acute exacerbation is <5 months.
D. Mortality increases as GAP score increases (Stage 1 = low mortality risk; Stage 3 = high mortality risk).
E. Death results from respiratory failure (ALS, 2022; Fabrellas et al., 2018; Kreuter et al., 2021).

NURSING INTERVENTIONS
A. Provide education on disease process and symptom management.
B. Teach patient importance of smoking cessation (see Appendices B-10 and C-9).
C. Teach patient to take all medications as prescribed.
D. Reposition for respiratory comfort.
E. Educate patient and caregiver(s) on disease trajectory.
F. Teach pursed-lip breathing.
G. Teach energy conservation techniques.
H. Implement infection control measures.
I. Provide mechanical ventilation and/or suctioning as needed.
J. Assess and address symptoms of depression and anxiety.
K. Provide assistance with activities of daily living (ADLs) as needed.
L. Provide education on oxygen therapy.
M. Encourage routine vaccination (influenza, pneumococcal, COVID-19).
N. Provide spiritual support.
O. Assess caregiver fatigue/burnout (see Appendix B-5).
P. Encourage completion of advance directives.
Q. Discuss wishes regarding withholding or withdrawing of life-sustaining interventions in late stage of disease with patient (if possible) and/or primary caregiver (see Appendices C-2, C-3, and C-4).
R. Educate patient and family regarding availability of palliative care.
S. Educate patient and family regarding availability of hospice services (when appropriate).
T. Provide referral to community support groups, as needed.

REFERENCES
Brashers, V. L., & Huether, S. E. (2019). Alterations in pulmonary function. In K. L. McCance & S. E. Huether (Eds.), *Pathophysiology: The biologic basis for disease in adults and children* (8th ed., pp. 1163–1201). Elsevier.

Doane, J. J., Hirsch, K. S., Baldwin, J. O., Wurfel, M. M., Pipavath, S. N., & West, T. E. (2021). Progressive pulmonary fibrosis after non-critical COVID-19: A case report. *The American Journal of Case Reports, 22*, e933458-1. https://www.ncbi.nlm.nih.gov/pmc/articles/PMC8650386/

Fabrellas, E.F., Peris Sánchez, R., Sabater Abad, C., & Juan Samper, G. (2018). Prognosis and follow-up of idiopathic pulmonary fibrosis. *Medical Sciences, 6*(2), 51. https://www.mdpi.com/2076-3271/6/2/51

Huang, X., Mu, X., Deng, L., Fu, A., Pu, E., Tang, T., & Kong, X. (2019). The etiologic origins for chronic obstructive pulmonary disease. *International Journal of Chronic Obstructive Pulmonary Disease, 14*, 1139. https://doi.org/10.2147%2FCOPD.S203215

Kiddle, S. J., Whittaker, H. R., Seaman, S. R., & Quint, J. K. (2020). Prediction of five-year mortality after COPD diagnosis using primary care records. *PLoS one, 15*(7), e0236011. https://journals.plos.org/plosone/article?id=10.1371/journal.pone.0236011

Kreuter, M., Müller-Ladner, U., Costabel, U., Jonigk, D., & Heussel, C. P. (2021). The diagnosis and treatment of pulmonary fibrosis. *Deutsches Ärzteblatt International, 118*(9), 152. https://www.ncbi.nlm.nih.gov/pmc/articles/PMC8212400/

Leader, D. (2022). *Understanding the differential diagnosis of COPD. Why the exclusion of other causes is needed.* https://www.verywellhealth.com/differential-diagnosis-of-copd-914739#:~:text=In%20the%20course%20of%20a,causes%20may%20also%20be%20explored.

López-Ramírez, C., Suarez Valdivia, L., & Rodríguez Portal, J. A. (2018). Causes of pulmonary fibrosis in the elderly. *Medical Sciences, 6*(3), 58. doi:10.3390/medsci6030058

Mosinfar, Z. (2022). *Chronic obstructive pulmonary disease (COPD) differential diagnoses.* https://emedicine.medscape.com/article/297664-differential

Rai, D. K., Sharma, P., & Kumar, R. (2021). Post-covid 19 pulmonary fibrosis. Is it real threat? *Indian Journal of Tuberculosis, 68*(3), 330–333. https://www.sciencedirect.com/science/article/pii/S0019570720302134

Sayf, A.A. (2021). *Idiopathic pulmonary fibrosis: Differential diagnoses.* https://emedicine.medscape.com/article/301226-differential

Vogelmeier, C. F., Román-Rodríguez, M., Singh, D., Han, M. K., Rodríguez-Roisin, R., & Ferguson, G. T. (2020). Goals of COPD treatment: Focus on symptoms and exacerbations. *Respiratory Medicine, 166*, 105938. https://doi.org/10.1016/j.rmed.2020.105938

Walker, Z., Possin, K. L., Boeve, B. F., & Aarsland, D. (2015). Lewy body dementias. *The Lancet, 386*(10004), 1683–1697. https://doi.org/10.1016/S0140-6736(15)00462-6

APPENDIX

TABLE 16A.1   DIAGNOSTIC TESTS FOR PULMONARY DISORDERS

TYPE	NOTES
Physical examination	• Thorough physical exam • Detailed medical history • Respiratory examination
Imaging	• CT scan • Chest x-ray
Laboratory tests	• Complete blood count • Arterial blood gas • Rheumatic factor (pulmonary fibrosis) • Antinuclear antibodies (pulmonary fibrosis)
Pathology	• Pulmonary function test • Spirometry • COPD is staged according to GOLD guidelines (see https://goldcopd.org/2023-gold-report-2/) • Pulmonary fibrosis is staged according to GAP model (see Figure 16.6)

COPD, chronic obstructive pulmonary disease.

Sources: Boss, J. B., & Huether, S. E. (2019). Alternations in cognitive systems, cerebral hemodynamics, and motor function. In K. L. McCance & S. E. Huether (Eds.), *Pathophysiology: The biologic basis for disease in adults and children* (8th ed., pp. 504–549). Elsevier; Centers for Centers for Disease Control and Prevention. (2022). *National Amyotrophic Lateral Sclerosis (ALS) registry.* https://www.cdc.gov/als/dashboard/index.html; Kreuter et al., 2021; Sommers, M. S. (2019). *Davis's diseases and disorders: A nursing therapeutics manual.* F.A. Davis. https://www.fadavis.com/product/nursing-fundamentals-med-surg-diseases-disorders-nursing-therapeutics-manual-sommers-6

TABLE 16A.2   PALLIATIVE INTERVENTIONS/SYMPTOM MANAGEMENT FOR PULMONARY DISORDERS

SYMPTOM	INTERVENTION
Anxiety and depression	• Antidepressants, anxiolytics, or benzodiazepines as indicated by patient's condition, age, and life expectancy (see Appendix D-1) • Non-pharmacological interventions (see Appendix D-2)
Anorexia	• Use of appetite stimulants (see Appendix D-1) • Offer small, frequent meals and snacks • Offer nutritional supplements
Caregiver burden	• Support of interdisciplinary hospice or palliative team • Non-pharmacological interventions for caregivers (see Appendix D-2)
Dyspnea	• Corticosteroids for reducing inflammation (see Appendix D-1) • Opioids to reduce inspiratory effort and tachypnea (see Appendix D-1) • Bronchodilators for opening airways (mechanism of action of relaxation of muscular bands that surround bronchi, thus widening the airway; see Appendix D-1) • Diuretics to reduce systemic congestion (see Appendix D-1) • Anticholinergics to reduce secretions, especially at the end of life (see Appendix D-1) • Use of fans • Lower temperature in the room

(continued)

TABLE 16A.2   PALLIATIVE INTERVENTIONS/SYMPTOM MANAGEMENT FOR PULMONARY DISORDERS (*CONTINUED*)

SYMPTOM	INTERVENTION
Fatigue and somnolence	• Alternate periods of rest with periods of activity • Utilize energy conversation techniques • Psychostimulants (see Appendix D-1)
Frequent infection	• Avoid crowds or large gatherings • Wear mask when in the company of others • Wash hands frequently • Use of antibiotics or anti-infectives as indicated • Avoid animals and live plants • Avoid dental work • Avoid vaccines unless otherwise directed • Avoid raw foods
Immobility	• Encourage active participation in repositioning, when possible • Implement use of bed mobility devices such as a bed hoist, bed ladder, grab rail, or trapeze bar • Frequently reposition patient to relieve pressure on bony surfaces • Use pillows, cushions, anti-pressure mattresses to alleviate pressure wound risk • If patient is at risk for falls, safety measures such as nonskid slippers, shoes, or socks, bed or chair alarms, floor sensor, or fall mat
Insomnia	• Use of benzodiazepines, antidepressants, or antihistaminic agents, as indicated by patient's condition, age, and life expectancy (see Appendix D-1) • Provide proper sleep hygiene • Use non-pharmacological interventions for relaxation (see Appendix D-2) • Address underlying anxiety and depression
Psychosocial distress and body image changes	• Antidepressants (see Appendix D-1) • Non-pharmacological interventions (see Appendix D-2)

Sources: Fusco, F. (2021). Mouth care. In E. Bruera, I. J. Higginson, C. F. von Gunten, & T. Morita (Eds.), *Textbook of palliative medicine and supportive care.* Taylor & Francis Group; Guyer, D. L., Almhanna, K., & McKee, K. Y. (2020). Palliative care for patients with esophageal cancer: A narrative review. *Annals of Translational Medicine, 8*(17). https://doi.org/10.21037/atm-20-3676; Khan, F., Amatya, B., Bensmail, D., & Yelnik, A. (2019). Non-pharmacological interventions for spasticity in adults: An overview of systematic reviews. *Annals of Physical and Rehabilitation Medicine, 62*(4), 265–273. https://pubmed.ncbi.nlm.nih.gov/29042299/; Kluger, B. M., Ney, D. E., Bagley, S. J., Mohile, N., Taylor, L. P., Walbert, T., & Jones, C. A. (2020). Top ten tips palliative care clinicians should know when caring for patients with brain cancer. *Journal of Palliative Medicine, 23*(3), 415–421. https://doi.org/10.1089/jpm.2019.0507; Sommers, M. S. (2019). *Davis's diseases and disorders: A nursing therapeutics manual.* F.A. Davis. https://www.fadavis.com/product/nursing-fundamentals-med-surg-diseases-disorders-nursing-therapeutics-manual-sommers-6; Tariq, R., & Singal, A. K. (2020). Management of hepatorenal syndrome: A review. *Journal of Clinical and Translational Hepatology, 8*(2), 192. https://www.ncbi.nlm.nih.gov/pmc/articles/PMC7438356/; Walker, Z., Possin, K. L., Boeve, B. F., & Aarsland, D. (2015). Lewy body dementias. *The Lancet, 386*(10004), 1683–1697. https://doi.org/10.1016/S0140-6736(15)00462-6

CHAPTER **17**

RENAL DISORDERS

CHRONIC GLOMERULONEPHRITIS

DEFINITION/CHARACTERISTICS
A. An umbrella term used to describe:
    1. Disorders that affect the glomeruli (see Figure 17.1).
    2. Glomerular disorders that can progress to chronic kidney disease (CKD; Huether, 2019).

INCIDENCE AND PREVALENCE
A. Third leading cause of CKD.
B. Accounts for 10% of all patients on dialysis.
C. Incidence is roughly 2.5/100,000/year (McGrogan et al., 2011; Salifu, 2022).

ETIOLOGY
A. Exact cause is not known (Salifu, 2022).

PATHOPHYSIOLOGY
A. Inflammatory processes lead to:
    1. Hyperfiltration.
    2. Kidney atrophy.
    3. Atrophy of renal cortex.
    4. Scar tissue formation on and in kidneys.
B. Renal insufficiency develops within 10 to 20 years.
C. Glomerular damage progresses to CKD (Hinkle & Cheever, 2018; Huether, 2019).

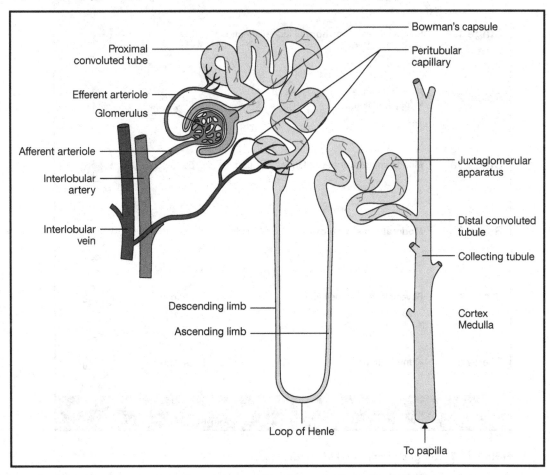

FIGURE 17.1   Structure of nephron.

PREDISPOSING FACTORS

A. Hypercholesterolemia.

B. Proteinuria.

C. Diabetes.

D. Systemic lupus erythematosus (SLE).

E. Episodes of acute glomerulonephritis.

F. Hypertensive nephrosclerosis.

G. Chronic tubulointerstitial injury.

H. Goodpasture syndrome (Hinkle & Cheever, 2018; Huether, 2019).

SUBJECTIVE DATA

A. Decreased physical endurance.

B. Irritability.

C. Headaches.

D. Dizziness.

E. Gastrointestinal distress.

F. Altered mentation.

G. Nausea.

H. Muscle cramps.

I. Fatigue (Hinkle & Cheever, 2018; Mayo Clinic, 2022).

OBJECTIVE DATA

A. Weight loss.

B. Nocturia.

C. Urinary frequency.

D. Hematuria.

E. Anemia.

F. Hypertension.

G. Peripheral neuropathy.

H. Metabolic acidosis.

I. Proteinuria.

J. Edema (Hinkle & Cheever, 2018; Mayo Clinic, 2022).

DIAGNOSTIC TESTS

A. See Appendix Table 17A.1 for listing of common diagnostic tests.

B. See Figure 17.2 for staging.

STAGES OF CHRONIC KIDNEY DISEASE		GFR*	% OF KIDNEY FUNCTION
Stage 1	Kidney damage with **normal** kidney function	90 or higher	90–100%
Stage 2	Kidney damage with **mild loss** of kidney function	89 to 60	89–60%
Stage 3a	**Mild to moderate** loss of kidney function	59 to 45	59–45%
Stage 3b	**Moderate to severe** loss of kidney function	44 to 30	44–30%
Stage 4	**Severe** loss of kidney function	29 to 15	29–15%
Stage 5	Kidney **failure**	Less than 15	Less than 15%

* Your GFR number tells you how much kidney function you have. As kidney disease gets worse, the GFR number goes down.

FIGURE 17.2 Stages of chronic kidney disease.

Source: Adapted from National Kidney Foundation. (2022). *Stages of chronic kidney disease.* https://www.kidney.org/content/kidney-failure-risk-factor-estimated-glomerular-filtration-rate-egfr

DIFFERENTIAL DIAGNOSES

A. Azotemia.
B. CKD.
C. Uremia.
D. Acute glomerulonephritis (Salifu, 2022).

POTENTIAL COMPLICATIONS

A. CKD.
B. Cardiac dysfunction (Hinkle & Cheever, 2018).

DISEASE-MODIFYING TREATMENTS

A. Dialysis.
B. Blood pressure management.
C. Diuretics.
D. Control of diabetes (Hinkle & Cheever, 2018; Huether, 2019).

PALLIATIVE INTERVENTIONS/SYMPTOM MANAGEMENT

A. See Appendix Table 17A.2 for listing of palliative interventions and symptom management.
B. See Appendix D-3 for overview of common symptoms.

PROGNOSIS

A. Prognosis is dependent on extent of kidney damage (Figure 17.3).
B. Cause of death is related to renal failure (see Figure 17.3; Salifu, 2022).

NURSING INTERVENTIONS

A. Provide education on disease process and symptom management.
B. Teach patient importance of renal dietary restrictions (see www.niddk.nih.gov/health-information/kidney-disease/chronic-kidney-disease-ckd/eating-nutrition).
C. Teach patient to take all medications as prescribed.
D. Monitor daily weight.
E. Encourage lifestyle modifications specific to renal disease (see Table 17.1).
F. Educate patient and caregiver(s) on disease trajectory.
G. Promptly treat symptoms of urinary tract infection.
H. Assess and address symptoms of depression and anxiety.

Prognosis of CKD by GFR and albuminuria categories				Albuminuria categories Description and range		
				A1	**A2**	**A3**
				Normal to mildly increased	Moderately increased	Severely increased
				<30 mg/g <3 mg/mmol	30–299 mg/g 3–29 mg/mmol	≥300 mg/g ≥30 mg/mmol
GFR categories (ml/min/1.73 m²) Description and range	**G1**	Normal or high	≥90			
	G2	Mildly decreased	60–90			
	G3a	Mildly to moderately decreased	45–59			
	G3b	Moderately to severely decreased	30–44			
	G4	Severely decreased	15–29			
	G5	Kidney failure	<15			

FIGURE 17.3 Prognosis of chronic kidney disease.

Source: Adapted from Kidney Disease: Improving Global Outcomes CKD Work Group. (2013). KDIGO 2012 Clinical practice guideline for the evaluation and management of chronic kidney disease. *Kidney International Supplement, 3,* 1–150. https://kdigo.org/wp-content/uploads/2017/02/KDIGO_2012_CKD_GL.pdf

TABLE 17.1 LIFESTYLE MODIFICATION

	EFFECT ON CHRONIC KIDNEY DISEASE PROGRESSION	EFFECT ON CARDIOVASCULAR DISEASE AND MORTALITY	COMMENTS	RECOMMENDATIONS
Physical activity	Slower decline in kidney function	Lower risk of adverse cardiovascular outcomes and mortality	Evidence on physical activity and progression of kidney disease and cardiovascular outcomes is largely based on observational studies. Small trials of physical activity show improvements in kidney function and blood pressure in people with chronic kidney disease not receiving dialysis. Small trials in patients receiving dialysis show improvements in physical function and health-related quality of life.	Target of 150 minutes/week of moderate intensity physical activity for patients with chronic kidney disease. Exercise should be individualized for patients according to comorbidities and functional status (mixed data in patients dependent on dialysis)
Smoking cessation of avoidance	Smoking is associated with a greater risk of incident chronic kidney disease	Smoking is associated with increased risk of all-cause mortality, including vascular causes and cancer, in people with chronic kidney disease.	Smoking cessation should be prioritized in all individuals for numerous recognized health benefits.	Smoking cessation for all patients with behavioral counselling and pharmacological therapies as required, with appropriate dose adjustment for patients with chronic kidney disease
Dietary sodium restriction	Reduced albuminuria and improved fluid status in people with and without chronic kidney disease	Reduces blood pressure and improves arterial stiffness in people with and without chronic kidney disease	People with chronic kidney disease are more likely to have salt-sensitive hypertension.	Limit sodium intake to a maximum of 2–3 g/day (<100 mmol) according to the American Heart Association.
Higher proportion of plant-based protein in the diet	Higher proportion of plant-based protein and fiber intake might improve acidosis, mitigate inflammation, reduce phosphorus burden, slow progression of chronic kidney disease, and create less uremic toxins.	Higher red meat intake might be associated with atherosclerosis due to higher carnitine generation via gut microbiota.	Reducing dietary protein intake can increase the risk of muscle mass loss and frailty. Protein intake recommendations vary depending on chronic kidney disease stage, acute kidney injury, and need for dialysis.	Higher intake of complex carbohydrates and fresh fruits and vegetables as opposed to processed carbohydrates

(continued)

TABLE 17.1 LIFESTYLE MODIFICATION (*CONTINUED*)

	EFFECT ON CHRONIC KIDNEY DISEASE PROGRESSION	EFFECT ON CARDIOVASCULAR DISEASE AND MORTALITY	COMMENTS	RECOMMENDATIONS
Weight reduction	Improved cardiometabolic health, potentially slower decline in kidney function, and improved albuminuria	Improves blood pressure	Little evidence from randomized controlled trials to guide the dietetic management of people with overweight and obesity and chronic kidney disease	Multidisciplinary approach to weight loss in overweight and obese individuals with chronic kidney disease with involvement of a renal dietitian. Mixed data in dialysis patients related to the obesity paradox

Source: Kalantar-Zadeh, K., Jafar, T. H., Nitsch, D., Neuen, B. L., & Perkovic, V. (2021). Chronic kidney disease. *The Lancet, 398*(10302), 786–802. https://doi.org/10.1016/S0140-6736(21)00519-5

I. Provide assistance with activities of daily living (ADLs) as needed.
J. Provide spiritual support.
K. Assess caregiver fatigue/burnout (see Appendix B-5).
L. Encourage completion of advance directives.
M. Discuss wishes regarding withholding or withdrawing of life-sustaining interventions in late stage of disease with patient (if possible) and/or primary caregiver (see Appendices C-2, C-3, and C-4).
N. Educate patient and family regarding availability of palliative care.
O. Educate patient and family regarding availability of hospice services (when appropriate).
P. Provide referral to community support groups, as needed.

CHRONIC KIDNEY DISEASE

DEFINITION/CHARACTERISTICS
A. An umbrella term used to describe:
   1. Progressive renal deterioration.
   2. Diminished kidney function lasting 3 months or longer (Hinkle & Cheever, 2018; Huether, 2019).

INCIDENCE AND PREVALENCE
A. Leading cause of death in the United States.
B. In the United States, 37 million adults have chronic kidney disease (CKD).
C. Among those who have renal dysfunction, 40% have undiagnosed CKD (Centers for Disease Control and Prevention, 2022).

ETIOLOGY
A. Diabetes and heart disease account for 75% of new cases.

B. Other causes of CKD include:
   1. Hypertension.
   2. Glomerulonephritis.
   3. Pyelonephritis.
   4. Polycystic, hereditary, or congenital disorders.
   5. Renal cancers (Hinkle & Cheever, 2018; Sommers, 2019).

PATHOPHYSIOLOGY
A. Prolonged inflammation leads to:
   1. Diminished kidney function.
   2. Decreased glomerular filtration rate (GFR; see Figure 17.4)
   3. Reduced tubular function (see Figure 17.1; Hinkle & Cheever, 2018; Huether, 2019).

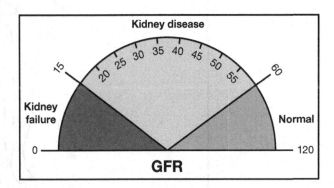

FIGURE 17.4 Glomerular filtration rate.

Source: Adapted from National Institute of Diabetes and Digestive and Kidney Diseases. (2023). *Chronic kidney disease.* https://www.niddk.nih.gov/health-information/kidney-disease/chronic-kidney-disease-ckd

PREDISPOSING FACTORS

A. Hypertension.
B. Diabetes mellitus.
C. Cardiovascular disease.
D. Obesity.
E. Systemic lupus erythematosus (SLE).
F. Intrinsic kidney disease.
G. Acute kidney disease.
H. Chronic glomerulonephritis.
I. Chronic pyelonephritis.
J. Obstructive uropathies.
K. Vascular disorders.
L. Coronavirus disease 2019 (COVID-19; Hinkle & Cheever, 2018; Huether, 2019; Sommers, 2019).

SUBJECTIVE DATA

A. Nausea.
B. Pruritus.
C. Neuropathies.
D. Pain.
E. Confusion.
F. Apathy.
G. Irritability.
H. Fatigue (Hinkle & Cheever, 2018; Huether, 2019; Sommers, 2019).

OBJECTIVE DATA

A. Azotemia (see Figure 17.5).
B. Uremia.
C. Hypertension.
D. Constipation.
E. Weight loss.
F. Edema.
G. Anemia.
H. Fever.
I. Reduced GFR.
J. Increased creatinine.
K. Increased blood urea nitrogen (BUN).
L. Tachycardia.
M. Atrial fibrillation.
N. Jugular vein distention (JVD; see Figure 9.4 in Chapter 9).
O. Distant heart sounds.
P. Orthopnea.
Q. Pulmonary congestion.
R. Rales.
S. Jaundice.
T. Uremic frost (see Figure 17.6).
U. Dry skin (Hinkle & Cheever, 2018; Huether, 2019; Sommers, 2019).

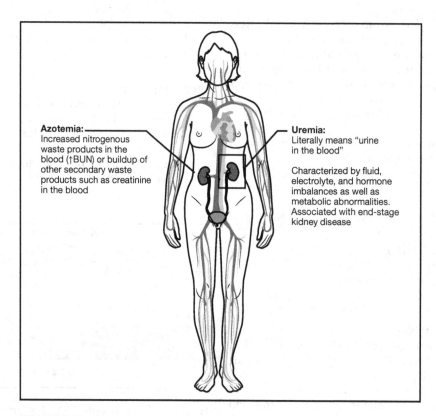

Azotemia:
Increased nitrogenous waste products in the blood (↑BUN) or buildup of other secondary waste products such as creatinine in the blood

Uremia:
Literally means "urine in the blood"

Characterized by fluid, electrolyte, and hormone imbalances as well as metabolic abnormalities. Associated with end-stage kidney disease

FIGURE 17.5 Azotemia versus uremia.

Sources: Adapted from Tyagi, A., & Aeddula, N. R. (2019). *Azotemia.* https://europepmc.org/article/NBK/nbk538145; Zemaitis, M. R., Foris, L. A., Katta, S., & Bashir, K. (2022). *Uremia.* https://www.ncbi.nlm.nih.gov/books/NBK441859/#_NBK441859_pubdet_

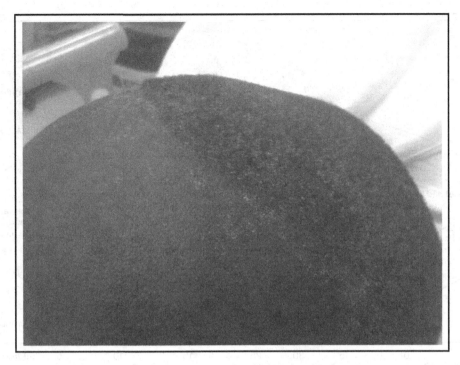

FIGURE 17.6 Uremic frost on the forehead and scalp of a young man.

Source: Fythrion. (2012). *Uremic frost on forehead and scalp of young Afro-Caribbean male.*

DIAGNOSTIC TESTS
A. See Appendix Table 17A.1 for listing of common diagnostic tests.

DIFFERENTIAL DIAGNOSES
A. SLE.
B. Renal artery stenosis.
C. Urinary tract obstruction.
D. Granulomatosis (Arora, 2021).

POTENTIAL COMPLICATIONS
A. Congestive heart failure.
B. Electrolyte imbalances.
C. Intractable hypertension.
D. Premature death (Hinkle & Cheever, 2018).

DISEASE-MODIFYING TREATMENTS
A. Dialysis.
B. Kidney transplantation.
C. Prevention of complications through:
   1. Blood pressure management.
   2. Control of diabetes.
   3. Management of heart disease.
   4. Management of anemia.
   5. Smoking cessation.
   6. Weight loss.
   7. Decreased sodium intake.
   8. Reduced alcohol intake (Figure 17.7; Hinkle & Cheever, 2018).

PALLIATIVE INTERVENTIONS/SYMPTOM MANAGEMENT
A. See Appendix Table 17A.2 for listing of palliative interventions and symptom management.
B. See Appendix D-3 for overview of common symptoms.

PROGNOSIS
A. Prognosis is dependent on extent of kidney damage:
   1. Stage 3 = 24 to 28 years.
   2. Stage 4 = 14 to 16 years.
   3. Stage 5 = 7 to 14 years (see Figure 17.3).
B. Kidney transplantation results in normal life span (LeBrun, 2020).

NURSING INTERVENTIONS
A. Provide education on disease process and symptom management.
B. Teach patient importance of renal dietary restrictions (see www.niddk.nih.gov/health-information/kidney-disease/chronic-kidney-disease-ckd/eating-nutrition).
C. Teach patient to take all medications as prescribed.
D. Monitor daily weight.
E. Encourage lifestyle modifications specific to renal disease (see Table 17.1).
F. Educate patient and caregiver(s) on disease trajectory.
G. Promptly treat symptoms of urinary tract infection.
H. Encourage smoking cessation (see Appendices B-10 and C-9).

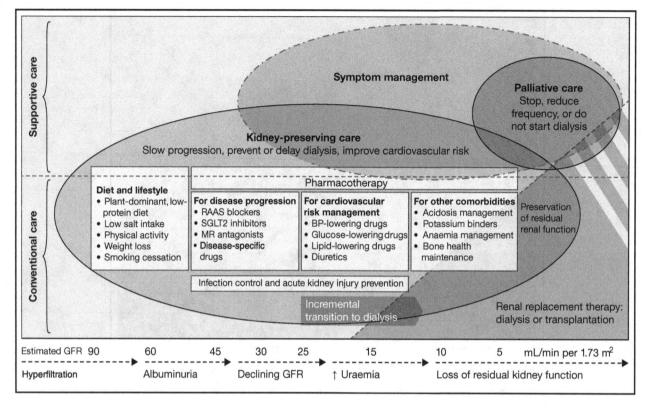

FIGURE 17.7 Management of chronic kidney disease.

Note: This chart highlights the role of preservative management and its goals within the overall conservative management of chronic kidney disease without dialysis, juxtaposing renal replacement therapy including dialysis and kidney transplantation. The X axis (showing chronic kidney disease progression) should be read exclusively from left to right. The bottom half of the chart represents conventional (life-prolonging and kidney-prolonging) strategies, whereas the top half represents supportive care, including palliative and hospice care, in which dialysis is often avoided or withdrawn. The oblique dotted line between the two main zones (conservative management vs. renal replacement therapy) suggests that there is variability in transitioning to dialysis therapy (moving from bottom left to top right), including timing (early vs. late vs. never), level of care (life-prolonging vs. supportive care), and type of dialysis (conventional vs incremental). The symptom management domain provides wide ranges of interventions to encompass the goals of care under both kidney-preserving care and palliative and hospice care. Preservative management can preserve residual kidney function for longer, especially after incremental transition to dialysis.

BP, blood pressure; GFR, glomerular filtration rate; MR, mineralocorticoid receptor; RAAS, renin–angiotensin–aldosterone system.

Source: Adapted from Kalantar-Zadeh, K., Jafar, T. H., Nitsch, D., Neuen, B. L., & Perkovic, V. (2021). Chronic kidney disease. *The Lancet, 398*(10302), 786–802. https://doi.org/10.1016/S0140-6736(21)00519-5

I. Assess and address symptoms of depression and anxiety.

J. Provide assistance with activities of daily living (ADLs) as needed.

K. Provide spiritual support.

L. Assess caregiver fatigue/burnout (see Appendix B-5).

M. Encourage completion of advance directives.

N. Discuss wishes regarding withholding or withdrawing of life-sustaining interventions in late stage of disease with patient (if possible) and/or primary caregiver (see Appendices C-2, C-3, and C-4).

O. Educate patient and family regarding availability of palliative care

P. Educate patient and family regarding availability of hospice services (when appropriate).

Q. Provide referral to community support groups, as needed.

REFERENCES

Arora, P. (2021). *Chronic kidney disease (CKD) differential diagnoses.* https://emedicine.medscape.com/article/238798-differential

Centers for Disease Control and Prevention. (2022). *Chronic kidney disease basics.* https://www.cdc.gov/kidneydisease/basics.html

Hinkle, J. L., & Cheever, K. H. (2018). *Brunner & Siddarth's textbook of medical-surgical nursing* (14th ed., pp. 1377–1427). Wolters Kluwer.

Huether, S. E. (2019). Alternations of renal and urinary tract function. In K. L. McCance & S. E. Huether (Eds.), *Pathophysiology:*

The biologic basis for disease in adults and children (8th ed., pp. 1246–1277). Elsevier.

LeBrun, N. (2020). *Kidney disease prognosis and life expectancy.* https://www.healthgrades.com/right-care/kidney-disease/kidney-disease-prognosis-and-life-expectancy

Mayo Clinic. (2022). *Glomerulonephritis.* https://www.mayo-clinic.org/diseases-conditions/glomerulonephritis/symptoms-causes/syc-20355705

McGrogan, A., Franssen, C. F., & de Vries, C. S. (2011). The incidence of primary glomerulonephritis worldwide: A systematic review of the literature. *Nephrology Dialysis Transplantation, 26*(2), 414–430. https://academic.oup.com/ndt/article/26/2/414/1895374

Salifu, M. O. (2022). *Chronic glomerulonephritis.* https://emedicine.medscape.com/article/239392-overview

Sommers, M. S. (2019). *Davis's diseases and disorders: A nursing therapeutics manual.* F.A. Davis. https://www.fadavis.com/product/nursing-fundamentals-med-surg-diseases-disorders-nursing-therapeutics-manual-sommers-6

APPENDIX

TABLE 17A.1 DIAGNOSTIC TESTS FOR RENAL DISORDERS

TYPE	NOTES
Physical examination	• Thorough physical examination with detailed medical history and urological examination
Imaging	• CT scan • MRI • Ultrasound of kidneys • Chest x-ray (chronic glomerulonephritis) • Electrocardiogram (chronic glomerulonephritis)
Laboratory tests	• Complete blood count • Blood urea nitrogen • Serum creatinine • Urinalysis • Lipid profile • Urine albumin • Glomerular filtration rate (see www.kidney.org/professionals/kdoqi/gfr_calculator) • Albumin-to-creatinine ratio (see www.omnicalculator.com/health/acr; chronic kidney disease)
Pathology	• Kidney biopsy • Renal disease is staged according to progression (see Figure 17.2)

Sources: Hinkle, J.L., & Cheever, K.H. (2018). *Brunner & Siddarth's textbook of medical-surgical nursing* (14th ed., pp. 1377–1427). Wolters Kluwer; Salifu, M. O. (2022). *Chronic glomerulonephritis.* https://emedicine.medscape.com/article/239392-overview

TABLE 17A.2 PALLIATIVE INTERVENTIONS/SYMPTOM MANAGEMENT FOR PULMONARY DISORDERS

SYMPTOM	INTERVENTION
Anemia	• Pharmacological interventions (see Appendix D-1) ■ Epoetin (Procrit) ■ Darbepoetin (Aranesp) ■ Iron supplementation
Anorexia	• Use of appetite stimulants (see Appendix D-1) • Offer small, frequent meals and snacks • Offer nutritional supplements
Anxiety and depression	• Antidepressants, anxiolytics, or benzodiazepines as indicated by patient's condition, age, and life expectancy (see Appendix D-1) • Non-pharmacological interventions (see Appendix D-2)
Caregiver burden	• Support of interdisciplinary hospice or palliative team • Non-pharmacological interventions for caregivers (see Appendix D-2)

(continued)

TABLE 17A.2 PALLIATIVE INTERVENTIONS/SYMPTOM MANAGEMENT FOR PULMONARY DISORDERS (*CONTINUED*)

SYMPTOM	INTERVENTION

Dysrhythmias	• Treatment depends on underlying cause (see section on dysrhythmias; CKD)
	• Possible interventions for CKD include:
	  ▪ Medications (e.g., adenosine, atropine, beta-blockers, calcium channel blockers, epinephrine, amiodarone, anticoagulants, lidocaine; see Appendix D-1)
	  ▪ Pacemaker placement
	  ▪ Cardioversion (as indicated by patient preference and disease progression)
	  ▪ Cardiac ablation

Edema	• Use of diuretics as indicated (see Appendix D-1) • Elevation of extremity • Compression
Fatigue and somnolence	• Alternate periods of rest with periods of activity • Utilize energy conversation techniques • Psychostimulants (see Appendix D-1)

Gastrointestinal symptoms	• Pharmacological interventions (see Appendix D-1)
	  ▪ Antacids
	  ▪ Antiemetics
	  ▪ Promotility agents
	  ▪ Laxatives
	  ▪ Antidiarrheals

Immobility/poor physical endurance	• Encourage active participation in repositioning, when possible • Implement use of bed mobility devices such as a bed hoist, bed ladder, grab rail, or trapeze bar • Frequently reposition patient to relieve pressure on bony surfaces • Use pillows, cushions, anti-pressure mattresses to alleviate pressure wound risk • If patient is at risk for falls, safety measures such as nonskid slippers, shoes, or socks, bed or chair alarms, floor sensor, or fall mat
Intractable hematuria	• Orally administered epsilon-aminocaproic acid • Intravesical formalin • Alum or prostaglandin irrigation • Hydrostatic pressure • Urinary diversion • Radiation therapy • Embolization • Intra-arterial mitoxantrone perfusion

(continued)

TABLE 17A.2   PALLIATIVE INTERVENTIONS/SYMPTOM MANAGEMENT FOR PULMONARY DISORDERS (*CONTINUED*)

SYMPTOM	INTERVENTION
Muscle spasm	<ul><li>Stretching</li><li>Exercise as tolerated</li><li>Alternate activity with periods of rest</li><li>Massage</li><li>Heat therapy</li><li>Frequent position change</li><li>Joint splinting</li><li>Pharmacological interventions (see Appendix D-1)<ul><li>Antispasmodics</li><li>Benzodiazepines</li><li>Muscle relaxants</li><li>Calcium channel blockers</li></ul></li></ul>
Nausea	<ul><li>Antiemetics (see Appendix D-1)</li><li>Non-pharmacological interventions (see Appendix D-2)</li></ul>
Neuropathy	<ul><li>Pharmacological interventions (see Appendix D-1)<ul><li>Antidepressants</li><li>Anticonvulsants (i.e., gabapentin)</li><li>Anesthetics (i.e., ketamine)</li><li>Opioids</li></ul></li></ul>
Pruritus	<ul><li>Thorough dermatological exam to establish cause (CKD)</li><li>Depending on cause, topical agents such as ointments, barrier creams, or soaks can be trialed (e.g., calamine, menthol, oatmeal bath, antihistamine cream; CKD)</li><li>Systemic antihistamines may be used but are not recommended for older adults (see Appendix D-1; CKD)</li><li>Maintain short fingernails (CKD)</li></ul>
Psychosocial	<ul><li>Antidepressants (see Appendix D-1)</li><li>Non-pharmacological interventions (see Appendix D-2)</li></ul>

CKD, chronic kidney disease.

Sources: Düll, M. M., & Kremer, A. E. (2019). Treatment of pruritus secondary to liver disease. *Current Gastroenterology Reports, 21*(9), 1–9. https://link.springer.com/article/10.1007/s11894-019-0713-6#Sec9; Fusco, F. (2021). Mouth care. In E. Bruera, I. J. Higginson, C. F. von Gunten, & T. Morita (Eds.), *Textbook of palliative medicine and supportive care.* Taylor & Francis Group; Guyer, D. L., Almhanna, K., & McKee, K. Y. (2020). Palliative care for patients with esophageal cancer: A narrative review. *Annals of Translational Medicine, 8*(17), 1103. https://doi.org/10.21037/atm-20-3676; Khan, F., Amatya, B., Bensmail, D., & Yelnik, A. (2019). Non-pharmacological interventions for spasticity in adults: An overview of systematic reviews. *Annals of Physical and Rehabilitation Medicine, 62*(4), 265–273. https://pubmed.ncbi.nlm.nih.gov/29042299/; Kluger, B. M., Ney, D. E., Bagley, S. J., Mohile, N., Taylor, L. P., Walbert, T., & Jones, C. A. (2020). Top ten tips palliative care clinicians should know when caring for patients with brain cancer. *Journal of Palliative Medicine, 23*(3), 415–421. https://doi.org/10.1089/jpm.2019.0507; Sommers, M. S. (2019). *Davis's diseases and disorders: A nursing therapeutics manual.* F.A. Davis. https://www.fadavis.com/product/nursing-fundamentals-med-surg-diseases-disorders-nursing-therapeutics-manual-sommers-6; Tariq, R., & Singal, A. K. (2020). Management of hepatorenal syndrome: A review. *Journal of Clinical and Translational Hepatology, 8*(2), 192. https://www.ncbi.nlm.nih.gov/pmc/articles/PMC7438356/; Walker, Z., Possin, K. L., Boeve, B. F., & Aarsland, D. (2015). Lewy body dementias. *The Lancet, 386*(10004), 1683–1697. https://doi.org/10.1016/S0140-6736(15)00462-6

APPENDIX A

PROGNOSTICATION TOOLS

APPENDIX A-1: MEASURING MID-ARM CIRCUMFERENCE AND BODY MASS INDEX

Measuring the Mid-Arm Circumference

Why should I get a mid-arm circumference?

Mid-arm circumference (MAC) is an important measure of nutritional status. Following a patient's nutritional status is key for establishing eligibility for hospice care. This measurement should be taken at the time of admission and then on a monthly basis or PRN. The MAC should be obtained even when you are able to obtain a weight as, in many cases, patients later reach a point where obtaining a weight is no longer possible. Having a MAC for comparison can sometimes be the key element in ensuring that the patient remains eligible for hospice services.

Taking the measurement

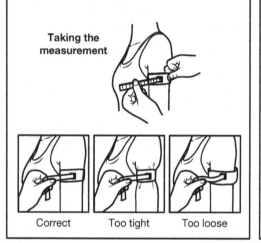

Correct | Too tight | Too loose

Measuring the Mid-Arm Circumference

How do I measure the mid-arm circumference?

- Always measure on the right arm unless there is a specific reason why this is not possible (i.e. lymphedema following mastectomy.) At the time of the first measurement, note the side used and use the same side for all subsequent measurements.
- Locate the olecranon process, the tip of the elbow.
- Locate the acromial process, the tip of the shoulder.
- Measure on the posterior aspect of the arm between these two points, being careful to keep the tape straight.
- Divide the length by 2 and mark this midpoint on the arm with a pen.
- Ask the patient to relax the arm at their side with the palm facing inward. Make certain that the patient is not flexing the muscles in the arm.
- Place the measuring tape around the arm at this midpoint, holding the tape perpendicular to the length of the arm.
- The tape should be touching the skin continuously and should follow the contours of the tissue but it should not compress the skin or tissue. Do not attempt to compress skin folds, just lay the tape measure gently around the arm.
- Record measurement in centimeters using a decimal point if the measurement does not fall on an exact number.
- Repeat the circumference measurement a total of 3 times and take an average of the 3 to get the most accurate mid-arm circumference measurement.
- Report the MAC at IDT and record your measurement in a consistent place in the patient's chart.
- Include the MAC from admission, the most current MAC, and the trend on the reassessment for eligibility form.

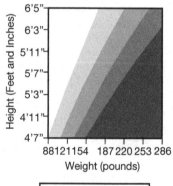

Acromion process of scapula

Olecranon process

Body Mass Index (BMI)

Body mass index (BMI) is a measure of body fat based on height and weight that applies to adult men and women.

Under weight < 18.5 | Normal weight 18.5–24.9 | Over weight 25.0–29.9

Obese (Class I) 30.0–34.9 | Obese (Class II) 35.0–39.9 | Obese (Class III) > 40

Calculating Body Mass Index

Go to the NIH (National Heart, Lung, and Blood Institute) website below to calculate the body mass index. Simply enter the height and weight (in standard or metric) and then click on the tab "Compute BMI."

http://www.nhlbi.nih.gov/health/educational/lose_wt/BMI/bmicalc.htm

You can also download the BMI calculator app to your iPhone or Android phone.

Height [ ] [ ] ft in
Weight [ ] lbs
[Compute BMI]
Your BMI [ ]

You will also be able to view the following on the website:

- View 2 BMI tables
- Limitations of the BMI
- Assessing your risk
- Controlling your weight
- Recipes

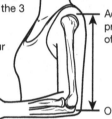

Height (Feet and Inches)
6'5"
6'3"
5'11"
5'7"
5'3"
4'11"
4'7"

88 121 154 187 220 253 286
Weight (pounds)

Key
☐ Under weight
☐ Normal weight
☐ Over weight
☐ Obese
☐ Morbidly obese

Source: Adapted from Home Health VNA. (n.d). *Measuring mid-arm circumference and body mass index (BMI).* http://www.hhvna.com/files/SkillsFair2016/Hospice_Arm_Circumference_and_BMI.pdf

APPENDIX A-2: THE KARNOFSKY SCALE

KS	DEFINITION
100	Normal; no complaints; no evidence of disease
90	Able to carry on normal activity; minor signs or symptoms of disease
80	Normal activity with effort; some sign or symptoms of disease
70	Cares for self; unable to carry on normal activity or do active work
60	Requires occasional assistance, but is able to care for most personal needs
50	Requires considerable assistance and frequent medical care
40	Disabled; requires special care and assistance
30	Severely disabled; hospitalization is indicated, although death not imminent
20	Very sick; hospitalization necessary; active support treatment is necessary
10	Moribund; fatal processes progressing rapidly
0	Dead

KS, Karnofsky score.

Source: Karnofsky, D. A., & Burchenal, J. H. (1949). *The clinical evaluation of chemotherapeutic agents.* Columbia University Press.

APPENDIX A-3: PALLIATIVE PERFORMANCE SCALE

PPS LEVEL	AMBULATION	ACTIVITY AND EVIDENCE OF DISEASE	SELF-CARE	INTAKE	CONSCIOUS LEVEL
100%	Full	Normal activity and work No evidence of disease	Full	Normal	Full
90%	Full	Normal activity and work Some evidence of disease	Full	Normal	Full
80%	Full	Normal activity with effort Some evidence of disease	Full	Normal or reduced	Full
70%	Reduced	Unable to do normal job/work Significant disease	Full	Normal or reduced	Full
60%	Reduced	Unable to do hobby/house work Significant disease	Occasional assistance necessary	Normal or reduced	Full or confusion
50%	Mainly sit/lie	Unable to do any work Extensive disease	Considerable assistance required	Normal or reduced	Full or confusion
40%	Mainly in bed	Unable to do most activity Extensive disease	Mainly assistance	Normal or reduced	Full or drowsy +/- confusion
30%	Totally bed bound	Unable to do any activity Extensive disease	Total care	Normal or reduced	Full or drowsy +/- confusion
20%	Totally bed bound	Unable to do any activity Extensive disease	Total care	Minimal to sips	Full or drowsy +/- confusion
10%	Totally bed bound	Unable to do any activity Extensive disease	Total care	Mouth care only	Drowsy or coma +/- confusion
0%	Death	-	-	-	-

INSTRUCTIONS FOR USE OF PPS (SEE ALSO DEFINITION OF TERMS)

1. PPS scores are determined by reading horizontally at each level to find a "best fit" for the patient which is then assigned as the PPS% score.

2. Begin at the left column and read downwards until the appropriate ambulation level is reached, then read across to the next column and downwards again until the activity/evidence of disease is located. These steps are repeated until all five columns are covered before assigning the actual PPS for that patient. In this way, "leftward" columns (columns to the left of any specific column) are "stronger" determinants and generally take precedence over others.

> Example 1: A patient who spends the majority of the day sitting or lying down due to fatigue from advanced disease and requires considerable assistance to walk even for short distances but who is otherwise fully conscious level with good intake would be scored at PPS 50%.

> Example 2: A patient who has become paralyzed and quadriplegic requiring total care would be PPS 30%. Although this patient may be placed in a wheelchair (and perhaps seem initially to be at 50%), the score is 30% because he or she would be otherwise totally bed bound due to the disease or complication if it were not for caregivers providing total care including lift/transfer. The patient may have normal intake and full conscious level.

> Example 3: However, if the patient in example 2 was paraplegic and bed bound but still able to do some self-care such as feed themselves, then the PPS would be higher at 40% or 50% since he or she is not "total care."

3. PPS scores are in 10% increments only. Sometimes, there are several columns easily placed at one level but one or two which seem better at a higher or lower level. One then needs to make a "best fit" decision. Choosing a "half-fit" value of PPS 45%, for example, is not correct. The combination of clinical judgment and "leftward precedence" is used to determine whether 40% or 50% is the more accurate score for that patient.

4. PPS may be used for several purposes. First, it is an excellent communication tool for quickly describing a patient's current functional level. Second, it may have value in criteria for workload assessment or other measurements and comparisons. Finally, it appears to have prognostic value.

DEFINITION OF TERMS FOR PPS

As noted below, some of the terms have similar meanings with the differences being more readily apparent as one reads horizontally across each row to find an overall "best fit" using all five columns.

1. AMBULATION

The items **"mainly sit/lie,"** **"mainly in bed,"** and **"totally bed bound"** are clearly similar. The subtle differences are related to items in the self-care column. For example, "totally bed bound" at PPS 30% is due to either profound weakness or paralysis such that the patient not only can't get out of bed but is also unable to do any self-care. The difference between "sit/lie" and "bed" is proportionate to the amount of time the patient is able to sit up vs. needs to lie down.

"Reduced ambulation" is located at the PPS 70% and PPS 60% level. By using the adjacent column, the reduction of ambulation is tied to inability to carry out their normal job, work occupation or some hobbies or housework activities. The person is still able to walk and transfer on their own but at PPS 60% needs occasional assistance.

2. ACTIVITY AND EXTENT OF DISEASE

"Some," **"significant,"** and **"extensive"** disease refer to physical and investigative evidence which shows degrees of progression. For example in breast cancer, a local recurrence would imply "some" disease, one or two metastases in the lung or bone would imply "significant" disease, whereas multiple metastases in lung, bone, liver, brain, hypercalcemia, or other major complications would be "extensive" disease. The extent may also refer to progression of disease despite active treatments. Using PPS in AIDS, "some" may mean the shift from HIV to AIDS, "significant" implies progression in physical decline, new or difficult symptoms and laboratory findings with low counts. "Extensive" refers to one or more serious complications with or without continuation of active antiretrovirals, antibiotics, etc.

The above extent of disease is also judged in context with the ability to maintain one's work and hobbies or activities. Decline in activity may mean the person still plays golf but reduces from playing 18 holes to 9 holes, or just a par 3, or to backyard putting. People who enjoy walking will gradually reduce the distance covered, although they may continue trying, sometimes even close to death (e.g., trying to walk the halls).

3. SELF-CARE

"Occasional assistance" means that most of the time patients are able to transfer out of bed, walk, wash, toilet, and eat by their own means, but that on occasion (perhaps once daily or a few times weekly) they require minor assistance.

"Considerable assistance" means that regularly every day the patient needs help, usually by one person, to do some of the activities noted above. For example, the person needs help to get to the bathroom but is then able to brush his or her teeth or wash at least hands and face. Food will often need to be cut into edible sizes but the patient is then able to eat of their own accord.

"Mainly assistance" is a further extension of "considerable." Using the above example, the patient now needs help getting up but also needs assistance washing his face and shaving, but can usually eat with minimal or no help. This may fluctuate according to fatigue during the day.

"Total care" means that the patient is completely unable to eat without help, toilet or do any self-care. Depending on the clinical situation, the patient may or may not be able to chew and swallow food once prepared and fed to them.

4. INTAKE

Changes in intake are quite obvious with **"normal intake"** referring to the person's usual eating habits while healthy. **"Reduced"** means any reduction from that and is highly variable according to the unique individual circumstances. **"Minimal"** refers to very small amounts, usually pureed or liquid, which are well below nutritional sustenance.

5. CONSCIOUS LEVEL

"Full consciousness" implies full alertness and orientation with good cognitive abilities in various domains of thinking, memory, etc. **"Confusion"** is used to denote presence of either delirium or dementia and is a reduced level of consciousness. It may be mild, moderate, or severe with multiple possible etiologies. **"Drowsiness"** implies either fatigue, drug side effects, delirium or closeness to death and is sometimes included in the term stupor. **"Coma"** in this context is the absence of response to verbal or physical stimuli; some reflexes may or may not remain. The depth of coma may fluctuate throughout a 24-hour period.

Source: Adapted from Victoria Hospice. (2001). *Palliative performance scale (PSv2)*. https://victoriahospice.org/wp-content/uploads/2019/12/PPSv2-English-Sample.pdf. Used with permission.

APPENDIX A-4: THE EASTERN COOPERATIVE ONCOLOGY GROUP PERFORMANCE STATUS

ECOG
PERFORMANCE
SCALE

Rating a patient's well-being

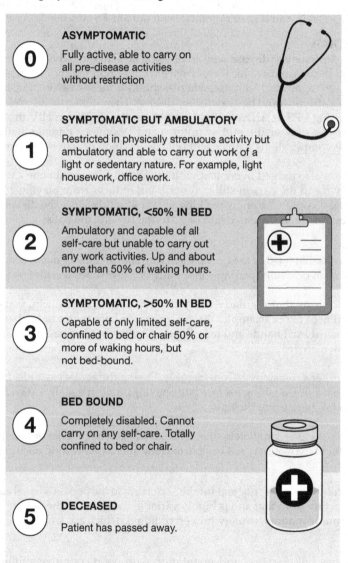

0

ASYMPTOMATIC

Fully active, able to carry on all pre-disease activities without restriction

1

SYMPTOMATIC BUT AMBULATORY

Restricted in physically strenuous activity but ambulatory and able to carry out work of a light or sedentary nature. For example, light housework, office work.

2

SYMPTOMATIC, <50% IN BED

Ambulatory and capable of all self-care but unable to carry out any work activities. Up and about more than 50% of waking hours.

3

SYMPTOMATIC, >50% IN BED

Capable of only limited self-care, confined to bed or chair 50% or more of waking hours, but not bed-bound.

4

BED BOUND

Completely disabled. Cannot carry on any self-care. Totally confined to bed or chair.

5

DECEASED

Patient has passed away.

Source: Adapted from Ginamisra. (2020). *The definitions of each level of the ECOG scale.*

APPENDIX A-5: FUNCTIONAL ASSESSMENT STAGING TOOL

FAST	
1	No difficulty either subjectively or objectively.
2	Complains of forgetting location of objects. Subjective work difficulties.
3	Decreased job functioning evident to coworkers. Difficulty in traveling to new locations. Decreased organizational capacity.[a]
4	Decreased ability to perform complex task (e.g., planning dinner for guests, handling personal finances, such as forgetting to pay bills, etc.).
5	Requires assistance in choosing proper clothing to wear for the day, season, or occasion (e.g., patient may wear the same clothing repeatedly, unless supervised).[a]
6	Occasionally or more frequently over the past weeks[a] for the following: A) Improperly putting on clothes without assistance or cueing. B) Unable to bathe properly (not able to choose proper water temperature). C) Inability to handle mechanics of toileting (e.g., forget to flush the toilet, does not wipe properly or properly dispose of toilet tissue). D) Urinary incontinence. E) Fecal incontinence.
7	A) Ability to speak limited to approximately ≤6 intelligible different words in the course of an average day or in the course of an intensive interview. B) Speech ability is limited to the use of a single intelligible word in an average day or in the course of an intensive interview. C) Ambulatory ability is lost (cannot walk without personal assistance). D) Cannot sit up without assistance (e.g., the individual will fall over if there are not lateral rests [arms] on the chair). E) Loss of ability to smile. F) Loss of ability to hold up head independently.

[a]Scored primarily on information obtained from a knowledgeable informant.

FAST, functional assessment staging tool.

Source: Reisberg, B. (1987). Functional assessment staging (FAST). *Psychopharmacology Bulletin, 24*(4), 653–659. https://www.researchgate.net/journal/0048-5764_Psychopharmacology_bulletin.

APPENDIX A-6: THE CLINICAL FRAILTY SCALE

1 VERY FIT People who are robust, active, energetic and motivated. They tend to exercise regularly and are among the fittest for their age.

2 FIT People who have **no active disease symptoms** but are less fit than category 1. Often, they exercise or are very **active occasionally,** e.g., seasonally.

3 MANAGING WELL People whose **medical problems are well controlled,** even if occasionally symptomatic, but often are **not regularly active** beyond routine walking.

4 LIVING WITH VERY MILD FRAILTY Previously "vulnerable," this category marks early transition from complete independence. While **not dependent** on others for daily help, often **symptoms limit activities.** A common complaint is being "slowed up" and/or being tired during the day.

5 LIVING WITH MILD FRAILTY People who often have **more evident slowing,** and need help with **high order instrumental activities of daily living** (finances, transportation, heavy housework). Typically, mild frailty progressively impairs shopping and walking outside alone, meal preparation, medications and begins to restrict light housework.

6 LIVING WITH MODERATE FRAILTY People who need help with **all outside activities** and with **keeping house.** Inside, they often have problems with stairs and need **help with bathing** and might need minimal assistance (cuing, standby) with dressing.

7 LIVING WITH SEVERE FRAILTY **Completely dependent for personal care,** from whatever cause (physical or cognitive). Even so, they seem stable and not at high risk of dying (within ~6 months).

8 LIVING WITH VERY SEVERE FRAILTY Completely dependent for personal care and approaching end of life. Typically, they could not recover even from a minor illness.

9 TERMINALLY ILL Approaching the end of life. This category applies to people with a **life expectancy <6 months,** who are **not otherwise living with severe frailty.** (Many terminally ill people can still exercise until very close to death.)

SCORING FRAILTY IN PEOPLE WITH DEMENTIA

The degree of frailty generally corresponds to the degree of dementia. Common **symptoms in mild dementia** include forgetting the details of a recent event, though still remembering the event itself, repeating the same question/story and social withdrawal.

In **moderate dementia,** recent memory is very impaired, even though they seemingly can remember their past life events well. They can do personal care with prompting.

In **severe dementia,** they cannot do personal care without help.

In **very severe dementia** they are often bedfast. Many are virtually mute.

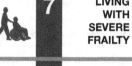

DALHOUSIE UNIVERSITY

Source: Adapted from Dalhousie University. (2005). *Clinical frailty score.*

APPENDIX A-7: THAMER RISK SCORE

Sample risk assessment questionnaire for clinicians and patients' use for those who initiate dialysis

PATIENT'S CONDITION	SCORE IF "YES"
Age category	
<70 y	0
70–74 y	1
75–79 y	1
80–84 y	1

(continued)

APPENDIX A-7: THAMER RISK SCORE (*CONTINUED*)

PATIENT'S CONDITION	SCORE IF "YES"
85–89 y	2
≥90 y	3
Albumin level is low (<3.5 g/dL) or unknown?	1
Needs assistance in daily living?	1
Lives in nursing home?	1
Had or has cancer?	1
Had or has heart failure?	1
Hospitalized more than once or >1 mo in last year?	1
Total score (range, 0–9)	

Disclaimer: This risk assessment tool is not intended as medical advice or to suggest treatment. Patients should always consult with their physician or other healthcare professional for advice.

Source: Thamer, M., Kaufman, J. S., Zhang, Y., Zhang, Q., Cotter, D. J., & Bang, H. (2015). Predicting early death among elderly dialysis patients: Development and validation of a risk score to assist shared decision making for dialysis initiation. *American Journal of Kidney Diseases, 66*(6), 1024–1032. https://doi.org/10.1053/j.ajkd.2015.05.014.

APPENDIX A-8: NYHA CLASSIFICATION OF FUNCTIONAL STATUS

NYHA CLASS	SYMPTOMS
I	Patients with heart disease but without limitation of physical activity
II	Patients with heart disease resulting in slight limitation of physical activity Comfortable at rest
III	Patients with heart disease resulting in marked limitation of physical activity. Comfortable at rest. Less than ordinary activity causes fatigue, dyspnea, palpitations, anginal pain
IV	Patients with heart disease resulting in inability to carry out any physical activity without discomfort. Symptoms of cardiac insufficiency or of the anginal syndrome may be present even at rest. If any physical activity is undertaken, discomfort increases.

NYHA, New York Heart Assocation.

Source: Lammers, A. E., Adatia, I., del Cerro, M. J., Diaz, G., Freudenthal, A. H., Freudenthal, F., Harikrishnan, S., Ivy, D., Lopes, A. A., Raj, J. U., Sandoval, J., Stenmark, K., & Haworth, S. G. (2011). Functional classification of pulmonary hypertension in children: Report from the PVRI pediatric taskforce, Panama 2011. *Pulmonary Circulation, 1*(2), 280–285. https://doi.org/10.4103/2045-8932.83445

APPENDIX B

PATIENT TEACHING RESOURCES

APPENDIX B-1: TREATMENT DISCUSSION AND PLANNING WORKSHEETS FOR CANCER DIAGNOSIS

QUESTIONS TO ASK MY PROVIDER	ANSWER	DIAGNOSTIC TESTS NEEDED	TREATMENT OPTIONS
Type of cancer			
Stage or grade			
How rare is this cancer?			
What is the location of the cancer?			
Has the cancer spread and if so, where?			

APPENDIX B-2: PATIENT GUIDE TO THE POLST FORM

National POLST:
Patient Guide to the POLST Portable Medical Order

This guide was created to help patients and caregivers learn more about the POLST form. There is a National POLST Form but most states still use their own state version of POLST. This map shows which states use the national version. While this guide uses images from the National POLST Form, your state form is likely very similar. Also, there are multiple names for POLST (MOLST, MOST, POST, etc.) so your state may call it something else (see https://polst.org/state-programs/).

Table of Contents

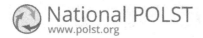

National POLST
www.polst.org

The POLST Form: 3 Treatment Decisions

POLST is a voluntary process that lets people who are seriously ill or have advanced frailty[1] choose certain health care treatments for when they cannot speak for themselves.

The POLST form is a special kind of medical document that turns your decisions about your care and treatment preferences into medical orders that travel with you. Patients, their legal surrogates, and health care providers discuss a patient's medical condition, treatment options and the patient's goals and care preferences. Health care providers fill out the POLST form with the patient/surrogate care preferences. The POLST form travels with the patient across health facilities and can be honored by every health care provider. POLST forms are voluntary meaning that no one should be forced or required to complete one.

To know if POLST will benefit you, talk with your health care provider about:
- Your current medical condition (diagnosis);
- What is likely to happen as your condition progresses (prognosis);
- Your goals of care, what you want to do, what you enjoy doing; and
- Treatment options, along with how each option effects what you want to be doing.
- What kind of care you would want to receive, especially if you have a medical emergency and cannot communicate.

The goal or purpose of talking with your health care provider is to understand what treatments you want to receive, what kinds of care that might work well or not work well for you, and to make decisions about:
- Going to the hospital or staying where you are, if possible.
- Being in the intensive care unit (ICU) and possibly being on a breathing machine.
- Having surgery.
- Attempting to restart your heart if it stops and your chances to return to living the kind of like you consider acceptable.

As you talk, you will be working with your provider to make important treatment decisions that your provider will put on the POLST form. Here are the three major treatment decisions you will be asked to make:
- Whether or not you want a provider to attempt to restart your heart if it has stopped beating (Section A);
- Whether or not you want to go to the hospital and what treatments you want there if your heart is beating or you are breathing (Section B); and
- Whether or not you want artificial nutrition (Section C).

---

[1] indicating a combination of advanced chronic disease and/or advanced age with functional decline with or without significant weight loss

	A. Cardiopulmonary Resuscitation Orders. Follow these orders if patient has no pulse and is not breathing.	
Pick 1	☐ YES CPR: Attempt Resuscitation, including mechanical ventilation, defibrillation and cardioversion. (Requires choosing Full Treatments in Section B)	☐ NO CPR: Do Not Attempt Resuscitation. (May choose any option in Section B)

In a medical emergency, the first thing medical provider will do is see if you have a pulse or are breathing. If you do not have a pulse and are not breathing, the provider wants to know if you want them to try cardiopulmonary resuscitation or CPR to restart your heart. The POLST form uses the word "attempted" because CPR does not always work. Getting CPR means that a provider may try some or all of these procedures to get your heart beating again:

- **Chest Compressions**: a provider will push hard on your chest to try to circulate your blood.
- **Defibrillation**: a provider will give you an electrical shock to try to get your heart to start beating again.
- **Intubation**: if you are not breathing, the provider needs to get air into your lungs. If you are able to breathe, a provider may put a breathing tube down your throat to help. If you are not able to breathe on your own, a provider may put you on a ventilator, which is a machine that pushes air into your lungs through a breathing tube. This is what is meant by "mechanical ventilation" in this Section.
- **Cardioversion**: a provider will try to return an abnormal heartbeat to a normal rhythm, usually with an electric shock.

If "YES CPR" is checked, this means you want a provider to provide whatever treatments above are medically appropriate to try and restart your heart. You are not able to pick and choose among these treatments using the POLST form.

> **Note:** If you choose "Yes CPR" that means you **must** choose "Full Treatments" in Section B. In order for emergency providers to attempt CPR, they must be able to put a plastic tube down your throat (called "intubation") if needed and only "Full Treatments" allows this option. Additionally, if CPR is successful, you will need to go to the hospital and probably be in the intensive care unit (ICU) on a breathing machine. Again, these treatments are only provided under "Full Treatments" below. If you like you can talk about Section B first with your health care provider to help with a decision about CPR.

If "NO CPR" is checked, this means you do not want the provider to try CPR and are okay in allowing natural death. In most states, having a POLST Form that says "No CPR" in Section A means it is a do-not-resuscitate (DNR) order.

Ask your health care provider if CPR is likely to work for you. If you do not want to make a decision about CPR, that is okay and a POLST form is not appropriate for you. In an emergency, without a POLST form, a provider will almost always try CPR (and the treatments listed under "YES CPR") to restart your heart.

Section B: Goals of Care and Medical Treatments

B. Initial Treatment Orders. Follow these orders if patient has a pulse and/or is breathing.	

Reassess and discuss interventions with patient or patient representative regularly to ensure treatments are meeting patient's care goals. Consider a time-trial of interventions based on goals and specific outcomes.

<table>
<tr><td rowspan="3">Pick 1</td><td>☐ Full Treatments (required if choose CPR in Section A). <u>Goal: Attempt to sustain life by all medically effective means.</u> Provide appropriate medical and surgical treatments as indicated to attempt to prolong life, including intensive care.</td></tr>
<tr><td>☐ Selective Treatments. <u>Goal: Attempt to restore function while avoiding intensive care and resuscitation efforts (ventilator, defibrillation and cardioversion).</u> May use non-invasive positive airway pressure, antibiotics and IV fluids as indicated. Avoid intensive care. Transfer to hospital if treatment needs cannot be met in current location.</td></tr>
<tr><td>☐ Comfort-focused Treatments. <u>Goal: Maximize comfort through symptom management; allow natural death.</u> Use oxygen, suction and manual treatment of airway obstruction as needed for comfort. Avoid treatments listed in full or select treatments unless consistent with comfort goal. Transfer to hospital only if comfort cannot be achieved in current setting.</td></tr>
</table>

Each option in this section provides a statement explaining the care goal for those treatments. Since your care goal will help with the rest of the decisions on this form, your provider will likely start the conversation with this section. This is not the first section on the form, however, because it is most important for emergency providers to know whether you want CPR attempted if your heart has stopped.

If you have a pulse or are breathing, the next most important questions for a provider are **do you want to go to the hospital** and, if yes, **what treatments do you want there**. Section B on provides this information.

This is where you talk about what different treatment options mean **for you,** given your current medical condition and goals of care. For example, going to the intensive care unit (ICU) doesn't mean the same thing to everyone. People have different treatments there, spend different amounts of time in the ICU and have different results.

Regardless of what box is checked in this section, you will be given treatments to keep you as comfortable as possible.

If "Full Treatments" is checked, it means you want to have **everything done** that is medically appropriate and possible to attempt to keep alive. If necessary, you are okay going to the ICU, having a breathing tube, and being on a ventilator. Your provider must choose this option if you want CPR but if this is still a choice if you choose No CPR.

If "Selective Treatments" is checked, if means you want to **treat medical problems that can be reversed**. You are okay going to the hospital to get antibiotics and other drugs through an IV tube, or a tube placed in a vein if these cannot be done elsewhere. You would not want major surgery, to be in the ICU, or on a breathing machine.

If "Comfort-Focused Treatments" is checked, you want to **be as comfortable as possible and allow death to happen naturally.** You *only* want to go to the hospital if you cannot be made comfortable where you are now.

Note: If you are in a hospital, a long-term care facility (nursing home, skilled nursing facility, assisted living facility, etc), or hospice, your provider will periodically confirm your choice in Section B still makes sense for you given your current care goals and medical condition.

Section D: Medically Assisted Nutrition (Tube Feeding)

D. Medically Assisted Nutrition (Offer food by mouth if desired by patient, safe and tolerated)	
☐ Provide feeding through new or existing surgically-placed tubes	☐ No artificial means of nutrition desired
☐ Trial period for artificial nutrition but no surgically-placed tubes	☐ Not discussed or no decision made (provide standard of care)

(Pick 1)

It is very helpful for health care providers to know your wishes about feeding tubes, called medically assisted nutrition. Some feeding tubes require a surgery to place them, usually if you are going to be on a feeding tube for longer than two weeks. Please watch the video at www.polst.org/form to learn more about tube feeding options.

Sections A and B share important orders that providers need to know during a medical emergency. Section D is not for emergencies but is on the POLST form because it can help guide decisions about non-emergency care in consultation with a patient's surrogate. Since POLST is a tool to provide care centered on the patient, this section exists on the POLST form to encourage conversations about this potentially critical treatment decision. It was important to national POLST leaders that patients and families be given an opportunity to make informed decisions about this treatment in the context of decision making about other potentially life-sustaining treatment.

Since this is not an emergent order, the National POLST form includes a box for "not discussed or no decision made (provide standard of care)" so that this section is not left blank.

Other POLST Form Sections

Most other sections on the National POLST form are instructions to make sure your provider uses the form the right way and to share other important information. Most state POLST forms have similar information. Below is information on some of the other sections.

Patient Information

Patient Information.	**Having a POLST form is always voluntary.**
This is a medical order, not an advance directive. For information about POLST and to understand this document, visit: www.polst.org/form	Patient First Name: _____ Middle Name/Initial: _____ Preferred name: _____ Last Name: _____ Suffix (Jr, Sr, etc): _____ DOB (mm/dd/yyyy): ___/___/___ State where form was completed:_____ Gender: ☐ M ☐ F ☐ X Social Security Number's last 4 digits (optional): xxx-xx-___ ___ ___ ___

This section:

- Reminds everyone that having a POLST form is *your choice* and that you should not be forced or required to have one.
- Reminds everyone that a POLST form is a *medical* order, not a legal document like an advance directive. See www.polst.org for more information. This matters because, in an emergency, emergency personnel are only able to follow medical orders.
- Has information to help providers make sure this is your POLST form.

Additional Orders

C. Additional Orders or Instructions. These orders are in addition to those above (e.g., blood products, dialysis).
[EMS protocols may limit emergency responder ability to act on orders in this section.]

Your provider may use this section to put in additional orders or instructions about your care or treatment. For example:

- Providing instructions about a pacemaker or other device;
- Stating you do not want any blood products; or
- Providing orders about dialysis.

Signatures

E. SIGNATURE: Patient or Patient Representative (eSigned documents are valid)			
I understand this form is voluntary. I have discussed my treatment options and goals of care with my provider. If signing as the patient's representative, the treatments are consistent with the patient's known wishes and in their best interest.			
✖ (required)			The most recently completed valid POLST form supersedes all previously completed POLST forms.
If other than patient, print full name:		Authority:	
F. SIGNATURE: Health Care Provider (eSigned documents are valid)		Verbal orders are acceptable with follow up signature.	
I have discussed this order with the patient or his/her representative. The orders reflect the patient's known wishes, to the best of my knowledge. [Note: Only licensed health care providers authorized by law to sign POLST form in state where completed may sign this order]			
✖ (required)		Date (mm/dd/yyyy): Required / /	Phone # : ( )
Printed Full Name:			License/Cert. #:
Supervising physician signature:	☐ N/A		License #:

The National POLST form, and almost all states, require you (or your surrogate) to sign the POLST form along with your provider. In signing the form, you are agreeing that you:

- Understand you do not need to have a POLST form. It is your choice to have one and
- Talked with your provider about what is important to you given your current medical condition and the decisions made on this form.

If you are the patient's surrogate, when you sign the form you are agreeing that you:

- Understand the patient does not need to have a POLST form;
- Talked with the patient's provider about what the patient would have chosen if they were able to communicate.

Other Important Information

Most of the back side form instructions are for your provider, but there are two things it is important for patients to know:

1. If you want **to change, or modify, your POLST form** you need to make an appointment with your provider. You <u>cannot</u> change your POLST form yourself. It is a medical order signed by your provider: just as you cannot change a prescription written by your provider, you cannot change the POLST form. Instead, your provider must void or cancel your current POLST form and fill out a new one. For example, here's Kathy's story:

It was important to Kathy to travel and see her grandchildren. She didn't want to be placed on a breathing machine or ventilator, but she was willing to go to the hospital, have IV fluids and antibiotics so her provider completed Kathy's first POLST form as DNR in Section A and Selective Treatments in Section B. During one of her trips she suddenly became ill and went to the hospital where the doctors told her she had cancer and that it had spread. They discussed her goals: Kathy really wanted to make sure she got to see her granddaughter get married in a couple of months. So the doctors kept her POLST as it was. After the wedding, she talked with her doctor again about what was important to her. This time, she said she wanted to focus on comfort and enjoying the last few months of her life; she did not want to go to the hospital. Her doctor completed a new POLST form ordering DNR in Section A and Comfort-Focused Treatments in Section B.

2. If you want **to void or cancel your POLST form** you can. Here are the steps to follow in most states:
   a. Write "VOID" in large letters across the form or destroy it.
   b. Tell your provider you have voided or cancelled your POLST form so they can remove it from your medical record. If your provider does not know you have voided your POLST form, they may think it is still what you want and provide those treatments if you cannot speak for yourself and need care. (Also, if your state has a POLST registry that keeps copies of POLST forms, your provider will need to tell the registry that you have canceled or voided your POLST form or emergency providers may also think the form still is what you want.)

For More Information
- Talk with your provider
- Look at our videos on www.polst.org/form
- Review advance care planning, advance directives and POLST form information, starting at www.polst.org

Note: Please see the website for the most updated information.

POLST, physician order for life-sustaining treatment.

Source: National POLST. (2021). *Patient guide to the POLST form.* https://polst.org/form-guide-patients-pdf.

APPENDIX B-3: PORTABLE MEDICAL ORDERS: WHAT TO KNOW BEFORE TALKING ABOUT POLST

Portable Medical Orders: What to Know Before Talking About POLST

Advance care planning is about making decisions for the treatments you want if you become unable to communicate. The *National POLST Form* is a *portable medical order* that is an advance care planning tool. It tells health care personnel — and friends and family — which treatments you want and which ones you do not want.

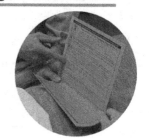

Like any advance care plan, you should not be required to have a POLST form. Using and having a POLST form is your choice.

Advance care planning: a process for throughout one's life

Most people (**Stage 1 and 2**) should use a legal document for advance care planning. This document may be called an *advance directive*, or may be a *living will* with a *health care power of attorney*.

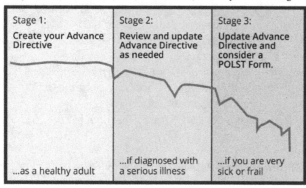

Stage 1: Create your Advance Directive	Stage 2: Review and update Advance Directive as needed	Stage 3: Update Advance Directive and consider a POLST Form.
...as a healthy adult	...if diagnosed with a serious illness	...if you are very sick or frail

What the legal document(s) are called varies from state to state. The document(s) tell health care providers who you want to speak for you if you can't speak for yourself and what types of treatments you may or may not want in case of a future, unknown medical emergency.

Regardless of age, if you are very sick or frail (**Stage 3**), a portable medical order is appropriate. A portable medical order tells emergency providers what to do during an emergency.

Learn more about POLST and advance directives	www.polst.org/advance-directives

How is a POLST form different from an advance directive?

An advance directive is not a medical order and does not provide specific directions about treatments. A POLST form gives medical orders. During an emergency, if you have a POLST form, emergency providers will give you the treatments listed on it. If you do not have a POLST form, emergency providers will attempt everything possible to keep you alive and take you to the hospital where your health care provider and surrogate will make a decision about what treatments to provide to you, based on your advance directive.

What is a POLST form?

A POLST form is a portable medical order that tells emergency providers what treatments you want to have during an emergency. (See What Your Completed Guide Means for details.) Additionally, a POLST form is meant to clarify your treatment goals, which can more broadly help health care providers understand how to treat you in a way that matches your goals and values.

Who should get a POLST form?

Anyone with a serious life-limiting condition or with advance frailty; someone who is really sick or very frail.

Where do you get a POLST form?

From your health care provider. It is a medical order that must be signed by a provider to be valid.

National POLST Patient Guide: Before Talking About POLST

Portable Medical Orders: What to Know Before Talking About POLST

Preparing for your POLST conversation

Your provider may schedule a separate appointment to discuss a POLST form, your treatment preferences and your goals of care. In order to prepare you for this conversation:

It may be helpful to

☐ Bring any advance care plan you've completed, such as an advance directive, living will, health care power of attorney.

☐ Invite your surrogate (or proxy or health care power of attorney), a family member, a friend, or spiritual advisor to the conversation.

To frame your thoughts, it may also help to

☐ Think about what makes a good day for you and what goals you have. Use the American Bar Association's tool to help.

☐ Play www.gowish.org online and bring the results with you.

☐ Look at Prepareforyourcare.org and complete and advance directive, if you don't have one (or start and bring your questions with you!).

☐ Read the free Conversation Starter Kit from *The Conversation Project.*

Online tools to help you get started	• www.americanbar.org/content/dam/aba/administrative/law_aging/tool4.pdf • www.gowish.org • prepareforyourcare.com • www.theconversationproject.org/starter-kits/

What should I expect from the POLST conversation?

During the conversation, you'll be talking about what your understanding is about your current medical condition and what is likely to happen to you. You'll discuss:

- *Your diagnosis* — Your disease(s) or condition(s).
- *Your prognosis* — How your disease(s) or condition(s) will likely affect you over time.
- *Your treatment options* — What are your options, how they could help, and what are potential the side effects.
- *Your goals of care* — What is important to you, what you enjoy doing, what a good day looks like for you.

You may be making decisions on the following things. It's okay if you don't know what these are or what they mean for you because your health care provider should explain what you need to know. This list is just to let you know some of what may be discussed:

- Whether you want cardiopulmonary resuscitation (CPR) if your heart stops beating.
- What kind of medical treatments you want:
    - Are you okay with surgery?
    - Are you okay being on a breathing machine?
    - Do you want a feeding tube (artificial nutrition)?

At the end of the conversation, you'll decide whether you want a POLST form. It is your choice about whether you want one or not. If you do, your health care provider will fill it out and ask you to sign it. Your provider will sign it and then give you the original to keep with you. You can always change your mind. And you can update the POLST at anytime by talking with your provider. For information about what the POLST form means and what to do with it, visit www.polst.org/form.

National POLST Patient Guide: Before Talking About POLST

The best way to learn about POLST is to contact your provider. For general information, go to www.polst.org.   page 2

Note: Please see the website for the most updated information.

Source: National POLST. (2021) *Portable medical orders: What to know before talking about POLST.* https://polst.org/patient-guide-before-pdf

APPENDIX B-4: WHAT YOUR COMPLETED POLST FORM MEANS

Portable Medical Orders: What Your Completed POLST Form Means

Your health care provider should have discussed your options with you before you signed the POLST form. This document is provided to help you remember your choices and explain what your POLST form means.

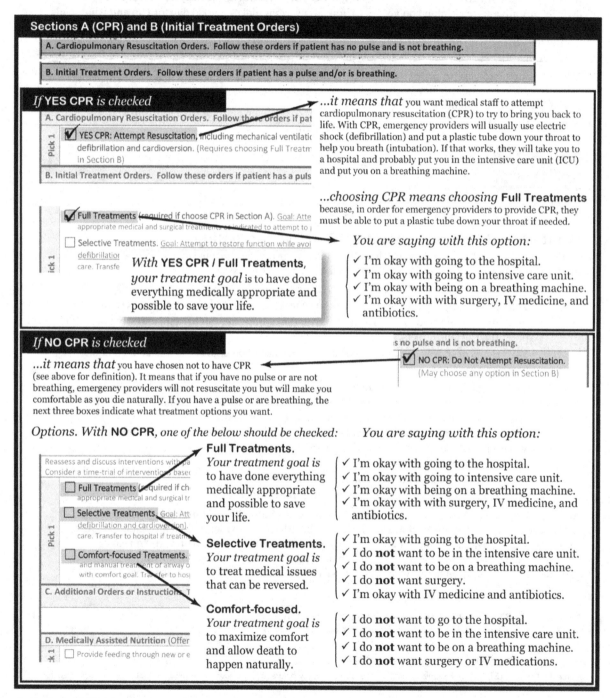

Sections A (CPR) and B (Initial Treatment Orders)

A. Cardiopulmonary Resuscitation Orders. Follow these orders if patient has no pulse and is not breathing.

B. Initial Treatment Orders. Follow these orders if patient has a pulse and/or is breathing.

If **YES CPR** *is checked*

A. Cardiopulmonary Resuscitation Orders. Follow these orders if pat

Pick 1 ☑ YES CPR: Attempt Resuscitation, including mechanical ventilatio defibrillation and cardioversion. (Requires choosing Full Treatm in Section B)

B. Initial Treatment Orders. Follow these orders if patient has a puls

☑ Full Treatments (required if choose CPR in Section A). Goal: Atte appropriate medical and surgical treatments as indicated to attempt to

☐ Selective Treatments. Goal: Attempt to restore function while avoi defibrillatio care. Transfe

...it means that you want medical staff to attempt cardiopulmonary resuscitation (CPR) to try to bring you back to life. With CPR, emergency providers will usually use electric shock (defibrillation) and put a plastic tube down your throat to help you breath (intubation). If that works, they will take you to a hospital and probably put you in the intensive care unit (ICU) and put you on a breathing machine.

...choosing CPR means choosing **Full Treatments** because, in order for emergency providers to provide CPR, they must be able to put a plastic tube down your throat if needed.

You are saying with this option:

- ✓ I'm okay with going to the hospital.
- ✓ I'm okay with going to intensive care unit.
- ✓ I'm okay with being on a breathing machine.
- ✓ I'm okay with with surgery, IV medicine, and antibiotics.

With **YES CPR / Full Treatments,** *your treatment goal* is to have done everything medically appropriate and possible to save your life.

If **NO CPR** *is checked*

☑ NO CPR: Do Not Attempt Resuscitation. (May choose any option in Section B)

...it means that you have chosen not to have CPR (see above for definition). It means that if you have no pulse or are not breathing, emergency providers will not resuscitate you but will make you comfortable as you die naturally. If you have a pulse or are breathing, the next three boxes indicate what treatment options you want.

Options. With **NO CPR,** *one of the below should be checked:*

Reassess and discuss interventions with pa Consider a time-trial of interventions based

☐ Full Treatments (required if ch appropriate medical and surgical tr

☐ Selective Treatments. Goal: Att defibrillation and cardioversion). care. Transfer to hospital if treatm

☐ Comfort-focused Treatments. and manual treatment of airway o with comfort goal. Transfer to hos

C. Additional Orders or Instructions. T

D. Medically Assisted Nutrition (Offer ☐ Provide feeding through new or e

Full Treatments.
Your treatment goal is to have done everything medically appropriate and possible to save your life.

Selective Treatments.
Your treatment goal is to treat medical issues that can be reversed.

Comfort-focused.
Your treatment goal is to maximize comfort and allow death to happen naturally.

You are saying with this option:

- ✓ I'm okay with going to the hospital.
- ✓ I'm okay with going to intensive care unit.
- ✓ I'm okay with being on a breathing machine.
- ✓ I'm okay with with surgery, IV medicine, and antibiotics.

- ✓ I'm okay with going to the hospital.
- ✓ I do **not** want to be in the intensive care unit.
- ✓ I do **not** want to be on a breathing machine.
- ✓ I do **not** want surgery.
- ✓ I'm okay with IV medicine and antibiotics.

- ✓ I do **not** want to go to the hospital.
- ✓ I do **not** want to be in the intensive care unit.
- ✓ I do **not** want to be on a breathing machine.
- ✓ I do **not** want surgery or IV medications.

Portable Medical Orders - What Your Completed POLST Form Means

Explanation of Additional Orders

Since no form can address every possible medical decision, the POLST form has space for your health care provider to order other treatments you may want. Your provider may have written additional orders in here based on your conversation.

> **C. Additional Orders or Instructions.** These orders are in addition to those above (e.g., blood products, dialysis).
> [EMS protocols may limit emergency responder ability to act on orders in this section.]

Explanation of Medically Assisted Nutrition Options

For every treatment option, health care providers will make reasonable attempts to give you food and fluids by mouth if you desire it, if it is safe and if you can tolerate it. If this is not possible, this section provides orders about what artificial nutrition you want. Options include temporary solutions or options requiring surgery, like a PEG tube. You can learn more by viewing this video about feeding tubes.

> **D. Medically Assisted Nutrition** (Offer food by mouth if desired by patient, safe and tolerated)
>
> **Pick 1**
> ☐ Provide feeding through new or existing surgically-placed tubes   ☐ No artificial means of nutrition desired
> ☐ Trial period for artificial nutrition but no surgically-placed tubes   ☐ Discussed but no decision made (standard of care provided)

Discussed but no decision made means you will receive the standard of care (as you will for any section not completed).

Explanation of Patient Signature

By signing the form, you acknowledged that you understand this is voluntary and that you have discussed your goals with your health care provider. You should not ever be required to have a POLST.

> ☐ Trial period for artificial nutrition but no surgically-placed tubes   ☐ Discussed but no decision made (standard of care provided)
>
> **E. SIGNATURE: Patient or Patient Representative** (eSigned documents are valid)
> I understand this form is voluntary. I have discussed my treatment options and goals of care with my provider. If signing as the patient's representative, the treatments are consistent with the patient's known wishes and in their best interest.
> (required)   The most recently completed valid

What if I change my mind?

You, as the patient, always have the right to change your mind about your POLST form. If you want to change to different options than the ones you selected, you need to have a new form created with your health care provider (you cannot modify the form yourself).

If you do not want to have a POLST form anymore, you have the right to void the form, too. If you want to void your form, be sure to: destroy the old form **and** contact your health care provider to void the orders in your medical records and also have the form voided in any POLST registries, if applicable. If the patient lacks capacity, the patient's representative should follow these steps on behalf of the patient.

What do I do with my completed POLST form?

✓ **Carry your POLST with you** if you go to a facility.

✓ **If you are home, post it on your refrigerator or put it in your medicine cabinet.** Emergency personnel will look for it those places.

✓ **Tell your family and friends** you have a POLST form so they can tell emergency personnel to look for it.

✓ **If you are traveling**, keep a copy in your purse or wallet near your ID. Emergency personnel will look there to find it.

National POLST Patient Guide: Your Completed Form
The best way to learn about POLST is to contact your provider. For general information, go to www.polst.org/form   page 2

Note: Please see the website for the most updated information.

Source: National POLST. (2021). *What your completed POLST form means.* https://polst.org/patient-guide-after-pdf.

APPENDIX B-5: BEING A CAREGIVER

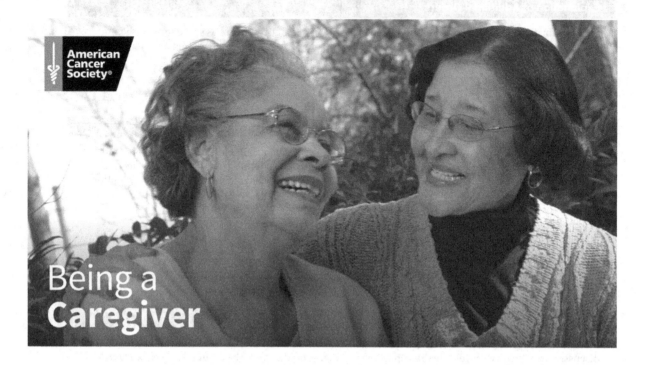

American Cancer Society®

Being a
Caregiver

A caregiver is the person who helps the person with cancer most often – without being paid to do so. In most cases, the main caregiver is a spouse, partner, or an adult child. Sometimes close friends, co-workers, or neighbors may fill this role. The caregiver is a key part of the cancer patient's care.

What does a caregiver do?

The caregiver is part of the cancer care team, which also includes the patient and the medical staff. Caregivers do many things, like:

- Help feed, dress, and bathe the patient.

- Make sure the patient eats and gets rest.

- See that the patient takes medicines as they were told to.

- Keep track of appointments.

- Take care of insurance problems.

- Drive the patient.

- Help with other family members' needs.

- Talk to the cancer care team about how the patient is doing.

- Help the patient live as normal a life as possible.

How to be a good caregiver

A good caregiver is often the one person who knows everything that's going on with the patient. Don't be afraid to ask questions and take notes during doctor visits. Learn who the members of the cancer care team are and know how to contact them.

- Keep the patient involved in planning their care. Help the patient do their part to get better.

- Let the person with cancer make decisions. If the patient is making poor choices, talk to them about their choices. Then talk it over with the cancer care team and get their help. (Things like not taking medicines or not following activity limits may be poor choices that should not be ignored.)

- Sometimes you might need to set limits with the patient. For example, have the patient care for themselves as much as they can, and encourage them to talk about things other than cancer and illness.

- Remember that professional help is there for you, too. It's normal to feel frustrated, upset, and stressed when caring for someone with cancer. Ask the cancer care team for help when you need it.

- Take care of your own needs. While you're helping your loved one, you must also take care of yourself. Be sure to keep your own doctor appointments, get enough sleep, exercise, eat healthy foods, and keep your normal routine as much as you can.

- Don't try to do it all yourself! Reach out to others. Involve them in your life and in the things you must do for your loved one.

When others want to help

Asking for help or letting others help can take some of the pressure off and allow you time to take care of yourself. Family and friends often want to help but may not know how or what you need. Here are some tips for working with family and friends:

- Look for areas where you need help. Make a list.

- Hold regular family meetings to keep everyone up to date. Use these meetings as a time to plan the patient's care. Include the patient.

- Ask family and friends when they can help and what jobs they think they can do. Be very clear about what you need.

- When you hear back from each person, note it on your list to make sure they have taken care of what you needed.

What if I mess up?

No matter what you do, you'll likely come to a point where you feel that you have failed your loved one in some way. Even though you do the best you can, there may be times you'll feel that you could have done better. Try not to blame yourself. Find a way to forgive yourself and move on. It helps to bear in mind that you'll keep making mistakes, and try to keep a sense of humor about it. Focus on those things that you do well.

Caring for someone going through cancer treatment is a demanding job, but being good at it can give you a sense of meaning and pride. These positive feelings can give you the strength to go on for as long as you're needed.

It's not easy to be a caregiver, but it can be rewarding.

For more information about being a caregiver, call the American Cancer Society at **1-800-227-2345** or visit us online at **cancer.org.**

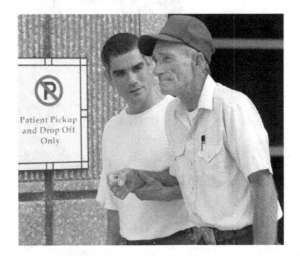

cancer.org | 1.800.227.2345

LANGUAGE
©2018, American Cancer Society, Inc.
No. 213400 Rev. 11/18
Models used for illustrative purposes only.

Source: American Cancer Society. (2020). *Being a caregiver.* https://www.cancer.org/content/dam/cancer-org/cancer-control/en/booklets-flyers/being-a-caregiver.pdf

APPENDIX B-6: SEEKING ALCOHOL ABUSE TREATMENT

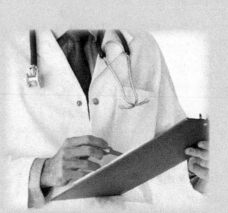

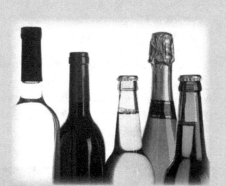

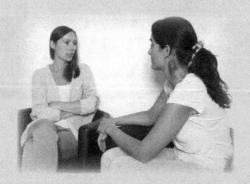

Treatment for Alcohol Problems:
Finding and Getting Help

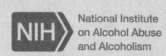

National Institute
on Alcohol Abuse
and Alcoholism

This guide is written for individuals, and their family and friends, who are looking for options to address alcohol problems. It is intended as a resource to understand what treatment choices are available and what to consider when selecting among them.

Table of Contents

When Is It Time for Treatment?

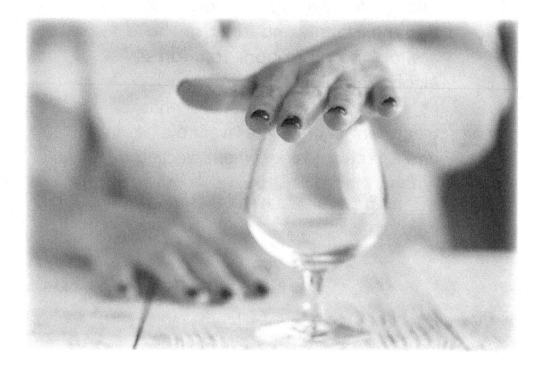

Alcohol-related problems—which result from drinking too much, too fast, or too often—are among the most significant public health issues in the United States.

Many people struggle with controlling their drinking at some time in their lives. More than **14 million adults ages 18 and older have alcohol use disorder (AUD)**, and 1 in 10 children live in a home with a parent who has a drinking problem.

Does Treatment Work?

The good news is that no matter how severe the problem may seem, most people with AUD can benefit from some form of treatment.

Research shows that about one-third of people who are treated for alcohol problems have no further symptoms 1 year later. Many others substantially reduce their drinking and report fewer alcohol-related problems.

Signs of an Alcohol Problem

Alcohol use disorder (AUD) is a medical condition that doctors diagnose when a patient's drinking causes distress or harm. The condition can range from mild to severe and is diagnosed when a patient answers "yes" to two or more of the following questions.

In the past year, have you:

❏ Had times when you ended up drinking **more, or longer** than you intended?

❏ More than once wanted to **cut down or stop drinking,** or tried to, but couldn't?

❏ Spent a **lot of time** drinking? Or being sick or getting over the aftereffects?

❏ Experienced **craving**—a strong need, or urge, to drink?

❏ Found that drinking—or being sick from drinking—often **interfered with taking care** of your **home** or **family**? Or caused **job** troubles? Or **school** problems?

❏ Continued to drink even though it was causing **trouble** with your **family** or **friends**?

❏ **Given up** or **cut back** on **activities** that were important or interesting to you, or gave you pleasure, in order to drink?

❏ More than once gotten into situations while or after drinking that **increased your chances of getting hurt** (such as driving, swimming, using machinery, walking in a dangerous area, or having unsafe sex)?

❏ Continued to drink even though it was making you feel **depressed or anxious** or adding to **another health problem**? Or after having had a **memory blackout**?

❏ Had to **drink much more** than you once did to **get the effect** you want? Or found that your **usual number** of drinks had **much less effect** than before?

❏ Found that when the effects of alcohol were wearing off, you **had withdrawal symptoms,** such as trouble sleeping, shakiness, irritability, anxiety, depression, restlessness, nausea, or sweating? Or sensed things that were not there?

If you have any of these symptoms, your drinking may already be a cause for concern. The more symptoms you have, the more urgent the need for change. A health professional can conduct a formal assessment of your symptoms to see if AUD is present. For an online assessment of your drinking pattern, go to **https://RethinkingDrinking.niaaa.nih.gov**.

Options for Treatment

When asked how alcohol problems are treated, people commonly think of 12-step programs or 28-day inpatient rehab but may have difficulty naming other options. In fact, there are a variety of treatment methods currently available, thanks to significant advances in the field over the past 60 years.

Ultimately, there is no one-size-fits-all solution, and what may work for one person may not be a good fit for someone else. Simply understanding the different options can be an important first step.

Types of Treatment

Behavioral Treatments

Behavioral treatments are aimed at changing drinking behavior through counseling. They are led by health professionals and supported by studies showing they can be beneficial.

Medications

Three medications are currently approved in the United States to help people stop or reduce their drinking and prevent relapse. They are prescribed by a primary care physician or other health professional and may be used alone or in combination with counseling.

Mutual-Support Groups

Alcoholics Anonymous (AA) and other 12-step programs provide peer support for people quitting or cutting back on their drinking. Combined with treatment led by health professionals, mutual-support groups can offer a valuable added layer of support.

Due to the anonymous nature of mutual-support groups, it is difficult for researchers to determine their success rates compared with those led by health professionals.

Starting With a Primary Care Doctor

For anyone thinking about treatment, talking to a primary care physician is an important first step—he or she can be a good source for treatment referrals and medications. A primary care physician can also:

- Evaluate a patient's drinking pattern
- Help craft a treatment plan
- Evaluate overall health
- Assess if medications for alcohol may be appropriate

Types of Professionals Involved in Care

Many health professionals can play a role in treatment. Below is a list of providers and the type of care they may offer.

Provider Type	Degrees & Credentials	Treatment Type
Primary Care Provider	**M.D., D.O.** (Doctor of Osteopathic Medicine); additionally you may see a **Nurse Practitioner** or **Physician's Assistant**	Medications, Brief Behavioral Treatment, Referral to Specialist
Psychiatrist	**M.D., D.O.**	Medications, Behavioral Treatment
Psychologist	**Ph.D., Psy.D., M.A.**	Behavioral Treatment
Social Worker	**M.S.W.** (Master of Social Work), **L.C.S.W.** (Licensed Clinical Social Worker)	Behavioral Treatment
Alcohol Counselor	Varies—most States require some form of certification	Behavioral Treatment

Individuals are advised to talk to their doctors about the best form of primary treatment.

Treatments Led by Health Professionals

Professionally led treatments include:

Medications

Some are surprised to learn that there are medications on the market approved to treat alcohol dependence. The newer types of these medications work by offsetting changes in the brain caused by AUD.

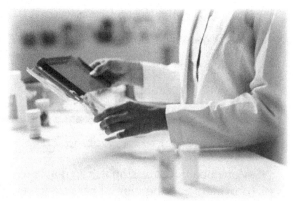

All approved medications are non-addictive and can be used alone or in combination with other forms of treatment. Learn more about these approved treatments on p. 8.

Behavioral Treatments

Also known as alcohol counseling, behavioral treatments involve working with a health professional to identify and help change the behaviors that lead to heavy drinking. Behavioral treatments share certain features, which can include:

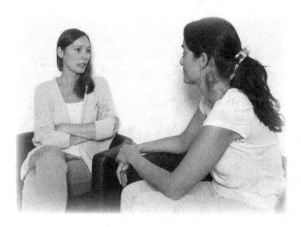

- Developing the skills needed to stop or reduce drinking

- Helping to build a strong social support system

- Working to set reachable goals

- Coping with or avoiding the triggers that might cause relapse

Types of Behavioral Treatments

- **Cognitive–Behavioral Therapy** can take place one-on-one with a therapist or in small groups. This form of therapy is focused on identifying the feelings and situations (called "cues") that lead to heavy drinking and managing stress that can lead to relapse. The goal is to change the thought processes that lead to alcohol misuse and to develop the skills necessary to cope with everyday situations that might trigger problem drinking.

- **Motivational Enhancement Therapy** is conducted over a short period of time to build and strengthen motivation to change drinking behavior. The therapy focuses on identifying the pros and cons of seeking treatment, forming a plan for making changes in one's drinking, building confidence, and developing the skills needed to stick to the plan.

- **Marital and Family Counseling** incorporates spouses and other family members in the treatment process and can play an important role in repairing and improving family relationships. Studies show that strong family support through family therapy increases the chances of maintaining abstinence (stopping drinking), compared with patients undergoing individual counseling.

- **Brief Interventions** are short, one-on-one or small-group counseling sessions that are time limited. The counselor provides information about the individual's drinking pattern and potential risks. After the client receives personalized feedback, the counselor will work with him or her to set goals and provide ideas for helping to make a change.

Ultimately, choosing to get treatment may be more important than the approach used, as long as the approach avoids heavy confrontation and incorporates empathy, motivational support, and a focus on changing drinking behavior.

What FDA-Approved Medications Are Available?

Certain medications have been shown to effectively help people stop or reduce their drinking and avoid relapse.

Current Medications

The U.S. Food and Drug Administration (FDA) has approved three medications for treating alcohol dependence, and others are being tested to determine whether they are effective.

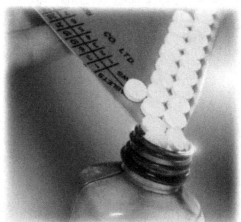

- **Naltrexone** can help people reduce heavy drinking.

- **Acamprosate** makes it easier to maintain abstinence.

- **Disulfiram** blocks the breakdown (metabolism) of alcohol by the body, causing unpleasant symptoms such as nausea and flushing of the skin. Those unpleasant effects can help some people avoid drinking while taking disulfiram.

It is important to remember that not all people will respond to medications, but for a subset of individuals, they can be an important tool in overcoming alcohol dependence.

Scientists are working to develop a larger menu of pharmaceutical treatments that could be tailored to individual needs. As more medications become available, people may be able to try multiple medications to find which they respond to best.

"Isn't taking medications just trading one addiction for another?"

This is not an uncommon concern, but the short answer is "no." All medications approved for treating alcohol dependence are non-addictive. These medicines are designed to help manage a chronic disease, just as someone might take drugs to keep their asthma or diabetes in check.

Looking Ahead: The Future of Treatment

Progress continues to be made as researchers seek out new and better treatments for alcohol problems. By studying the underlying causes of AUD in the brain and body, the National Institute on Alcohol Abuse and Alcoholism (NIAAA) is working to identify key cellular or molecular structures—called "targets"—that could lead to the development of new medications.

Personalized Medicine

Ideally, health professionals would be able to identify which AUD treatment is most effective for each person. NIAAA and other organizations are conducting research to identify genes and other factors that can predict how well someone will respond to a particular treatment. These advances could optimize how treatment decisions are made in the future.

Current NIAAA Research—Leading to Future Breakthroughs

Certain medications already approved for other uses have shown promise for treating alcohol dependence and problem drinking:

- The anti-smoking drug varenicline (marketed under the name Chantix) significantly reduced alcohol consumption and craving among people with AUD.

- Gabapentin, a medication used to treat pain conditions and epilepsy, was shown to increase abstinence and reduce heavy drinking. Those taking the medication also reported fewer alcohol cravings and improved mood and sleep.

- The anti-epileptic medication topiramate was shown to help people curb problem drinking, particularly among those with a certain genetic makeup that appears to be linked to the treatment's effectiveness.

Tips for Selecting Treatment

Professionals in the alcohol treatment field offer advice on what to consider when choosing a treatment program.

Overall, gather as much information as you can about the program or provider before making a decision on treatment. If you know someone who has first-hand knowledge of the program, it may help to ask about his or her personal experience.

Here are some questions you can ask that may help guide your choice:

❑ **What kind of treatment does the program or provider offer?**
It is important to gauge whether the facility provides all the currently available methods or relies on one approach. You may want to learn if the program or provider offers medication and if mental health issues are addressed together with addiction treatment.

❑ **Is treatment tailored to the individual?**
Matching the right therapy to the individual is important to its success. No single treatment will benefit everyone. It may also be helpful to determine whether treatment will be adapted to meet changing needs as they arise.

❑ **What is expected of the patient?**
You will want to understand what will be asked of you in order to decide what treatment best suits your needs.

❑ **Is treatment success measured?**
By assessing whether and how the program or provider measures success, you may be able to better compare your options.

❑ **How does the program or provider handle relapse?**
Relapse is common, and you will want to know how it is addressed. For more information on relapse, see p. 12.

When seeking professional help, it is important that you feel respected and understood and that you have a feeling of trust that this person, group, or organization can help you. Remember, though, that relationships with doctors, therapists, and other health professionals can take time to develop.

Additional Considerations

Treatment Setting—Inpatient or Outpatient?

In addition to choosing the type of treatment that's best for you, you'll also have to decide if that treatment is inpatient (you would stay at a facility) or outpatient (you stay in your home during treatment). Inpatient facilities tend to be more intensive and costly. Your healthcare provider can help you evaluate the pros and cons of each.

Cost may be a factor when selecting a treatment approach. Evaluate the coverage in your health insurance plan to determine how much of the costs your insurance will cover and how much you will have to pay. Ask different programs if they offer sliding scale fees—some programs may offer lower prices or payment plans for individuals without health insurance.

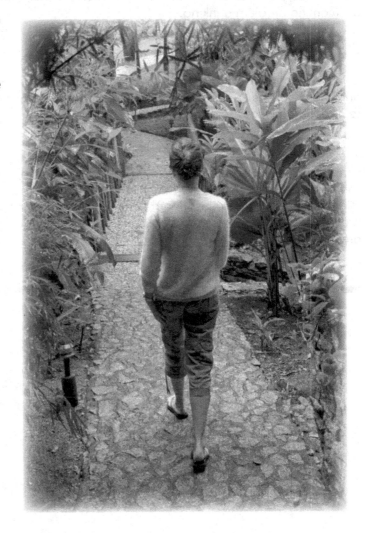

An Ongoing Process

Overcoming alcohol use disorder is an ongoing process, one which can include setbacks.

The Importance of Persistence

Because AUD can be a chronic relapsing disease, persistence is key. It is rare that someone would go to treatment once and then never drink again. More often, people must repeatedly try to quit or cut back, experience recurrences, learn from them, and then keep trying. For many, continued followup with a treatment provider is critical to overcoming problem drinking.

Relapse Is Part of the Process

Relapse is common among people who overcome alcohol problems. People with drinking problems are most likely to relapse during periods of stress or when exposed to people or places associated with past drinking.

Just as some people with diabetes or asthma may have flare-ups of their disease, a relapse to drinking can be seen as a temporary setback to full recovery and not a complete failure. Seeking professional help can prevent relapse—behavioral therapies can help people develop skills to avoid and overcome triggers, such as stress, that might lead to drinking. Most people benefit from regular checkups with a treatment provider. Medications also can deter drinking during times when individuals may be at greater risk of relapse (e.g., divorce, death of a family member).

Mental Health Issues and Alcohol Use Disorder

Depression and anxiety often go hand in hand with heavy drinking. Studies show that people who are alcohol dependent are two to three times as likely to suffer from major depression or anxiety over their lifetime. When addressing drinking problems, it's important to also seek treatment for any accompanying medical and mental health issues.

Advice For Friends and Family Members

Caring for a person who has problems with alcohol can be very stressful. It is important that as you try to help your loved one, you find a way to take care of yourself as well. It may help to seek support from others, including friends, family, community, and support groups. If you are developing your own symptoms of depression or anxiety, think about seeking professional help for yourself. Remember that your loved one is ultimately responsible for managing his or her illness.

However, your participation can make a big difference. Based on clinical experience, many health providers believe that support from friends and family members is important in overcoming alcohol problems. But friends and family may feel unsure about how best to provide the support needed. The groups for family and friends listed on p. 14 may be a good starting point.

Remember that changing deep habits is hard, takes time, and requires repeated efforts. We usually experience failures along the way, learn from them, and then keep going. AUD is no different. Try to be patient with your loved one. Overcoming this disorder is not easy or quick.

Pay attention to your loved one when he or she is doing better or simply making an effort. Too often we are so angry or discouraged that we take it for granted when things are going better. A word of appreciation or acknowledgement of a success can go a long way.

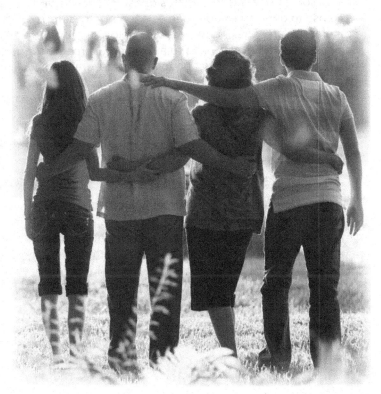

An Ongoing Process

Overcoming alcohol use disorder is an ongoing process, one which can include setbacks.

The Importance of Persistence

Because AUD can be a chronic relapsing disease, persistence is key. It is rare that someone would go to treatment once and then never drink again. More often, people must repeatedly try to quit or cut back, experience recurrences, learn from them, and then keep trying. For many, continued followup with a treatment provider is critical to overcoming problem drinking.

Relapse Is Part of the Process

Relapse is common among people who overcome alcohol problems. People with drinking problems are most likely to relapse during periods of stress or when exposed to people or places associated with past drinking.

Just as some people with diabetes or asthma may have flare-ups of their disease, a relapse to drinking can be seen as a temporary setback to full recovery and not a complete failure. Seeking professional help can prevent relapse—behavioral therapies can help people develop skills to avoid and overcome triggers, such as stress, that might lead to drinking. Most people benefit from regular checkups with a treatment provider. Medications also can deter drinking during times when individuals may be at greater risk of relapse (e.g., divorce, death of a family member).

Mental Health Issues and Alcohol Use Disorder

Depression and anxiety often go hand in hand with heavy drinking. Studies show that people who are alcohol dependent are two to three times as likely to suffer from major depression or anxiety over their lifetime. When addressing drinking problems, it's important to also seek treatment for any accompanying medical and mental health issues.

Research shows that most people who have alcohol problems are able to reduce their drinking or quit entirely.

There are many roads to getting better. What is important is finding yours.

Understanding the available treatment options—from behavioral therapies and medications to mutual-support groups—is the first step. The important thing is to remain engaged in whatever method you choose.

Ultimately, receiving treatment can improve your chances of success.

NATIONAL INSTITUTE ON ALCOHOL ABUSE AND ALCOHOLISM

NIH...Turning Discovery Into Health

NIH Publication No. 21–AA–7974
Revised August 2021

Source: National Institute on Drug Abuse. (2013). *Seeking drug abuse treatment: Know what to ask.* https://nida.nih.gov/sites/default/files/treatmentbrochure_web.pdf

APPENDIX B-7: HIV 101

(Page 1 is in English, Page 2 is in Spanish)

October 2022

HIV 101

Without treatment, HIV (human immunodeficiency virus) can make a person very sick and even cause death. Learning the basics about HIV can keep you healthy and prevent transmission.

HIV CAN BE TRANSMITTED BY

Sexual Contact

Sharing Needles to Inject Drugs

During Pregnancy, Birth, or Breast/Chestfeeding

HIV IS NOT TRANSMITTED BY

Air or Water

Saliva, Sweat, Tears, or Closed-Mouth Kissing

Insects or Pets

Sharing Toilets, Food, or Drinks

PROTECT YOURSELF FROM HIV

- Get tested at least once or more often if you have certain risk factors.
- Use condoms the right way every time you have anal or vaginal sex.
- Choose activities with little to no risk like oral sex.
- Don't inject drugs, or if you do, don't share needles, syringes, or other drug injection equipment.

- If you engage in behaviors that may increase your chances of getting HIV, ask your health care provider if pre-exposure prophylaxis (PrEP) is right for you.
- If you think you've been exposed to HIV within the last 3 days, ask a health care provider about post-exposure prophylaxis (PEP) right away. PEP can prevent HIV, but it must be started within 72 hours.
- Get tested and treated for other STDs.

KEEP YOURSELF HEALTHY AND PROTECT OTHERS IF YOU HAVE HIV

- Find HIV care and stay in HIV care.
- Take your HIV treatment as prescribed.
- Get and keep an undetectable viral load. This is the best way to stay healthy and protect others.
- If you have an undetectable viral load, you will not transmit HIV through sex.

- If your viral load is not undetectable—or does not stay undetectable—you can still protect your partners by using other HIV prevention options.
- Learn more at **www.cdc.gov/hiv/basics/ livingwithhiv.**

Scan to learn more!

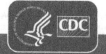

For more information, please visit **www.cdc.gov/hiv.**

INFORMACIÓN BÁSICA SOBRE EL VIH

Octubre de 2022

Sin tratamiento, el VIH (virus de la inmunodeficiencia humana) puede hacer que una persona esté muy enferma, e incluso causarle la muerte. Aprender lo básico sobre el VIH puede mantenerlo saludable y | revenir la transmisión de este virus.

EL VIH PUEDE SER TRANSMITIDO

Mediante el contacto sexual

Al compartir las agujas para inyectarse drogas

Durante el embarazo, el parto o el pecho/lactancia materna

EL VIH NO SE TRANSMITE

A través del aire o del agua

Mediante la saliva, el sudor, las lágrimas o los besos con la boca cerrada

Por los insectos o por las mascotas

Al compartir el inodoro, los alimentos o las bebidas

PROTÉJASE DEL VIH

- Hágase la prueba al menos una vez o con más frecuencia si tiene ciertos factores de riesgo.
- Use condones de la manera correcta cada vez que tenga relaciones sexuales anales o vaginales.
- Elija actividades que impliquen poco o nada de riesgo, como las relaciones sexuales orales.
- No se inyecte drogas, pero si lo hace, no comparta las agujas, jeringas, u otro equipo de inyección de drogas.

- Si tiene comportamientos que pueden aumentar sus posibilidades de contraer el VIH, pregúntele a su proveedor de atención médica si la profilaxis preexposicíon (PrEP) es adecuada para usted.
- Si cree que se ha expuesto al VIH dentro delos últimos 3 días, pregúntele de inmediato a un proveedor de atención médica acerca de la profilaxis posexposición (PEP). La PEP puede prevenir el VIH, pero debe comenzarse dentro de las 72 horas de la posible exposición.
- Hágase las pruebas de detección de otras ETS y reciba el tratamiento necesario.

SI TIENE EL VIH, MANTÉNGASE SALUDABLE Y PROTEJA A LOS DEMÁS

- Busque atención médica para el VIH y no deje de recibir la atención médica para el VIH.
- Tomar el tratamiento para el VIH según las indicaciones.
- Obtenga y mantenga una carga viral indetectable. Esta es la mejor manera de mantenerse saludable y proteger a los demás.
- Si tiene una carga viral indetectable, no transmitirá el VIH a su pareja sexual.

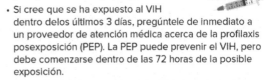

- Si su carga viral no es indetectable, o no permanece indetectable, aún puede proteger a sus parejas utilizando otras opciones de prevención del VIH.
- Obtenga más información en **www.cdc.gov/hiv/spanish/basics/livingwithhiv**.

¡Escanea para obtener más información!

Para obtener más información, visite la página
www.cdc.gov/hiv/spanish.

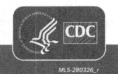

MLS-280326_r

Source: Centers for Disease Control and Prevention. (2022). *HIV 101.* https://www.cdc.gov/hiv/pdf/library/consumer-info-sheets/cdc-hiv-consumer-info-sheet-hiv-101.pdf

APPENDIX B-8: COVID TRANSMISSION EDUCATION

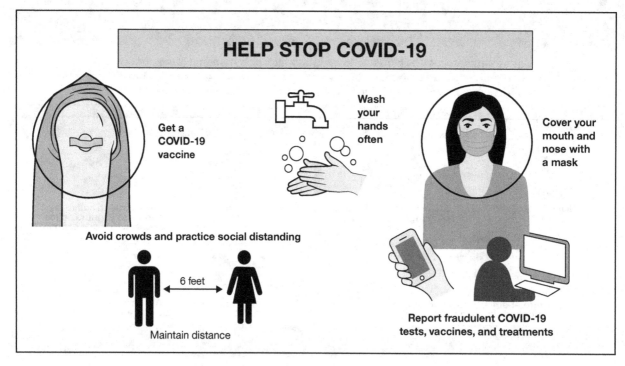

Source: Adapted from U.S. Food & Drug Administration. (2022). *Help stop the spread of coronavirus and protect your family.* https://www.fda.gov/consumers/consumer-updates/help-stop-spread-coronavirus-and-protect-your-family

APPENDIX B-9: KNOW STROKE

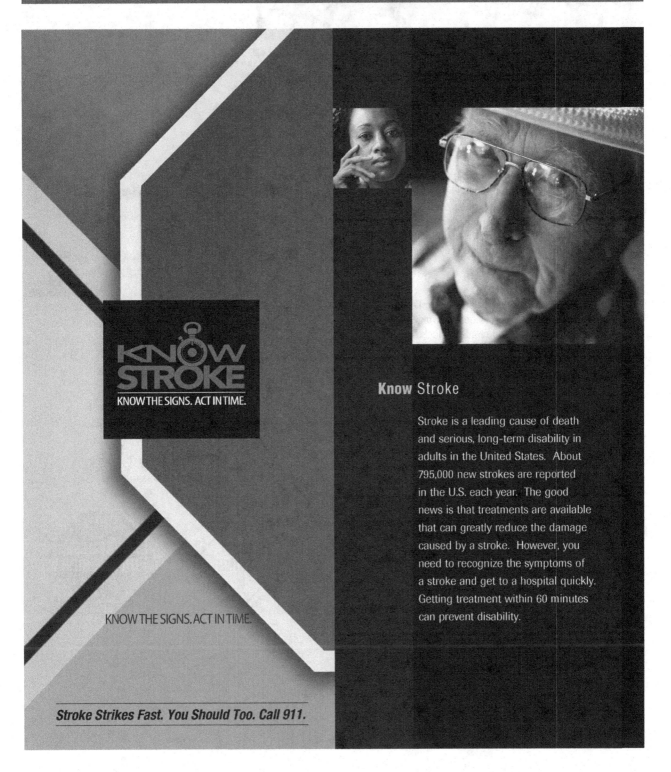

KNOW
STROKE
KNOW THE SIGNS. ACT IN TIME.

KNOW THE SIGNS. ACT IN TIME.

Stroke Strikes Fast. You Should Too. Call 911.

Know Stroke

Stroke is a leading cause of death and serious, long-term disability in adults in the United States. About 795,000 new strokes are reported in the U.S. each year. The good news is that treatments are available that can greatly reduce the damage caused by a stroke. However, you need to recognize the symptoms of a stroke and get to a hospital quickly. Getting treatment within 60 minutes can prevent disability.

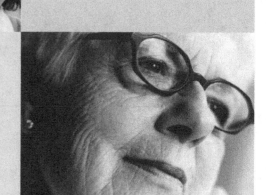

WHAT IS A
STROKE?

A stroke, sometimes called a "brain attack," occurs when blood flow to the brain is interrupted. When a stroke occurs, brain cells in the immediate area begin to die because they stop getting the oxygen and nutrients they need to function.

What causes a stroke?

There are two major kinds of stroke. The first, called an ischemic stroke, is caused by a blood clot that blocks or plugs a blood vessel or artery in the brain. About 80 percent of all strokes are ischemic. The second, known as a hemorrhagic stroke, is caused by a blood vessel in the brain that breaks and bleeds into the brain. About 20 percent of strokes are hemorrhagic.

What disabilities can result from a stroke?

Although stroke is a disease of the brain, it can affect the entire body. The effects of a stroke range from mild to severe and can include paralysis, problems with thinking, problems with speaking, and emotional problems. Patients may also experience pain or numbness after a stroke.

Know the Signs

Because stroke injures the brain, you may not realize that you are having a stroke. To a bystander, someone having a stroke may just look unaware or confused. Stroke victims have the best chance if someone around them recognizes the symptoms and acts quickly.

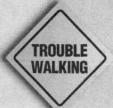

TROUBLE WALKING

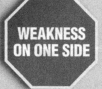

WEAKNESS ON ONE SIDE

WHAT ARE THE
SYMPTOMS
OF A STROKE?

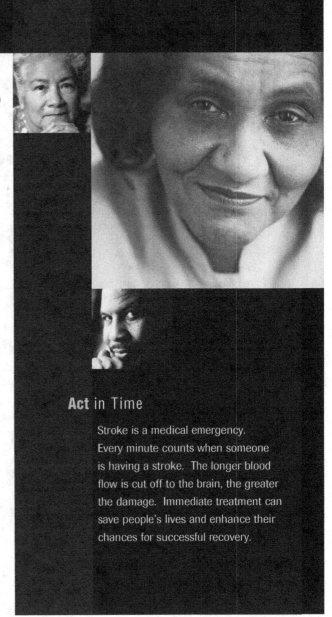

The symptoms of stroke are distinct because they happen quickly:

- Sudden numbness or weakness of the face, arm, or leg (especially on one side of the body)
- Sudden confusion, trouble speaking or understanding speech
- Sudden trouble seeing in one or both eyes
- Sudden trouble walking, dizziness, loss of balance or coordination
- Sudden severe headache with no known cause

What should a bystander do?

If you believe someone is having a stroke – if he or she suddenly loses the ability to speak, or move an arm or leg on one side, or experiences facial paralysis on one side – call 911 immediately.

TROUBLE SEEING

TROUBLE SPEAKING

Act in Time

Stroke is a medical emergency. Every minute counts when someone is having a stroke. The longer blood flow is cut off to the brain, the greater the damage. Immediate treatment can save people's lives and enhance their chances for successful recovery.

WHY IS THERE A NEED TO ACT FAST?

There are several treatments for stroke. All of them are delivered on an emergency basis. Many ischemic strokes can be treated with a clot-busting drug called t-PA that is most effective within 4.5 hours of stroke onset. There are devices that can extend that window by applying the medicine directly to the clot. There are now ways to mechanically remove blood clots, but again time is of the essence. Even after waking up with a stroke, don't delay; rush to the hospital to be evaluated for treatment. Even a small stroke — a transient ischemic attack — is something to have looked at immediately.

How can I reduce my risk of stroke?

The best treatment for stroke is prevention. Several factors increase your risk of having a stroke:

- High blood pressure
- Diabetes
- Heart disease
- High cholesterol
- Smoking
- Physical inactivity/ obesity

If you smoke – quit. If you have high blood pressure, heart disease, diabetes, or high cholesterol, get them under control. If you are overweight, start a healthy diet and exercise regularly.

www.stroke.nih.gov
1-800-352-9424

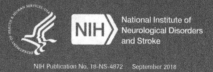

National Institute of
Neurological Disorders
and Stroke

NIH Publication No. 18-NS-4872   September 2018

Source: National Institutes of Health. (2022). *What you need to know about stroke.* https://www.stroke.nih.gov/materials/needtoknow.htm

APPENDIX B-10: REASONS TO QUIT SMOKING

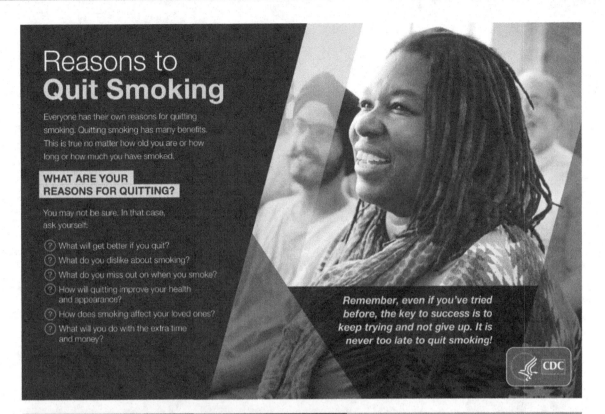

Reasons to
Quit Smoking

Everyone has their own reasons for quitting smoking. Quitting smoking has many benefits. This is true no matter how old you are or how long or how much you have smoked.

WHAT ARE YOUR REASONS FOR QUITTING?

You may not be sure. In that case, ask yourself:

- (?) What will get better if you quit?
- (?) What do you dislike about smoking?
- (?) What do you miss out on when you smoke?
- (?) How will quitting improve your health and appearance?
- (?) How does smoking affect your loved ones?
- (?) What will you do with the extra time and money?

Remember, even if you've tried before, the key to success is to keep trying and not give up. It is never too late to quit smoking!

CDC

HEALTH AND APPEARANCE REASONS

- Chance of cancer, heart disease, stroke, chronic obstructive pulmonary disease (COPD), and other diseases goes down
- Easier breathing and less coughing
- Look and feel younger
- Prevents stains on teeth and fingernails

Quitting smoking will improve your health and can add up to 10 years to your life!

FAMILY AND LOVED ONES REASONS

- More time to spend with family and loved ones
- Set a good example for your children
- Keep children and loved ones safe from the danger of secondhand smoke

Quitting smoking will help make sure you are around for special moments with your loved ones, like weddings, graduations, and the births of grandchildren!

LIFESTYLE REASONS

- More time to do the things you love
- More time and energy to exercise
- Food tastes better
- More money to spend
- Sense of smell improves

Quitting smoking will help you enjoy life!

Get Help Quitting

Quitting smoking can be hard and may require multiple tries. The good news is there are proven treatments – medications and counseling – that can improve your chances of quitting for good. Many of these treatments are available free of charge or are covered by insurance.

When you are ready to quit, call a quitline coach (1-800-QUIT-NOW) or talk to your doctor, nurse, or other healthcare professional about the best treatments and resources for you.

For More Information About Quitting

CDC.gov/quit
Call 1-800-QUIT-NOW
(1-800-784-8669)

July 2021

Source: Centers for Disease Control & Prevention. (2022). *Patient cessation materials.* https://www.cdc.gov/tobacco/patient-care/patient-resources/index.html

APPENDIX C

CLINICIAN RESOURCES

APPENDIX C-1: DISEASE TRAJECTORIES

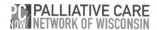
PALLIATIVE CARE
NETWORK OF WISCONSIN

FAST FACTS AND CONCEPTS #326
ILLNESS TRAJECTORIES: DESCRIPTION AND CLINICAL USE
Paige Comstock Barker, MD and Jennifer S. Scherer, MD

Illness trajectories can provide a framework for addressing patient and family expectations of what will happen with regards to their anticipated health. Distinct illness trajectories have been recognized in the medical literature (see Figure 1). This *Fast Fact* will review the medical evidence of these trajectories as well as their utility as a patient teaching tool.

General Evidence: A large observational study, described distinct illness trajectories at the end of life for frailty/dementia, cancer, and organ failure (1). Subsequent research has cast some controversy about the validity of these findings, particularly whether hospitalizations may have a more significant role on the pattern of decline than the specific illness itself (2-4).

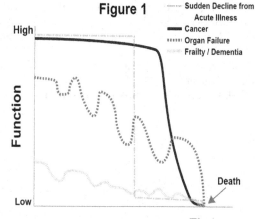

Figure 1

Illness Trajectories:
Frailty / Dementia: A pattern of dwindling cognitive and/or physical disability that may progress over several years (1). Seventy percent of dementia patients require assistance in ≥3 ADLs, in the last year of life, making these patients at heightened risk for nursing home placement and caregiver breakdown (2). Many clinicians and families may not recognize that dementia by itself is a terminal illness.

Cancer: A relatively stable period of physical function followed by an acute decline in the last few months of life. Multiple studies have supported this trajectory however, the timing of steep decline ranges between 1 to 5 months before death depending on the study (1,5-7). Cancer patients may also experience more predictable patterns of spiritual distress with peaks at diagnosis, disease recurrence, and the terminal phase of illness (8). Because the physical decline and psycho-spiritual distress can be better anticipated, especially in solid tumors, more accurate prognostication and implementation of specialized palliative care services can occur. One study of Medicare patients showed that cancer patients were more likely to utilize hospice in comparison to other chronic illnesses because of the more predictable trajectory (9). More research is needed to validate this trajectory in the face of new targeted treatment modalities.

Organ failure: A more erratic trajectory with punctuated periods of decline likely correlating with acute exacerbations (1). Each exacerbation may result in death but is often survived with gradual deterioration in health and functional status. Timing of death is less certain than in cancer. Perhaps as a result, patients with congestive heart failure (CHF) and chronic obstructive pulmonary disorder are more likely to die in the hospital and less likely to receive hospice services nor understand the likely progression of their illness (9-12). Other take home points regarding the organ failure trajectory include:
- The functional decline for CHF has been shown to be particularly heterogeneous (2,13). Some hypothesize this may be related to co-morbidities and/or research methodologies (13).
- Often prognosis is more centered around patient specific goals regarding acceptance or not of repeat hospitalizations and treatment of potentially reversible complications.
- Although observational studies have shown inconsistent findings, elderly end stage renal disease patients who forgo initiating hemodialysis may be more likely to have an illness trajectory similar to sudden death – stable function for months with a rapid end of life deterioration (14-16).

Sudden Death or Decline: An abrupt change from normal physical function to either death or significant medical disability, often as a result of trauma or an acute cardiopulmonary/neurologic event. Many times there is little or no prior interaction with the health system nor a recognizable pattern of functional decline preceding the event (1,9). Thus, intense displays of shock or anger are common from family members when clinicians break bad news. See *Fast Fact* #305. Loved ones are at increased risk for depression and complicated grief as they adjust to the new medical reality after the event (17,18).

Clinical Use: Although there is no known published data assessing the effectiveness of utilizing the illness trajectories as a clinical teaching tool, describing or even diagramming these illness trajectories with patients and families may be a concise communication technique to set expectations and offer guidance regarding the anticipated impact of chronic illness on daily life. Clinicians should be aware of the significant variability in the medical literature regarding the validity of these illness trajectories as well as the limitations in the way functional decline is measured between studies. Therefore, it is vital that illness trajectories are reevaluated as the condition evolves. In particular, certain patterns such as an abrupt functional decline or frequent hospitalizations may indicate the need to readdress goals of care.

References:

1. Lunney JR, Lynn J, Foley D, et al; Patterns of Functional Decline at the End of Life. *JAMA.* 2003;289(18): 2387-2392.
2. Gill TM, Gahbauer EA, Han L, et al; Trajectories of Disability in the Last Year of Life. *The New England Journal of Medicine.* 2010;362(13): 1173-1180.
3. Gill TM, Gahbauer EA, Han L, et al; The role of intervening hospital admission on trajectories of disability in the last year of life: prospective cohort study of older people. *BMJ.* 2015;350:1-8.
4. Steinhauser KE, Arnold RM, Olsen MK, et al. Comparing Three Life-Limiting Diseases: Does Diagnosis Matter or Is Sick, Sick? *J Pain Symptom Manage.* 2011; 42(3): 331-341.
5. Seow, H, Barbera L, Sutradhar R, et al. Trajectory of Performance Status and Symptom Scores for Patients With Cancer During the Last Six Months of Life. Journal of Oncology. 2011; 29(9): 1151 – 1158.
6. Tang ST, Liu LN, Lin KC, et al; Trajectories of the Multidimensional Dying Experience for Terminally Ill Cancer Patients. *Journal of Pain and Symptom Management.* 2014;48(5): 863-874.
7. Teno JM, Weitzen S, Fennell ML, et al. Dying Trajectory in the Last Year of Life: Does Cancer Trajectory Fit Other Diseases? Journal of Palliative Medicine. 2001; 4(4): 457 – 464.
8. Murray SA, Kendall M, Grant E, et al; Patterns of Social, Psychological, and Spiritual Decline Toward the End of Life in Lung Cancer and Heart Failure. *Journal of Pain and Symptom Management.* 2007;34(4): 393-402.
9. Lunney JR, Lynn J, Hogan C. Profiles of Older Medicare Decedents. *JAGS.* 2002;50:1108-1112.
10. Gavazzi, A, De Maria R, Manzoli L, et al. Palliative needs for heart failure or chronic obstructive pulmonary disease: Results of a multicenter observational registry. *International Journal of Cardiology.* 2015;184: 552-558.
11. Kendall M, Carduff E, Lloyd A, et al; Different Experiences and Goals in Different Advanced Diseases: Comparing Serial Interviews With Patients With Cancer, Organ Failure, or Frailty and Their Family and Professional Carers. Journal of Pain and Symptom Management. 2015;50(2): 216-224.
12. Levenson JW, McCarthy EP, Lynn J, et al; The Last Six Months of Life for Patients with Congestive Heart Failure. *JAGS.* 2000;48(5): S101-S109.
13. Kheribek RE, Alemi F, Citron BA, et al; Trajectory of Illness for Patients with Congestive Heart Failure. Journal of Palliative Medicine. 2013;16(5): 478-484.
14. Murtagh, FEM, Addington-Hall J, and Higginson IJ. End-Stage Renal Disease: A New Trajectory of Functional Decline in the Last Year of Life. *JAGS.* 2011; 59: 304-308.
15. Schell JO, Da Silva-Gane M, and Germain MJ. Recent insights into life expectancy with and without dialysis. *Current Opin Nephrol Hypertens.* 2013;22: 185-192.
16. Schell JO and O'Hare AM. Illness trajectories and their relevance to the care of adults with kidney disease. *Current Opin Nephrol Hypertens.* 2013;22: 316-324.
17. Burton, AM, Haley WE, Small BJ. Bereavement after caregiving or unexpected death: Effects on elderly spouses. *Aging and Mental Health.* 2006;10(3): 319-326.
18. Kristensen, P, Weisaeth L, Heir T. Bereavement and Mental Health after Sudden and Violent Losses: A Review. *Psychiatry.* 2012;75(1):76-97.

Author's Affiliations: New York University, New York, NY
Conflicts of Interest: None
Version History: Originally edited by Sean Marks MD; first electronically published in December 2016.

Source: Comstock, P., & Scherer J. S. (2016). *Fast facts and concepts #326: Illness trajectories: Description and clinical use.* https://www.mypcnow.org/fast-facts/.

See also: Ballentine, J. M. (2018). *The five trajectories: Supporting patients during serious illness.* CSU Shiley Institute for Palliative Care. https://csupalliativecare.org/wp-content/uploads/Five-Trajectories-eBook-02.21.2018.pdf (This ebook is a resource for clinicians but can also be used to teach patients and families about what to expect as the disease process unfolds. The five main trajectories of terminal disease progression are included as well as clinical tips, case studies, practice resources, and numerous links to online educational resources.)

APPENDIX C-2: SERIOUS ILLNESS CONVERSATION GUIDE

SERIOUS ILLNESS CONVERSATION GUIDE		
CONVERSATION FLOW		**PATIENT-TESTED LANGUAGE**

1. *Set up the conversation*
    Introduce the idea and benefits
    Ask permission
	SET UP	"I'm hoping we can talk about where things are with your illness and where they might be going—**is this okay?**"

2. Assess *illness understanding and information preferences*	ASSESS	"What is your **understanding** now of where you are with your illness?" "How much **information** about what is likely to be ahead with your illness would you like from me?"

3. *Share prognosis*
    Tailor information to patient preference
    Allow silence, explore emotion
	SHARE	**Prognosis:** "I'm worried that time may be short."
		    or "This may be as strong as you feel."

4. *Explore key topics*
    Goals
    Fears and worries
    Sources of strength
    Critical abilities
    Trade-offs
    Family
	EXPLORE	"What are your most important **goals** if your health situation worsens?"
		
		"What are your biggest **fears and worries** about the future with your health?"
		
		"What gives you **strength** as you think about the future with your illness?"
		
		"What **abilities** are so critical to your life that you can't imagine living without them?"
		
		"If you become sicker, **how much are you willing to go through** for the possibility of gaining more time?"
		
		"How much does your **family** know about your priorities and wishes?"

5. *Close the conversation*
    Summarize what you've heard
    Make a recommendation
    Affirm your commitment to the patient
	CLOSE	"**It sounds like** _____ is very important to you."
		
		"Given your goals and priorities and what we know about your illness at this stage, I **recommend . . .**"
		
		"**We're in this together.**"

6. *Document your conversation*		

(continued)

APPENDIX C-2: SERIOUS ILLNESS CONVERSATION GUIDE (*CONTINUED*)

SERIOUS ILLNESS CONVERSATION GUIDE
CONVERSATION FLOW

1. **Set up the conversation**
   Introduce the idea and benefits
   Ask permission
2. **Assess illness understanding and information preferences**
3. **Share prognosis**
   Tailor information to patient preference
   Allow silence, explore emotion
4. **Explore key topics**
   Goals
   Fears and worries
   Sources of strength
   Critical abilities
   Tradeoffs
   Family
5. **Close the conversation**
   Summarize what you've heard
   Make a recommendation
   Affirm your commitment to the patient
6. **Document your conversation**

	PATIENT-TESTED LANGUAGE
SET UP	"I'm hoping we can talk about where things are with your illness and where they might be going—**is this okay**?"
ASSESS	"What is your **understanding** now of where you are with your illness?" "How much **information** about what is likely to be ahead with your illness would you like from me?"
SHARE	**Prognosis:** "I'm worried that time may be short." *or* "This may be as strong as you feel."
EXPLORE	"What are your most important **goals** if your health situation worsens?" "What are your biggest **fears and worries** about the future with your health?" "What gives you **strength** as you think about the future with your illness?" "What **abilities** are so critical to your life that you can't imagine living without them?" "If you become sicker, **how much are you willing to go through** for the possibility of gaining more time?" "How much does your **family** know about your priorities and wishes?"
CLOSE	"**It sounds like** _____ is very important to you." "Given your goals and priorities and what we know about your illness at this stage, **I recommend** . . ." "**We're in this together**."

Source: Ariadne Labs. (2015). *Serious illness conversation guide.* http://www.instituteforhumancaring.org/documents/Providers/Serious-Illness-Guide-old.pdf.

APPENDIX C-3: BREAKING THE COMPASSION WALL

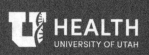

U HEALTH
UNIVERSITY OF UTAH

Four Ways to Break Through the Compassion Wall

Hospitalist Dr. Ryan Murphy is in the unique position of having experienced cared during the Covid-19 crisis from both sides – both as a patient's son and as an attending physician for admitted patients. His experience introduced four ways to break through the compassion wall—the barrier created by the extra precautions COVID-19 requires.

VALIDATE EMOTIONS TO CLOSE THE PHYSICAL DISTANCE

Whether you're in full protective gear or an ear loop mask, your eyes, body language, and attitude matter. Given these precautions, I try to validate patients' emotions by telling them that I recognize how scared they must feel. I spend time focusing on their emotions first, instead of diving straight into the medical details. I believe it is easier for patients to listen to the medical analysis if you address their emotions first. Then, I ask, "What is your understanding of what is going on?" Learning what a patient already understands about their care helps me tailor the conversation to their needs.

SHARE THE DECISION-MAKING

One of the hard things about COVID is the unknown. I've adopted a mindset similar to other clinical decisions that don't have clear answers. I embrace shared decision-making. I tell them, "Here are your options, here are the pros and cons of each." I say, "I would recommend this, or I would prefer that." Ultimately, you have to be transparent and honest with what we know and what we don't know.
Learn a simple model for shared decision-making: choice, option, and decision. It starts with eliciting what patients already know. Utah's palliative care physician Paige Patterson shares a conversation model for serious illness.

ANSWER THEIR QUESTIONS

Instead of saying, "Do you have other questions?" I ask, "What other questions do you have?" I ask this question multiple times before I leave the room. I also make sure they have a pen and paper, or their cell phone, to write down additional questions after I leave.

HELP PATIENTS STAY CONNECTED

Make sure that patients can communicate with their family and that they have a phone or an iPad and a charger. You can also set up a video call for patients to communicate with their family through myChart, InTouch or Zoom .

https://accelerate.uofuhealth.utah.edu/connect/breaking-dow-the-compassion-wall

Source: Murphy, R. (2020, April 24). *Breaking down the compassion wall.* https://accelerate.uofuhealth.utah.edu/connect/breaking-dow-the-compassion-wall.

APPENDIX C-4: SPIKES MODEL

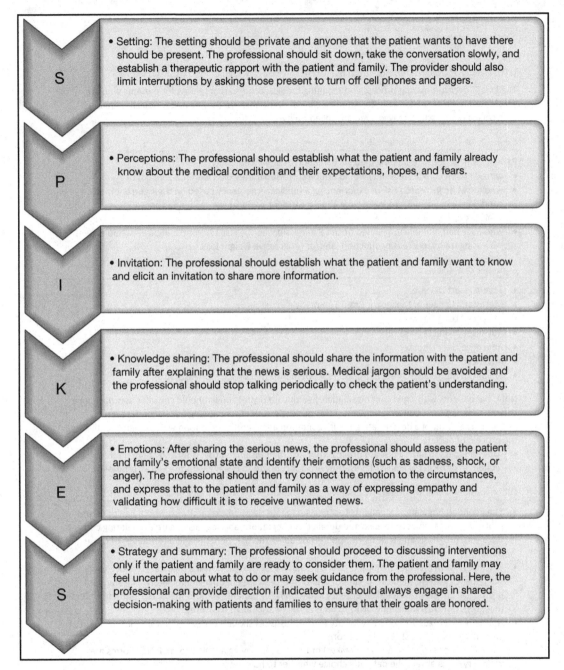

- **S** • Setting: The setting should be private and anyone that the patient wants to have there should be present. The professional should sit down, take the conversation slowly, and establish a therapeutic rapport with the patient and family. The provider should also limit interruptions by asking those present to turn off cell phones and pagers.

- **P** • Perceptions: The professional should establish what the patient and family already know about the medical condition and their expectations, hopes, and fears.

- **I** • Invitation: The professional should establish what the patient and family want to know and elicit an invitation to share more information.

- **K** • Knowledge sharing: The professional should share the information with the patient and family after explaining that the news is serious. Medical jargon should be avoided and the professional should stop talking periodically to check the patient's understanding.

- **E** • Emotions: After sharing the serious news, the professional should assess the patient and family's emotional state and identify their emotions (such as sadness, shock, or anger). The professional should then try connect the emotion to the circumstances, and express that to the patient and family as a way of expressing empathy and validating how difficult it is to receive unwanted news.

- **S** • Strategy and summary: The professional should proceed to discussing interventions only if the patient and family are ready to consider them. The patient and family may feel uncertain about what to do or may seek guidance from the professional. Here, the professional can provide direction if indicated but should always engage in shared decision-making with patients and families to ensure that their goals are honored.

Source: Adapted from Baile, W. F., Buckman, R., Lenzl, R., Global, G., Beale, E. A., & Kudelka, A. P. (2000). SPIKES: A six-step protocol for delivering bad news: Application to the patient with cancer. *The Oncologist, 5*(4), 302–311. https://doi.org/10.1634/theoncologist:5-4-302. http://theoncologist.alphamedpress.org/

APPENDIX C-5: INTENDED POLST POPULATION AND GUIDANCE

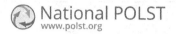

National POLST
www.polst.org

Intended Population & Guidance for Health Care Professionals[1]

The POLST decision-making process and resulting medical orders are intended for patients who are considered to be at risk for a life-threatening clinical event because they have a serious life-limiting medical condition, which may include advanced frailty.

Examples of appropriate patients for engagement in POLST conversations

Patients with serious life-limiting medical condition or advanced frailty:

- whose health care professional would not be surprised if they died within 1-2 years; or
- who are at an increased risk of experiencing a medical emergency based on their current medical condition and who wish to make clear their treatment preferences, including about CPR, mechanical ventilation, ICU; or
- who have had multiple unplanned hospital admissions in the last 12 months, typically coupled with increasing frailty, decreasing function, and/or progressive weight loss.

Examples of medical conditions (**not** an exhaustive list)

- Severe Heart Disease
- Metastatic Cancer or Malignant Brain Tumor
- Advanced Lung Disease
- Advanced Renal Disease
- Advanced Liver Disease
- Advanced Frailty[2]
- Advanced Neurodegenerative Disease (e.g., Dementia, Parkinson's Disease, ALS)

Note: For patients with significant disabilities, health care professionals should consider approaching a patient about a POLST conversation only if this patient's level of functioning has become severely impaired as a result of a deteriorating health condition and when intervention will not significantly impact the process of decline.

- Does the person have a disease process (not just their disability) that is an end-stage medical condition or terminal illness? If yes, they are appropriate to engage with the POLST process.

Other considerations for identifying appropriate patients for engagement in POLST conversations

- The intended population is patients (or their surrogate decision-makers) with whom health care professionals can initiate specific and detailed conversations about goals of care considering current diagnosis, prognosis and treatment options (including the risk, benefits and alternatives of those options).
- The POLST form provides medical orders for what happens right now if a medical crisis occurs given the patient's current medical condition; the form orders are effective immediately. The standard protocol in an out-of-hospital emergency situation is for patients without medical treatment orders (e.g., DNR or POLST indicating DNR) to receive full resuscitative measures.
- Neither age nor admission to any facility (except hospice) should serve as an automatic indication of patient appropriateness for a POLST form.
  The patient (or surrogate decision-maker) must agree to having a POLST form. **POLST forms are voluntary – it is always the patient's choice whether to have one.**

---

[1] State law varies about which health care professionals are able to sign a POLST form. Guidance is available at http://polst.org/state-signature-requirements-pdf; please check your state law to confirm.
[2] indicating a combination of advanced chronic disease and/or advanced age with significant weight loss and functional decline

Approved November 7, 2018. Revised January 14, 2019.

Note: Please see the website for the most updated information.

Source: National POLST. (2021). *Intended population & Guidance for health care professionals.* https://polst.org/guidance-appropriate-patients-pdf.

APPENDIX C-6: POLST FORM

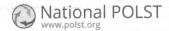 National POLST
www.polst.org

NOTICE

This is the National POLST Form and can only be *completed* in states that have adopted it (it is valid in most states). Check with your POLST Program (www.polst.org/map) to determine if your state uses this version.

National POLST Form

The National POLST Form is a portable medical order. Health care professionals should complete this form only after a conversation with their patient or the patient's representative. The POLST decision-making process is for patients who are at risk for a life-threatening clinical event because they have a serious life-limiting medical condition, which may include advanced frailty (www.polst.org/guidance-appropriate-patients-pdf).

This form should be obtained from a health care provider.
It should not be provided to patients or individuals to complete.

Printing the National POLST Form

1. **Do not alter this form**.

2. This national form must be adopted by the state before it can be completed in that state as a valid POLST form. Find your POLST Program contact at www.polst.org/map – this is because some states have added information on page 2, have added a border, or have requirements about the color of the form.

3. Print BOTH pages as a double-sided form on a single sheet of paper.

HIPAA PERMITS DISCLOSURE OF POLST ORDERS TO HEALTH CARE PROVIDERS AS NECESSARY FOR TREATMENT

SEND FORM WITH PATIENT WHENEVER TRANSFERRED OR DISCHARGED

Medical Record # (Optional)

National POLST Form: A Portable Medical Order

Health care providers should complete this form only after a conversation with their patient or the patient's representative. The POLST decision-making process is for patients who are at risk for a life-threatening clinical event because they have a serious life-limiting medical condition, which may include advanced frailty (www.polst.org/guidance-appropriate-patients-pdf).

Patient Information.	Having a POLST form is always voluntary.
This is a medical order, not an advance directive. For information about POLST and to understand this document, visit: www.polst.org/form	Patient First Name: _____ Middle Name/Initial: _____ Preferred name: _____ Last Name: _____ Suffix (Jr, Sr, etc): _____ DOB (mm/dd/yyyy): ____/____/_____ State where form was completed:_____ Gender: ☐ M ☐ F ☐ X Social Security Number's last 4 digits (optional): xxx-xx-___ ___ ___ ___

A. Cardiopulmonary Resuscitation Orders. Follow these orders if patient has no pulse and is not breathing.

Pick 1

☐ YES CPR: Attempt Resuscitation, including mechanical ventilation, defibrillation and cardioversion. (Requires choosing Full Treatments in Section B)

☐ NO CPR: Do Not Attempt Resuscitation. (May choose any option in Section B)

B. Initial Treatment Orders. Follow these orders if patient has a pulse and/or is breathing.

Reassess and discuss interventions with patient or patient representative regularly to ensure treatments are meeting patient's care goals. Consider a time-trial of interventions based on goals and specific outcomes.

Pick 1

☐ Full Treatments (required if choose CPR in Section A). Goal: Attempt to sustain life by all medically effective means. Provide appropriate medical and surgical treatments as indicated to attempt to prolong life, including intensive care.

☐ Selective Treatments. Goal: Attempt to restore function while avoiding intensive care and resuscitation efforts (ventilator, defibrillation and cardioversion). May use non-invasive positive airway pressure, antibiotics and IV fluids as indicated. Avoid intensive care. Transfer to hospital if treatment needs cannot be met in current location.

☐ Comfort-focused Treatments. Goal: Maximize comfort through symptom management; allow natural death. Use oxygen, suction and manual treatment of airway obstruction as needed for comfort. Avoid treatments listed in full or select treatments unless consistent with comfort goal. Transfer to hospital **only** if comfort cannot be achieved in current setting.

C. Additional Orders or Instructions. These orders are in addition to those above (e.g., blood products, dialysis).

[EMS protocols may limit emergency responder ability to act on orders in this section.]

D. Medically Assisted Nutrition (Offer food by mouth if desired by patient, safe and tolerated)

Pick 1

☐ Provide feeding through new or existing surgically-placed tubes

☐ Trial period for artificial nutrition but no surgically-placed tubes

☐ No artificial means of nutrition desired

☐ Not discussed or no decision made (provide standard of care)

E. SIGNATURE: Patient or Patient Representative (eSigned documents are valid)

I understand this form is voluntary. I have discussed my treatment options and goals of care with my provider. If signing as the patient's representative, the treatments are consistent with the patient's known wishes and in their best interest.

✖ (required)

If other than patient, print full name:		Authority:	The most recently completed valid POLST form supersedes all previously completed POLST forms.

F. SIGNATURE: Health Care Provider (eSigned documents are valid)   Verbal orders are acceptable with follow up signature.

I have discussed this order with the patient or his/her representative. The orders reflect the patient's known wishes, to the best of my knowledge. [Note: Only licensed health care providers authorized by law to sign POLST form in state where completed may sign this order]

✖ (required)

	Date (mm/dd/yyyy): Required / /	Phone # : ( )
Printed Full Name:		License/Cert. #:
Supervising physician signature: ☐ N/A		License #:

A copied, faxed or electronic version of this form is a legal and valid medical order. This form does not expire.

2019

National POLST Form – Page 2   *****ATTACH TO PAGE 1*****

Patient Full Name:

Contact Information (Optional but helpful)

Patient's Emergency Contact. (Note: Listing a person here does **not** grant them authority to be a legal representative. Only an advance directive or state law can grant that authority.)

Full Name:	☐ Legal Representative ☐ Other emergency contact	Phone #: Day: ( ) Night: ( )
Primary Care Provider Name:		Phone: ( )
☐ Patient is enrolled in hospice	Name of Agency: Agency Phone: ( )	

Form Completion Information (Optional but helpful)

Reviewed patient's advance directive to confirm no conflict with POLST orders: (A POLST form does not replace an advance directive or living will)	☐ Yes; date of the document reviewed:_____ ☐ Conflict exists, notified patient (if patient lacks capacity, noted in chart) ☐ Advance directive not available ☐ No advance directive exists
Check everyone who participated in discussion:	☐ Patient with decision-making capacity ☐ Court Appointed Guardian ☐ Parent of Minor ☐ Legal Surrogate / Health Care Agent ☐ Other: _____

Professional Assisting Health Care Provider w/ Form Completion (if applicable): Full Name:	Date (mm/dd/yyyy): / /	Phone #: ( )

This individual is the patient's: ☐ Social Worker ☐ Nurse ☐ Clergy ☐ Other: _____

Form Information & Instructions

- **Completing a POLST form:**
  - Provider should document basis for this form in the patient's medical record notes.
  - Patient representative is determined by applicable state law and, in accordance with state law, may be able execute or void this POLST form only if the patient lacks decision-making capacity.
  - Only licensed health care providers authorized to sign POLST forms in their state or D.C. can sign this form. See www.polst.org/state-signature-requirements-pdf for who is authorized in each state and D.C.
  - Original (if available) is given to patient; provider keeps a copy in medical record.
  - Last 4 digits of SSN are optional but can help identify / match a patient to their form.
  - If a translated POLST form is used during conversation, attach the translation to the signed English form.
- **Using a POLST form:**
  - Any incomplete section of POLST creates no presumption about patient's preferences for treatment. Provide standard of care.
  - No defibrillator (including automated external defibrillators) or chest compressions should be used if "No CPR" is chosen.
  - For all options, use medication by any appropriate route, positioning, wound care and other measures to relieve pain and suffering.
- **Reviewing a POLST form:** This form does not expire but should be reviewed whenever the patient:
  - (1) is transferred from one care setting or level to another;
  - (2) has a substantial change in health status;
  - (3) changes primary provider; or
  - (4) changes his/her treatment preferences or goals of care.
- **Modifying a POLST form:** This form cannot be modified. If changes are needed, void form and complete a new POLST form.
- **Voiding a POLST form:**
  - **If a patient or patient representative (for patients lacking capacity) wants to void the form:** destroy paper form and contact patient's health care provider to void orders in patient's medical record (and POLST registry, if applicable). State law may limit patient representative authority to void.
  - **For health care providers:** destroy patient copy (if possible), note in patient record form is voided and notify registries (if applicable).
- **Additional Forms.** Can be obtained by going to www.polst.org/form
- As permitted by law, this form may be added to a secure electronic registry so health care providers can find it.

State Specific Info	For Barcodes / ID Sticker

For more information, visit www.polst.org or email info@polst.org   Copied, faxed or electronic versions of this form are legal and valid.   2019

APPENDIX C-7: ACUTE COMPLICATIONS OF ADVANCED CANCER

COMPLICATION	DESCRIPTION	SYMPTOMS	DIAGNOSIS	INTERVENTIONS
TLS[a]	Occurs when the by-products of tumor cell breakdown cannot be cleared quickly enough by the kidneys and remain in the bloodstream. This causes a buildup of metabolites, resulting in hyperkalemia, hyperphosphatemia, hyperuricemia, and hypocalcemia. TLS can result from cancer treatment and can be fatal.	Nausea, vomiting, diarrhea Weakness/fatigue Neuralgias Dysrhythmias Confusion/ delirium/ hallucinations Restlessness/ irritability Seizures	CBC Chem 14 Uric acid levels Urinalysis	Allopurinol to reduce uric acid production IV hydration Diuresis Hemodialysis may be required.
DIC[b]	Results from the formation of blood clots in the body's small vessels. This can lead to organ damage. Because the platelets coagulate in the small vessels, fewer remain in circulation, which can lead to severe bleeding.	Chest pain, shortness of breath, dyspnea, myocardial infarction DVT, gangrene Headache, aphasia, paralysis Oliguria Hemorrhage	CBC Blood smear PT/PTT Serum fibrinogen	Supplemental oxygen Fluid replacement Whole blood or blood products, as indicated Heparin as indicated
Hyperleukocytosis and leukocytosis[c,d]	Most commonly seen in patients who have acute leukemia or chronic myeloid leukemia. It is a blood abnormality characterized by a leukocyte count $>50 \times 10^9$/L to 100 $\times 10^9$/L (normal range = 4×10^9/L– 11×10^9/L). This is caused by excessive proliferation of leukocytes and puts patients at risk for DIC and TML.	Respiratory distress Neurological deficits	Leukocyte count $>50 \times 10^9$/L to 100×10^9/L	Prevention of tumor lysis Cytoreduction Blood or platelet transfusion, as indicated Anticoagulant therapy, as indicated Allopurinol to decrease uric acid IV hydration CBC BID

(continued)

APPENDIX C-7: ACUTE COMPLICATIONS OF ADVANCED CANCER (*CONTINUED*)

COMPLICATION	DESCRIPTION	SYMPTOMS	DIAGNOSIS	INTERVENTIONS
Neutropenia[e]	Neutropenia occurs when the ANC falls below 1,000/mm^3 (normal range 1,500–8,000/mm^3). Neutropenia increases the risk of infection. Chemotherapy is the most common cause.	Many be asymptomatic Fever Fatigue Lethargy	ANC below 1,000/mm^3 Anemia	Treatment with broad-spectrum antibiotics Hospitalization may be required.
Metastatic spinal cord compression[f]	The spread of bony metastasis into the spine causes displacement of the spinal nerves and/or vertebral collapse.	Acute-onset back pain Paraplegia or tetraplegia Cauda equina syndrome (neurological deficits in the lower extremities, bowel or bladder incontinence, lower back or leg pain, saddle anesthesia)	MRI	Corticosteroids Analgesia Palliative management is often the treatment of choice.
Superior vena cava syndrome[h]	Occurs when the superior vena cava is compressed by an extrinsic tumor or metastatic lymph nodes	Facial edema, venous dilation across chest and in upper extremities, dyspnea, hoarseness, and dysphagia. Patient may report feeling of constriction in the neck or throat area. Neurological complications may include increased intracranial pressure, confusion, coma, brainstem herniation, and death.	May be diagnosed empirically Chest x-ray or CT scan are useful for determining size and location of tumor or malignant lymph nodes.	Reducing intracranial pressure, airway management, steroids to decrease edema Chemotherapy and radiation may be options to decrease size of tumors or malignant lymph nodes if consistent with goals of care.

(continued)

APPENDIX C-7: ACUTE COMPLICATIONS OF ADVANCED CANCER (*CONTINUED*)

COMPLICATION	DESCRIPTION	SYMPTOMS	DIAGNOSIS	INTERVENTIONS
Septic shock[i,j]	Cancer and cancer treatments deplete the immune system, which can lead to overwhelming systemic infection.	Severe hypotension, hypoxia, tachycardia, fluctuating temperature, restlessness, changes in mentation, tachypnea that can lead to ARDS	Often diagnosed empirically. The patient may have increased white cell count, lactic acidosis, and impaired coagulation. Cultures should be obtained.	Consistent with goals of care, artificial ventilation, cardiac support, and antibiotics are options.
Cardiac tamponade[g,h]	Accumulation of fluid in the pericardial sac that causes compression of the cardiac muscle	Beck's triad: hypotension, increased jugular vein pressure and distention, muffled heart sounds Tachycardia, pulsus paradoxus (drop in systolic BP >10 mmHg with inspiration) New-onset cardiomegaly on x-ray, low voltage on EKG Shortness of breath, chest pain, orthopnea, and general weakness	Chest x-ray, EKG, 2D echocardiogram	Pericardiocentesis, percutaneous pericardiostomy If consistent with goals of care, indwelling pericardial catheter, VATS pericardial window, intrapericardial instillation of antineoplastic and sclerosing agents
SIADH[h]	Characterized by hyponatremia that results from the production of arginine vasopressin by the tumor	Many patients are asymptomatic. Early symptoms include anorexia, nausea, irritability or depression, muscle cramps, peripheral edema, lethargy, weakness, and behavioral changes.	Low serum sodium, normal CO_2, normal potassium, low urine osmolality	Fluid restriction to 0.5 to 1 L/day with increased sodium and protein intake. In severe cases, and when consistent with the patient's goals of care, serum sodium level can be corrected cautiously with 3% saline solution.

(continued)

APPENDIX C-7: ACUTE COMPLICATIONS OF ADVANCED CANCER (*CONTINUED*)

COMPLICATION	DESCRIPTION	SYMPTOMS	DIAGNOSIS	INTERVENTIONS
		If sodium levels drop below 110 mEq/l, depressed deep tendon reflexes, seizures, and coma may occur.		
Hypercalcemia of malignancy[g]	Increased serum calcium levels due to the breakdown of bone tissue from metastasis	Use the mnemonic "moans, stones, groans, bones, thrones, psychiatric overtones" (p. 136; muscle pains, renal calculi, bone pain, constipation polyuria, confusion/depression/lethargy).	Serum calcium levels 12 mg/dL to ≥14 mg/dL Median survival is 30 days without intervention; only a few days if serum calcium level is >16 mg/dL	Treat symptoms in accordance with the patient's goals of care. Interventions to reduce serum calcium may include isotonic saline hydration, calcitonin, biphosphates, loop diuretics, glucocorticoids, denosumab, and/or hemodialysis. Avoid medication that increase serum calcium such as theophylline and calcium supplements (including antacids).

ANC, absolute neutrophil count; ARDS, adult respiratory distress syndrome; CBC, complete blood count; DIC, disseminated intravascular coagulation; DVT, deep vein thrombosis; IV, intravenous; PT, prothrombin time; PTT, partial thromboplastin time; SIADH, syndrome of inappropriate secretion of antidiuretic hormone; TLS, tumor lysis syndrome; TML, tumor mutation load; VATS, video-assisted thoracoscopic surgery.

[a]Sekeres, M. (2010). *Oncologic emergencies.* http://www.clevelandclinicmeded.com/medicalpubs/diseasemanagement/hematology-oncology/oncologic-emergencies/

[b]National Heart, Lung, and Blood Institute. (2017). *Disseminated intravascular coagulation.* https://www.nhlbi.nih.gov/health-topics/disseminated-intravascular-coagulation

[c]Röllig, C. & Ehninger, G. (2015). How I treat hyperleukocytosis in acute myeloid leukemia. *Blood, 125,* 3246–3252. doi: https://doi.org/10.1182/blood-2014-10-551507

[d]Riggiero, A., Rizzo, D., Amato, M. & Riccardi, R. (2016). Management of hyperleukocytosis. *Current Treatment Options in Oncology, 17*(7), 1–10. https://doi.org/ 10.1007/s11864-015-0387-8

[e]Lustberg, M. (2012). Management of neutropenia in cancer patients. *Advances in Hematology and Oncology.* https://www.ncbi.nlm.nih.gov/pmc/articles/PMC4059501/

[f]Al-Qurainy, R. (2016). Metastatic spinal cord compression: Diagnosis and management. *BMJ, 353.* doi: https://doi.org/10.1136/bmj.i2539

[g]Bodtke, S. & Ligon, K. (2016). *Hospice and palliative medicine handbook: A clinical guide.* http://www.hpmhandbook.com/

[h]Borooah, B. (2018). Oncologic emergencies: A review. *International Journal of Research in Medical Sciences, 6*(5), 1484–1490. http://dx.doi.org/10.18203/2320-6012.ijrms20181492

[i]Canadian Cancer Society. (2018). *Septic shock.* http://www.cancer.ca/en/cancer-information/diagnosis-and-treatment/managing-side-effects/septic-shock/?region=sk

[j]Martin, L., Cheek, D.J., & Morris, S. E. (2014). Shock, multiple organ dysfunction syndrome, and burns in adults. In K.L. McCance, S.E. Huether, V.L. Brashers, & N.S. Rote (Eds.), *Pathophysiology: The biologic basis for diseases in adults and children* (pp. 1669–1698). Elsevier Mosby.

APPENDIX C-8: TUMOR STAGING

PRIMARY TUMOR (T)	REGIONAL LYMPH NODE (N)	DISTANT METASTASIS (M)
TX: Primary tumor cannot be measured.	**NX:** Cancer in nearby lymph nodes cannot be measured.	**MX:** Metastasis cannot be measured.
T0: No evidence of tumor	**N0:** No evidence of cancer in nearby lymph nodes	**M0:** No evidence that cancer has spread to other parts of the body
T1, T2, T3, T4: Refers to the size and/or extent of the main tumor. The higher the number after the T, the larger the tumor or the more it has grown into nearby tissues. T's may be further divided to provide more detail, such as T3a and T3b.	**N1, N2, N3:** Refers to the number and location of lymph nodes that contain cancer. The higher the number after the N, the more lymph nodes that contain cancer.	**M1:** There is evidence that the cancer has spread to other parts of the body.

Source: National Cancer Institute. (2015). *Cancer staging.* https://www.cancer.gov/about-cancer/diagnosis-staging/staging

APPENDIX C-9: ENCOURAGING SMOKING CESSATION

A Practical Guide to Help Your Patients Quit Using Tobacco

Tobacco dependence is a chronic condition driven by addiction to nicotine. No amount of tobacco use is safe, and treatment of tobacco use and dependence often requires multiple interventions and long-term support. Effective clinical interventions are available to help patients who use tobacco to quit.

This guide provides simple steps and suggested language that you can use to briefly (3 to 5 minutes) intervene with patients who use tobacco. These steps can be integrated into the routine clinical workflow and can be delivered by the entire clinical care team.

Key considerations for treating tobacco dependence:

▶ **Behavioral counseling** can benefit all patients.

▶ **Medication** can help patients quit and can be used with most patients, though special considerations may apply for some individuals. *See page 3.*

▶ **Combining behavioral counseling and medication** is more effective than either treatment alone.

▶ **Follow-up** is key to monitoring patients for treatment adherence, side effects, and efficacy, along with providing support and continued assistance.

Overview: Tobacco Cessation Brief Clinical Intervention

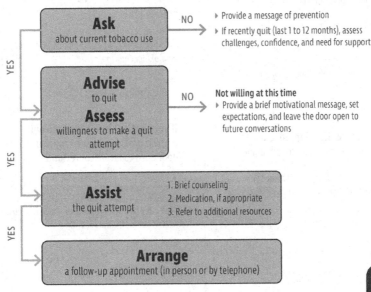

Ask about current tobacco use — NO →
▶ Provide a message of prevention
▶ If recently quit (last 1 to 12 months), assess challenges, confidence, and need for support

Advise to quit / **Assess** willingness to make a quit attempt — NO →
Not willing at this time
▶ Provide a brief motivational message, set expectations, and leave the door open to future conversations

Assist the quit attempt
1. Brief counseling
2. Medication, if appropriate
3. Refer to additional resources

Arrange a follow-up appointment (in person or by telephone)

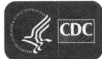

1

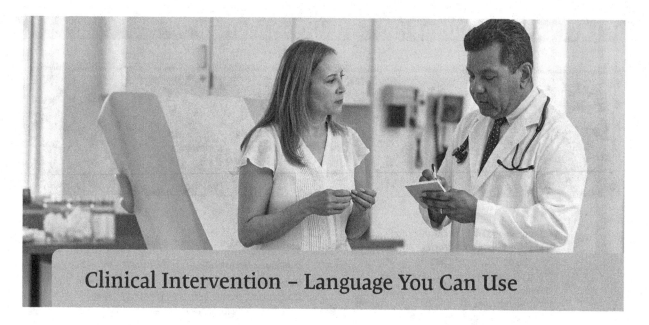

Clinical Intervention – Language You Can Use

Ask

Ask every patient about tobacco use at every visit.

"Do you use tobacco products, for example cigarettes or e-cigarettes?"

If your patient has recently quit (in the last 1 to 12 months), congratulate them and assess challenges, confidence, and need for support.

"The first few weeks after quitting can be hard. Have you felt the urge to use tobacco?"

"You are doing a great job. This is such an important step to take. Is there anything I can do to support you?"

If your patient has recently relapsed, provide encouragement and support to try to quit again.

"Quitting can be hard. It can often take someone several tries to quit successfully. Would you like to try again?"

Advise + Assess

Advise your patient to quit using tobacco, and assess their willingness to quit.

A clinician's advice to quit is an important motivator for patients. Using nonjudgmental language, deliver a message that is clear, strong, and personalized.

"Quitting [smoking, chewing, etc.] is the most important thing you can do for your health. As someone who cares about you and your health, I'd like to help you quit."

"I'd like to hear your thoughts about quitting [smoking, chewing, etc.]."

"Would you be willing to quit in the next 30 days?"

If your patient is not ready to quit, provide a brief motivational message, set expectations, and leave the door open to future conversation.

"I feel strongly about tobacco use and its effect on your health. I understand that quitting can be hard, but I am here to support you. I will ask you about it again the next time I see you."

Assist

If your patient is ready to make a quit attempt, assist with counseling, medications (if appropriate), and resources for support.

Provide and document brief tobacco cessation counseling. (1-3 minutes; 3-10 minutes)

- ▶ Set a quit date within 30 days
- ▶ Review past quit attempts, including counseling and medication used

- ▶ Discuss potential withdrawal symptoms and coping strategies — *see table on page 4*
- ▶ Discuss potential triggers and coping strategies — *see table on page 4*

Discuss, prescribe, and document tobacco cessation medication(s) unless medically contraindicated.

Populations for which there is insufficient evidence for the effectiveness of cessation medications include pregnant women (unless with medical clearance and patient consent); adolescents; people who smoke ≤5 cigarettes a day; and people who use tobacco products other than cigarettes, including smokeless tobacco and e-cigarettes.

- ▶ Nicotine replacement therapy (NRT) — patch, gum, lozenge, inhaler, and nasal spray
- ▶ Bupropion
- ▶ Varenicline

- ▶ Medication combinations: combining long-acting NRT (i.e., patch) with short-acting NRT (e.g., lozenge) increases the chances of quitting compared with using a single form of NRT

Make a referral to additional in-depth and free cessation help.

- ▶ State tobacco quitline (1-800-QUIT-NOW; 1-855-DÉJELO-YA)
- ▶ Tobacco cessation program based in the community, clinic, or healthcare system

- ▶ Web support: CDC.gov/quit; Smokefree.gov; becomeanex.org
- ▶ Text support: Smokefree.gov/SmokefreeTXT
- ▶ App support: Smokefree.gov/tools-tips/apps/quitstart

Arrange

Arrange follow-up with patients who are making a quit attempt.

Follow up either in person or by telephone within a week of the patient's quit date. A second follow-up is recommended within the first month.

"Before you leave today, we are going to schedule a follow-up appointment close to your quit date. We will check in to see how your quit attempt is going, ask if you have any questions, and see if there are ways we can support your quit attempt."

"Please feel free to contact us at any point. We are here to help and support you."

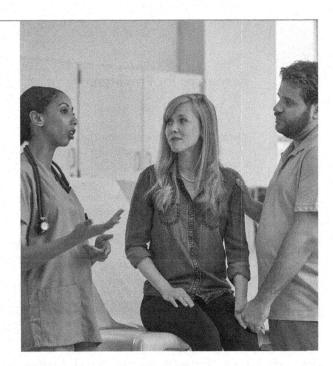

Withdrawal Symptoms and Coping Strategies

ANXIETY AND IRRITABILITY

▸ Exercise; even a 5-minute walk can help
▸ Contact a friend for support
▸ Take a few slow, deep breaths
▸ Chew sugar-free gum

INSOMNIA OR SLEEP PROBLEMS

▸ Avoid caffeine in the late afternoon and evening
▸ Exercise
▸ Go to sleep and wake up on a regular, consistent schedule

RESTLESSNESS

▸ Exercise
▸ Focus on an existing hobby, or try something new like cooking, drawing, or hiking
▸ Clean the house, garage, basement, or attic

HUNGER

▸ Eat plenty of fruits and vegetables
▸ Exercise regularly
▸ Avoid high-calorie foods and beverages
▸ Carry sugar-free gum or toothpicks
▸ Drink more water

Triggers and Coping Strategies

SITUATIONS

▸ Avoid people who use tobacco, or ask them not to use tobacco around you
▸ Establish friendships with people who don't use tobacco
▸ Avoid smoke breaks and other social situations where you use tobacco
▸ Avoid other situations where you usually use tobacco

THINGS

▸ Get rid of cigarettes, matches, lighters, ashtrays, and any other objects that are cues or triggers for smoking or using other tobacco products
▸ Avoid alcohol (at least for the first month) as it may trigger a desire to smoke
▸ Develop new ways to manage stress, such as going for a walk

PLACES

▸ Avoid places where you usually buy tobacco products
▸ Avoid locations where you usually use tobacco
▸ Take a different route to work or school

Resources for Providers

▸ CDC's Office on Smoking and Health — CDC.gov/TobaccoHCP
▸ National Cancer Institute: Help Others Quit (Smokefree.gov/help-others-quit/health-professionals)
▸ Million Hearts (available at millionhearts.hhs.gov)
  - Tobacco Cessation Protocol
  - Tobacco Cessation Clinical Action Guide
  - Tobacco Cessation Change Package

▸ Treating Tobacco Use and Dependence, Clinical Practice Guideline: 2008 Update (available at www.ahrq.gov)
▸ U.S. Preventive Services Task Force (USPSTF) Tobacco Cessation Recommendations (available at www.uspreventiveservicestaskforce.org)

Adapted from:
▸ Million Hearts Protocol for Identifying and Treating Patients Who Use Tobacco (https://millionhearts.hhs.gov/files/Tobacco-Cessation-Protocol.pdf)
▸ New York City Department of Health and Mental Hygiene Quit Smoking Coaching Guide (https://www1.nyc.gov/assets/doh/downloads/pdf/csi/smoke-quit-smoking-coaching-guide.pdf)

4

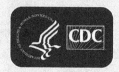

Source: Centers for Disease Control and Prevention. (2022). *Clinical cessation tools.* https://www.cdc.gov/tobacco/patient-care/clinical-tools/index.html

APPENDIX D

PHARMACOLOGICAL INTERVENTIONS FOR SYMPTOM MANAGEMENT IN ADVANCED DISEASE

APPENDIX D-1: PHARMACOLOGICAL INTERVENTIONS FOR SYMPTOM MANAGEMENT IN ADVANCED DISEASE

PHARMACOLOGICAL INTERVENTIONS		
MEDICATION	**DOSE/FREQUENCY (ADULTS ONLY)**	**COST[a]**
ANTACIDS		
Calcium carbonate (Maalox, Mylanta, Rolaids, Tums)	For treatment of dyspepsia: 750–3,000 mg PO prn. Maximum of 7,500 mg per 24 hours For treatment of chronic hypocalcemia: 1–2 g PO in divided doses (BID or TID)	649 mg tablet: 1.6¢ per tablet $16.71 for 1,000 tablets
Aluminum hydroxide (AlternaGEL, Amphojel, Nephrox)	For use as an antacid: 640 mg PO 5–6 times per day. Maximum of 3,840 mg per 24 hours For prevention of gastrointestinal bleeding: 1,920–3,840 mg PO q 1–2 hours prn	200 mg/5 mL: 11¢ per mL $322.64 for 3,000 mL
Simethicone (Mylicon)	For treatment of flatulence: 40–360 mg PO QID prn Maximum of 500 mg/24 hours	125 mg capsule: 60¢ per capsule $11.36 for 20 capsules
APPETITE STIMULANTS		
Megestrol (Megace)	For the treatment of cancer-related cachexia: 40 mg/mL oral suspension: 400–800 mg PO daily 125 mg/mL suspension: 625 mg PO daily	40 mg/mL oral suspension: 11¢ per mL $33.00 for 300 mL 625 mg/5 mL oral suspension $1.56 per mL $234.00 for 150 mL
ANTICHOLINERGIC AGENTS		
Atropine eye drops 1% (Isopto Atropine)	For treating end-of-life secretions: 1–2 drops sublingually q 8 hours prn For treating dysrhythmias (bradycardia): Initiate at 0.5–1 mg IV q 3–5 min prn to a maximum total dose of 3 mg per total dose	$17.68 per 5 mL of 1% solution $3.5 per mL
Glycopyrrolate (Robinul)	For treating end-of-life secretions: Initiate at 1 mg PO BID or TID prn. If necessary, may increase to 2 mg PO BID or TID. Maximum of 8 mg per day or 0.1–0.2 mg SQ q 4–8 hours prn. Maximum of 0.8 mg per day	2 mg tablets: $1.7 per tablet $106.16 for 60 tablets 0.2 mg/mL injectable solution: $5.10 per mL
Hyoscyamine (Levsin)	For treating end-of-life secretions: 0.4–0.6 mg SQ q 4 hours prn	0.5 mg/mL injectable solution: $51.74 per mL $258.70 for 5 mL

(continued)

APPENDIX D-1: PHARMACOLOGICAL INTERVENTIONS FOR SYMPTOM MANAGEMENT IN ADVANCED DISEASE (*CONTINUED*)

PHARMACOLOGICAL INTERVENTIONS		
MEDICATION	**DOSE/FREQUENCY (ADULTS ONLY)**	**COST**[a]
Scopolamine (Anti-muscarinic) (Transderm Scop, Scopace, Maldemar)	For treating end-of-life secretions: 1 mg patch q 72 hours	1 mg over 3 days patch: $8.43 per patch
ANTIDEPRESSANTS		
Tricyclic antidepressants (Generally, not first-line treatment for depression)	Examples of drugs in class: *Amitriptyline* (Elavil) <u>For depression or management of neuropathic pain:</u> Initiate at 25 to 50 mg PO at hs daily. If necessary, increase dose gradually, in increments of 25 mg every 5–7 days to a maximum of 100–200 mg per day (may divide doses). Full effect in 3–4 weeks. Decrease dose or discontinue if anticholinergic or sedative effects are not tolerated. *Doxepin* (Silenor) <u>For treatment of depression or anxiety:</u> Initiate at 25 mg daily. If necessary, increase dose gradually, in increments of 25 mg, every 5–7 days to a maximum of 200 mg per day. If daily dose exceeds 150 mg, divide dose and administer q 12 hours rather than daily. If prescribed as a single daily dose, this medication should be given at bedtime due its sedating effect. <u>For treatment of insomnia:</u> Initiate a single dose of 3 mg within 30 minutes of bedtime. If necessary, dose may be increased to 6 mg within 30 minutes of bedtime. *Imipramine* (Tofranil) <u>For treatment of major depression:</u> Initiate at 75 mg PO daily at hs. If necessary, increase dose gradually in increments of 25 mg every 5–7 days to a maximum of 200 mg per day (may divide doses). Full effect in 1–4 weeks. Decrease dose or discontinue if anticholinergic or sedative effects are not tolerated. For geriatric patients, initiate at 30–40 mg PO at hs and titrate, if needed, to a maximum dose of 100 mg per day. *Nortriptyline* (Allegron) <u>For depression or management of neuropathic pain:</u> Initiate at 25 mg PO every 6–8 hours daily. If necessary, increase dose gradually in increments of 25 mg every 5–7 days to a maximum of 150 mg (may divide doses). Full effect in 3–4 weeks. Decrease dose or discontinue if anticholinergic or sedative effects are not tolerated.	Examples of drugs in class: Amitriptyline 25 mg tablet: 15¢ per tablet $26.52 for 180 tablets Doxepin 25 mg tablet: 77¢ per tablet $22.99 for 30 tablets Doxepin 10 mg/mL oral solution: 23¢ per mL $27.62 for 120 mL $27.76 for 180 capsules Imipramine 25 mg tablets: 12.7¢ per tablet $22.68 for 180 tablets Nortriptyline 25 mg capsule: 15¢ per capsule $27.76 for 180 capsules

(continued)

APPENDIX D-1: PHARMACOLOGICAL INTERVENTIONS FOR SYMPTOM MANAGEMENT IN ADVANCED DISEASE (*CONTINUED*)

MEDICATION	DOSE/FREQUENCY (ADULTS ONLY)	COST[a]
PHARMACOLOGICAL INTERVENTIONS		
Selective serotonin reuptake inhibitors	Examples of drugs in class: *Citalopram* (Celexa) <u>For treatment of depression:</u> Initiate at 20 mg PO daily. If necessary, may increase daily dose to 40 mg after 1 week. Full effect may require 4 or more weeks of treatment. *Escitalopram* (Lexapro) <u>For treatment of depression:</u> Initiate at 10 mg PO daily. If necessary, may increase daily dose to 20 mg PO daily after 1 week. *Fluoxetine* (Prozac) <u>For treatment of depression:</u> Initiate at 20 mg PO daily. If necessary, may increase in increments of 10 mg every few weeks to a maximum daily dose of 80 mg per day. Full effect may require 4 or more weeks of treatment. *Paroxetine* (Paxil) <u>For treatment of depression:</u> Initiate at 20 mg PO in the a.m. If necessary, may increase daily dose by 10 mg weekly to a maximum of 40 mg per day. *Sertraline* (Zoloft) <u>For treatment of depression:</u> Initiate at 25 mg PO daily. If necessary, increase dose gradually by 25 mg at increments of no less than 7 days to a maximum of 150 mg per day (may divide doses). Partial mitigation of symptoms may be noted in 1 week of initiation of the medication. Full effect may require up to 6 weeks of treatment.	Examples of drugs in class: Citalopram 20 mg tablets: 7¢ per tablet $12.17 for 180 tablets Escitalopram 10 mg tablets: 12¢ per tablet $22.25 for 180 tablets Fluoxetine 10 mg tablets: 9¢ per tablet $16.36 for 180 tablets Paroxetine 20 mg tablets: 12¢ per tablet $21.60 for 180 tablets Sertraline 25 mg tablets: 12¢ per tablet $22.39 for 180 tablets
Serotonin–norepinephrine reuptake inhibitors	Examples of drugs in class: *Duloxetine* (Cymbalta) <u>For the treatment of major depression:</u> Initiate treatment at 20–30 mg PO BID. <u>For the treatment of musculoskeletal pain (including osteoarthritis):</u> Initiate treatment at 30 mg PO daily. If necessary, titrate to 60 mg PO daily after 1 week.	Examples of drugs in class: Duloxetine 20 mg tablets: 43¢ per tablet $77.83 for 180 tablets

(*continued*)

APPENDIX D-1: PHARMACOLOGICAL INTERVENTIONS FOR SYMPTOM MANAGEMENT IN ADVANCED DISEASE (*CONTINUED*)

MEDICATION	DOSE/FREQUENCY (ADULTS ONLY)	COST[a]
	Venlafaxine (Effexor) For treatment of depression, generalized anxiety disorder, panic disorder, fibromyalgia, or management of neuropathic pain: Initiate at 37.5 mg daily. If necessary, increase to 75 mg after 4–7 days. Titration may continue, if needed, in increments of 75 mg every 4–7 days to a maximum of 225 mg per day. Titrate cautiously as full effect of this medication may require 4–6 weeks of treatment.	Venlafaxine 37.5 mg tablets: 24¢ per tablet $43.39 for 180 tablets
Atypical antidepressants	Examples of drugs in class: *Trazodone* (Molipaxin) For the treatment of major depressive disorder: Initiate at 75–150 mg PO daily in divided doses. If necessary, may increase by 50 mg every 3–4 days to a maximum of 400 mg per day. Full effect may take 4–6 weeks. For treatment of insomnia: 25 to 50 mg PO at bedtime. *Mirtazapine* (Remeron) For the treatment of major depression: 15 mg PO daily at bedtime. If necessary, may gradually titrate every 1–3 weeks to a maximum of 45 mg per day. For the treatment of intractable pruritus: 15 to 30 mg PO daily *Bupropion* (Wellbutrin) For the treatment of major depression: Initiate at 100 mg PO twice daily. After 3 days and if necessary, may increase dose to 100 mg PO three times daily. No single dose should exceed 150 mg. Full effect may take up to 4 weeks. For the treatment of neuropathic pain: 150–300 mg PO daily in divided doses. Most patients experienced pain reduction within 2 weeks.	Examples of drugs in class: Trazodone 50 mg tablets: 9¢ per tablet $16.26 for 180 tablets Mirtazapine 15 mg tablets: 15¢ per tablet $27.30 for 180 tablets Bupropion 100 mg tablets: 20¢ per tablet $36.99 for 180 tablets
ANTIDIARRHEALS		
Bismuth subsalicylate (Pepto-Bismol)	For the treatment of acute diarrhea: 1–2 chewable tablets (262 mg) hourly *or* 30 mL of oral liquid (262 mg/15 mL) hourly up to a maximum of 4,200 mg	Oral liquid: 30¢ per ounce $4 for 12 ounces Oral chewable tablets: 19¢ per tablet $9 for 48 tablets

(continued)

APPENDIX D-1: PHARMACOLOGICAL INTERVENTIONS FOR SYMPTOM MANAGEMENT IN ADVANCED DISEASE (*CONTINUED*)

PHARMACOLOGICAL INTERVENTIONS		
MEDICATION	**DOSE/FREQUENCY (ADULTS ONLY)**	**COST**ᵃ
Diphenoxylate with atropine (Lomotil)	For the treatment of diarrhea: 2.5–5 mg PO BID to QID prn Maximum dose is 8 tablets per 24-hour period Decrease dose or discontinue use when symptoms subside. Discontinue use after 10 days if no improvement.	2.5 mg tablets: 26¢ per tablet $32 for 120 tablets
Loperamide (Imodium)	For the treatment of diarrhea: 4 mg PO x1, then 2 mg PO after each loose stool. Maximum of 16 mg per day	2 mg capsules: 20¢ per capsule $24.00 for 120 capsules
Octreotide (Sandostatin, Sandostatin LAR Depot)	For carcinoid tumor symptoms: 100–600 mcg per day SQ/IV divided BID to QID Maximum of 500 mg per dose. Maximum of 1,500 mg per day. Titrate dose based on patient's response For the treatment of secretory diarrhea: Initiate at 50 mcg SQ/IV BID to TID. If necessary, may increase by 100 mcg per dose q 48 hours. Maximum 500 mcg per dose. Maximum of 1,500 mcg per day Titrate dose based on patient's response.	Injectable solution (50 mcg/ml): $1.7 per mL $156.00 for 90 vials, 1 mL each Injectable solution (200 mcg/mL): $35 per mL $634.00 for 18 vials, 5 mL each
ANTIEMETICS		
Octreotide (Sandostatin, Sandostatin LAR Depot)	For the treatment of nausea and vomiting associated with bowel obstruction: 100–400 mcg SQ every 8 hours	$4.20 per mL (100 mcg/mL) $42.99 for 10 mL (100 mcg/mL)
Prokinetic agents	*Metoclopramide* (Reglan) For the treatment of chemotherapy-induced nausea and vomiting: 10–20 mg PO/SQ/IV every 4–6 hours up to 40 mg	4¢ per 5 mg tablet 4¢ per 10 mg tablet
Selective 5HT3 receptor antagonists	*Ondansetron* (Zofran) For preventing chemotherapy or radiation-induced nausea and vomiting: 4–8 mg PO/SQ/IV every 8 hours on day 1 of chemotherapy; 16–24 mg PO once, or 8–16 mg IV once (maximum dose of 16 mg).	41¢ per 4 mg tablet 25¢ per 8 mg tablet For ODT: 41¢ per 4 mg tablet For ODT: 49¢ per 8 mg tablet
Substance P antagonists (NK1 receptor antagonists)	*Aprepitant* (Emend) For the treatment of chemotherapy or radiation-induced nausea and vomiting: 125 mg PO once on day 1 of chemotherapy, then 80 mg PO every morning on days 2–3. Start 1 hour prior to chemotherapy on day 1. Give with a corticosteroid and a 5-HT3 antagonist. May be used in combination with ondansetron.	$89.32 per 40 mg tablet

(continued)

APPENDIX D-1: PHARMACOLOGICAL INTERVENTIONS FOR SYMPTOM MANAGEMENT IN ADVANCED DISEASE (*CONTINUED*)

PHARMACOLOGICAL INTERVENTIONS		
MEDICATION	**DOSE/FREQUENCY (ADULTS ONLY)**	**COST**[a]
ANTIEPILEPTIC MEDICATIONS		
Levetiracetam (Keppra)	<u>For treatment of partial-onset seizures:</u> 500–1500 mg PO/IV q 12 hours	100 mg/mL solution: 7¢ per mL $21.27 for 300 mL 250 mg tablet: 12¢ per tablet $21.84 for 180 tablets
Valproic acid (Depakote)	<u>For treatment of partial seizures, complex:</u> 30–60 mg/kg per day IV in divided doses, BID to TID <u>For treatment of absence seizures, simple and complex:</u> 30–60 mg/kg per day IV in divided doses, BID to TID	250 mg capsule: 20¢ per capsule $38.86 for 180 capsules 250 mg/5 mL solution: 4¢ per mL $48.71 for 1,200 mL
Benzodiazepines	Examples of drugs in class: *Lorazepam* (Ativan) <u>For treatment of status epilepticus:</u> 4 mg IV ×1; may repeat ×1 after 10–15 min *Diazepam* (Valium) <u>For treatment of seizure disorder (adjunct):</u> 2–10 mg PO BID to QID <u>For treatment of status epilepticus:</u> 5–10 mg IV q 5–10 min prn Max: 30 mg <u>For treatment of alcohol withdrawal:</u> 10 mg PO q 6–8 hours during the first 24 hours, then reduce to 5 mg PO q 6–8 hours prn	Examples of drugs in class: <u>Lorazepam</u> 1 mg tablet: 9¢ per tablet $11.43 or f120 tablets <u>Diazepam</u> 2 mg tablet: 8¢ per tablet $9.68 for 120 tablets
Ethosuximide (Emeside, Zarontin)	<u>For treatment of absence seizures:</u> 250–750 mg PO BID	250 mg capsule: $1.59 per capsule $159 for 100 capsules
Tiagabine (Gabitril)	<u>For treatment of partial seizures (adjunct):</u> 32–56 mg per day PO in divided doses BID to QID	5 mg tablet: $5.17 per tablet $155.13 for 30 tablets
Zonisamide (Zonegran)	<u>For treatment of partial seizures:</u> 100–600 mg per day PO in divided daily BID	25 mg capsule: 18¢ per capsule $32.95 for 180 capsules

(continued)

APPENDIX D-1: PHARMACOLOGICAL INTERVENTIONS FOR SYMPTOM MANAGEMENT IN ADVANCED DISEASE (*CONTINUED*)

PHARMACOLOGICAL INTERVENTIONS		
MEDICATION	**DOSE/FREQUENCY (ADULTS ONLY)**	**COST**[a]
ANTIHISTAMINIC AGENTS		
Diphenhydramine (Benadryl, Nytol) *Avoid use in those 65 and older*	For treatment of allergic reactions: 25–50 mg PO q 6–8 hours; not to exceed 300 mg per 24 hours For treatment of insomnia: 25–50 mg PO 30 minutes before bedtime For treatment of nausea: Diphenhydramine 25–50 mg PO/SQ/IV every 6 hours prn For treatment of cough: 25–50 mg PO q 4 hours prn. Not to exceed 150 mg per day	25 mg tablet: 96¢ per tablet 50 mg/mL IV solution: $1.1 per mL $27.77 for 25 mL
Cyclizine (Marezine, Valoid, Nausicalm)	For treatment of nausea: 50 mg PO every 4–6 hours prn Maximum of 200 mg daily	25 mg tablet: $2 per tablet
Meclizine (Antivert, Dramamine)	For treatment of nausea: 25–50 mg PO daily For treatment of vertigo: 25–100 mg daily, in divided doses Caution is advised for patients who have renal or hepatic disease.	12.5 mg tablet: 64¢ per tablet
ANTISPASMODIC AGENTS		
Cyclobenzaprine (Flexeril)	For treatment of muscle spasms: Immediate-release form: Initiate at 5–10 mg PO TID up to 3 weeks ER form: Initiate at 15 mg ER PO daily up to 3 weeks	5 mg immediate-release tablet: 7¢ per tablet $13.97 for 180 tablets
Onabotulinumtoxin A (Botox)	For treatment of muscle spasms: 1.25–7.5 units IM divided among affected muscles ×1	1 unit of powder for injection: $355.06 per unit

(*continued*)

APPENDIX D-1: PHARMACOLOGICAL INTERVENTIONS FOR SYMPTOM MANAGEMENT IN ADVANCED DISEASE (*CONTINUED*)

PHARMACOLOGICAL INTERVENTIONS		
MEDICATION	**DOSE/FREQUENCY (ADULTS ONLY)**	**COST**[a]
ANXIOLYTICS **(SEE ALSO ANTIDEPRESSANTS AND BENZODIAZEPINES FOR TREATMENT OF ANXIETY)**		
Buspirone (Buspar)	<u>For treatment of anxiety:</u> Initiate at 7.5 mg PO BID. If necessary, may increase by 5 mg daily every 2–3 days to a maximum of 60 mg per day	5 mg tablets: 23¢ per tablet $13.89 for 60 tablets
BENZODIAZEPINES		
Lorazepam (Ativan)	<u>For the treatment of anxiety:</u> 2–6 mg per day PO/IM/IV in divided doses BID to TID Maximum of 10 mg per day Use cautiously in geriatric patients. If necessary to use in this population, initiate at 1–2 mg per day PO/IM/IV in divided doses. Frequently reassess need for continued treatment. When discontinuing, taper dose down gradually. <u>For the treatment of insomnia (short-term use only):</u> 2–4 mg PO at hs prn When discontinuing, taper dose down gradually. <u>For the management of acute alcohol withdrawal:</u> 2–4 mg PO/IM/IV hourly prn <u>For the treatment of chemotherapy-related nausea and</u> <u>vomiting:</u> 0.5–2 mg PO/SQ/IV every 8–12 hours	0.5 mg tablet: 2¢ per tablet 2 mg/mL injectable solution: 90¢ per mL $22.66 for 25 mL
BETA-2 AGONISTS		
Short-acting beta-2 agonists	Examples of drugs in class: *Albuterol* (Proventil HFA and Proair HFA) <u>For the treatment of bronchospasm:</u> Immediate-release oral form: 2–4 mg PO TID–QID. Maximum of 32 mg per day ER oral form: 4–8 mg ER PO q 12 hours. Maximum of 32 mg per day ER Powder inhaler: 1–2 puffs (90 mcg per actuation) at onset of symptoms and q 4–6 hours as needed Use with or without spacer, as directed	<u>Albuterol</u> 2 mg oral tablet: $1 per tablet $91.00 for 90 tablets 4 mg oral tablets: 91¢ per tablet $55.00 for 60 tablets Inhalation aerosol: $44.00 per 90 mcg

(continued)

APPENDIX D-1: PHARMACOLOGICAL INTERVENTIONS FOR SYMPTOM MANAGEMENT IN ADVANCED DISEASE (*CONTINUED*)

	PHARMACOLOGICAL INTERVENTIONS	
MEDICATION	**DOSE/FREQUENCY (ADULTS ONLY)**	**COST**[a]
	Nebulized solution: 2.5–5 mg nebulized q 20 min × 3, then q 1–2 prn	Inhalation solution: $12.00 per 30 vials (2.5 mg/0.5 mL)
	Levalbuterol (Xopenex) <u>For the treatment of bronchospasm:</u> <u>Metered dose inhaler:</u> 1–2 puffs inhaled q 4–6 hours prn. Maximum of 12 puffs per day	Levalbuterol Inhalation aerosol: $57.00 per 1 inhaler (45 mcg/15 g)
	<u>Nebulized solution:</u> 0.63–1.25 mg nebulized TID prn	Inhalation solution: $74.00 per 60 vials (1.25/ 0.5 mL)
Long-acting beta-2 agonists	Examples of drugs in class: *Formoterol* (Symbicort) <u>For the treatment of COPD symptoms (maintenance):</u> 20 mcg nebulized q 12 hours. Maximum of 40 mcg per day	Formoterol Inhalation solution: $453.00 per 60 vials (20 mcg/2 mL)
	Salmeterol (Serevent) <u>For the treatment of bronchospasm (exercise-related):</u> 1 puff 30–60 min before exercise Maximum of 1 puff inhaled q 12 hours <u>For the treatment of COPD symptoms (maintenance):</u> 1 puff inhaled q 12 hours	Salmeterol $429 per diskus inhaler (60 blisters/50 mcg each)
Ultra-long-acting beta-agonists	Examples of drugs in class: *Indacaterol* (Arcapta Neohaler; not available in the United States) <u>For the treatment of COPD symptoms (maintenance):</u> 1 dose (75 mcg) daily via the Neohaler When initiating indacaterol therapy, discontinue use of short-acting beta-2 agonist medications. Avoid simultaneous use with β-adrenergic blocking agents. Use with extreme caution in those taking tricyclic antidepressants or MAO inhibitors.	Indacaterol, 75 mcg capsules: $9 per capsule $275 for 30 capsules
	Olodaterol (Striverdi, Respimat) <u>For the treatment of COPD symptoms (maintenance):</u> 2 inhalations (5 mcg) once a day	Olodaterol 2.5 mcg inhaler $253 per 4 g
	Vilanterol (Breo Ellipta, Relvar Ellipta) <u>For the treatment of COPD symptoms (maintenance):</u> Administered in combination with fluticasone Inhale 1 dose (fluticasone 100 mcg–vilanterol 25 mcg per dose powder) daily	Vilanterol 25 mcg/fluticasone 100 mcg powder for inhalation: $390.00 per 60 blisters

(*continued*)

APPENDIX D-1: PHARMACOLOGICAL INTERVENTIONS FOR SYMPTOM MANAGEMENT IN ADVANCED DISEASE (*CONTINUED*)

PHARMACOLOGICAL INTERVENTIONS		
MEDICATION	**DOSE/FREQUENCY (ADULTS ONLY)**	**COST**[a]
	For the treatment of asthma (maintenance): Administered in combination with fluticasone Inhale 1 dose (fluticasone 200 mcg–vilanterol 25 mcg per dose powder) daily	Vilanterol 25 mcg/fluticasone 200 mcg powder for inhalation: $390.00 per 60 blisters
BETA-BLOCKERS		
Atenolol (Tenormin)	For the treatment of angina: Initiate at 50 mg PO daily. If necessary, may gradually increase to a maximum daily dose of 200 mg PO daily. If discontinuing, taper dose down gradually.	50 mg tablet: 13¢ per tablet $12 for 90 tablets
Metoprolol succinate (Lopressor, Toprol)	For the treatment of angina: Initiate at 100 mg PO daily. If necessary, may gradually increase (weekly) to a maximum daily dose of 400 mg PO daily. Do not crush or chew tablet. If converting to an immediate-release preparation, use same total daily dose. For risk reduction in patients with heart failure: For NYHA Class II: Initiate at 25 mg PO daily. For NYHA Class III–IV., Initiate at 12.5 mg PO daily May gradually increase to a maximum daily dose of 200 mg PO daily. Do not crush or chew tablet.	25 mg tablet: 22¢ per tablet $20 for 90 tablets 100 mg tablets: 26¢ per tablet $24 for 90 tablets
Propranolol (Inderal)	For the treatment of angina: Initiate at 80 mg PO daily in divided doses given BID to QID. If necessary, may gradually increase (q 3–7 days) to a maximum daily dose of 328 mg PO daily. Alternate dosing: Initiate at 80 mg ER PO dosing. If necessary, may gradually increase (q 3–7 days). If discontinuing, taper dose down gradually.	Immediate release 80 mg tablets: 30¢ per tablet $18 for 60 tablets ER 80 mg tablets: 37¢ per tablet $34 for 90 tablets
BISPHOSPHONATES		
Zoledronic acid (Zometa, Reclast)	For bone metastasis: 4 mg IV q 3–4 weeks	4 mg/5 mL: $8.67 per mL $43.00 for 5 mL
Pamidronate (Aredia)	For bone metastasis: 90 mg IV × 1 q 3–4 weeks	3mg/mL: $2.67 per mL $26.70 for 10 mL

(continued)

APPENDIX D-1: PHARMACOLOGICAL INTERVENTIONS FOR SYMPTOM MANAGEMENT IN ADVANCED DISEASE (*CONTINUED*)

PHARMACOLOGICAL INTERVENTIONS		
MEDICATION	**DOSE/FREQUENCY (ADULTS ONLY)**	**COST**ᵃ
Calcium channel blockers		
Diltiazem (Cardizem)	For the treatment of angina: Initiate at 180–360 mg PO daily in divided doses given q 6–8 hours. If necessary, may gradually increase (q 1–2 days) to a maximum daily dose of 360 mg PO daily. If using ER preparation: Initiate at 120–180 mg daily. Titrate over 7–14 days to a maximum daily dose of 540 mg per day. Do not chew or crush. May open capsule. For treatment of muscle spasms: 180–360 mg per day PO in divided doses q 6–8 hours	Immediate release 90 mg tablet: 31¢ per tablet $56 for 180 tablets ER 90 mg tablet: 77¢ per tablet $70 for 90 tablets
CANNABINOIDS		
Dronabinol (Marinol)	For the treatment of nausea: 5–10 mg PO every 3–6 hours For the treatment of AIDS-related anorexia: 2.5–10 mg PO BID. Maximum of 20 mg per day Administer 1 hour before lunch and dinner. When discontinuing, gradually taper dose down for high-dose or prolonged use.	2.5 mg capsule: $16 per capsule $982.65 for 60 capsules
Nabilone (Cesamet)	For the treatment of nausea: 1–2 mg PO BID	1 mg capsule: $285 per capsule $8563.40 for 30 capsules
CORTICOSTEROIDS		
Dexamethasone (Decadron, Dexasone)	For reducing inflammation: 4–8 mg PO daily For the prevention of chemotherapy-related nausea and vomiting: Highly emetogenic parenteral chemotherapy: 12 mg PO ×1 on day 1, then 8 mg PO daily on days 2–4 Used as a component of a multidrug regimen. If given with olanzapine and palonosetron, administer only on day 1 of chemotherapy. Moderately emetogenic parenteral chemotherapy: 12 mg PO ×1 on day 1, then 8 mg PO daily on days 2–3 Used as a part of multidrug regimen. If given with olanzapine and palonosetron, administer only on day 1 of chemotherapy. Low-emetogenic parenteral chemotherapy: 8–12 mg PO ×1 on day 1 Used as a part of multidrug regimen	0.5 mg tablet: 9¢ per tablet $17.11 for 180 tablets

(*continued*)

APPENDIX D-1: PHARMACOLOGICAL INTERVENTIONS FOR SYMPTOM MANAGEMENT IN ADVANCED DISEASE (*CONTINUED*)

	PHARMACOLOGICAL INTERVENTIONS	
MEDICATION	**DOSE/FREQUENCY (ADULTS ONLY)**	**COST**[a]
Prednisone (Deltasone)	For reducing inflammation: 5–60 mg PO daily For the management of acute asthma: 40–60 mg per day PO in divided doses daily BID for 3–10 days Should be taken with food For the management of severe, persistent asthma: 7.5–60 mg per day PO in divided doses daily Should be taken with food For the management of acute gout: 0.5 mg/kg per day PO for 5–10 days Should be taken with food For the management of COPD exacerbation: 40 mg PO daily for 5 days Should be take	1 mg tablet 8¢ per tablet $15.99 for 180 tablets
Prednisolone (Flo-pred)	For reducing inflammation: 5–60 mg PO daily For management of aspiration pneumonia: 5–60 mg PO daily For management of acute asthma: 40–60 mg PO daily in two divided doses for 5–10 days For the management of asthma (maintenance): 7.5–60 mg PO daily or QOD For treatment of hypercalcemia of malignancy: 5–60 mg PO daily as single dose or in divided doses	15 mg/5 mL sol: 12¢ per mL $9.15 for 75 mL
Methylprednisolone (Medrol)	For reducing inflammation: 4–48 mg per day PO in divided doses daily QID Should be taken with food For management of acute asthma: 40–60 mg per day PO divided daily BID × 3–10 days Should be taken with food For the management of severe, persistent asthma: 7.5–60 mg PO daily QID Should be taken with food When discontinuing, taper dose down gradually if high dose or used for long-term treatment.	40 mg (powder for injection): 12¢ per mg $4.86 for 40 mg

(continued)

APPENDIX D-1: PHARMACOLOGICAL INTERVENTIONS FOR SYMPTOM MANAGEMENT IN ADVANCED DISEASE (*CONTINUED*)

PHARMACOLOGICAL INTERVENTIONS		
MEDICATION	**DOSE/FREQUENCY (ADULTS ONLY)**	**COST**ᵃ
Diuretics		
Furosemide (Lasix)	For treatment of edema: *Oral dosing:* Initiate at 20–80 mg PO × 1 dose. If necessary, increase dose in 20–40 mg increments q 6–8 hours up to a maximum of 600 mg per day. *Parenteral dosing:* Initiate at 20–40 mg IM/IV ×1 dose. If necessary, increase in increments of 20 mg q 2 hours	20 mg tablet: 6¢ per tablet $10.80 for 180 tablets 10 mg/mL injectable solution: 15 (2 mL) vials: $15.00
Spironolactone (Aldactone)	For treatment of edema: Initiate at 25–50 mg per day PO daily or BID. If necessary, the dose may be titrated every 5 days up to a maximum of 200 mg per day. For treatment of heart failure with reduced ejection fraction (NYHA Class III–IV): 12.5–50 mg per day PO divided daily BID. If necessary, may increase dose every 2 weeks to a maximum of 50 mg per day Hold of potassium level is >5 mEq/L	25 mg tablets: 10¢ per tablet $18.76 for 180 tablets
DOPAMINE RECEPTOR ANTAGONISTS		
Haloperidol (Haldol)	For the treatment of nausea: 0.5–2 mg PO/SQ/IV every 4–6 hours For the treatment of psychosis: *Moderate symptoms:* Initiate at 0.5–2 mg PO BID to TID *Severe symptoms:* 3–5 mg PO BID to TID For treatment of acute agitation: Initiate at 0.5 mg PO q 1–4 hours prn. Increase dose gradually up to 10 mg PO q 1–4 hours. Maximum of 100 mg per day; this dose should be used only for severe/refractory symptoms. When discontinuing after long-term use, taper dose to avoid symptoms of withdrawal. Discontinue use of this medication if WBC count decreases unexpectedly or if ANC <1,000. Not recommended for patients diagnosed with Lewy body dementia	0.5 mg tablet: 17¢ per tablet 5 mg/mL injectable solution: $19.66 per 10 mL

(continued)

APPENDIX D-1: PHARMACOLOGICAL INTERVENTIONS FOR SYMPTOM MANAGEMENT IN ADVANCED DISEASE (*CONTINUED*)

PHARMACOLOGICAL INTERVENTIONS		
MEDICATION	**DOSE/FREQUENCY (ADULTS ONLY)**	**COST**[a]
Prochlorperazine (Compazine)	For the treatment of nausea: 10–20 mg PO/SQ/IV every 6 hours or 25 mg rectally. Best for opioid-induced nausea	5 mg tablet: 14¢ per mL 10 mg tablet: 7¢ per tablet 5 mg/ml injectable solution: $10.13 per 10 mL
ERYTHROPOIESIS-STIMULATING AGENTS		
Epoetin alpha (Procrit)	For the treatment of anemia associated with CKD: Starting dose is 50–100 units/kg per dose SQ/IV 3 times per week. Dosage must be individualized based on patient's response. Goal of treatment is to reduce need for red blood cell transfusion. Treatment should be paused or dose reduced if Hgb reaches or exceeds 11 g/dL for patients on dialysis and 10g/dL for those not on dialysis. Iron supplementation should be considered. For the treatment of anemia associated with HIV: Starting dose is 100 units/kg per dose SQ/IV 3 times per week. Dosage must be individualized based on patient's response. Goal of treatment is to reduce need for red blood cell transfusion. If Hgb >12 g/dL, hold medication until Hgb <11 g/dL and then restart with a dose 25% lower than previous dose. Iron supplementation should be considered. For the treatment of anemia associated with chemotherapy: Starting dose is 40,000 units/kg per dose SQ/IV 3 times per week. Dosage must be individualized based on patient's response. Goal of treatment is to reduce need for red blood cell transfusion. If Hgb exceeds level to avoid red blood cell transfusion, pause therapy until Hgb drops and then restart with a dose 25% lower than previous dose. Iron supplementation should be considered. CAUTION: Use of this medication in patients who have cancer has been associated with tumor growth stimulation, blood clots, heart failure, and/or infarct.	Injectable solution: 10,000 units/mL (1 vial, 2 mL): $348.00

(continued)

APPENDIX D-1: PHARMACOLOGICAL INTERVENTIONS FOR SYMPTOM MANAGEMENT IN ADVANCED DISEASE (*CONTINUED*)

PHARMACOLOGICAL INTERVENTIONS		
MEDICATION	**DOSE/FREQUENCY (ADULTS ONLY)**	**COST**[a]
Darbepoetin alpha (Aranesp)	For the treatment of anemia associated with CKD: Starting dose is 0.45 mcg/kg per dose SQ/IV weekly. Dosage must be individualized based on patient's response. Goal of treatment is to reduce need for red blood cell transfusion. Treatment should be paused or dose reduced if Hgb reaches or exceeds 11 g/dL for patients on dialysis and 10 g/dL for those not on dialysis. For the treatment of anemia associated with chemotherapy: Starting dose is 2.25 mcg/kg per dose SQ weekly or 500 mcg SQ every 3 weeks. Dosage must be individualized based on patient's response. Goal of treatment is to reduce need for red blood cell transfusion. If Hgb exceeds level to avoid red blood cell transfusion, pause therapy until Hgb drops and then restart with a dose 40% lower than previous dose. Iron supplementation should be considered. CAUTION: Use of this medication in patients who have cancer has been associated with tumor growth stimulation, blood clots, heart failure, and/or infarct.	Injectable solution: 100 mcg/mL (1 carton, 4 vials): $3,168.00
LAXATIVES		
Bulk-forming	Examples of drugs in class: *Methylcellulose* (Citrucel) For the treatment of constipation: Tablets: Two tablets PO with 8 ounces of water up to a maximum of 6 tablets in a 24-hour period Powder: 30 mL of powder dissolved in 8 ounces of water up to three times in a 24-hour period Onset of action is 12–72 hours. *Polycarbophil* (FiberCon) For the treatment of constipation: Two tablets PO daily with 8 ounces of water. Maximum of 8 tabs PO daily Onset of action is 12–72 hours.	500 mg tablets: 6¢ per tablet $29.99 for 500 tablets 625 mg tablets: 20¢ per tablet $11.94 for 60 tablets

(*continued*)

APPENDIX D-1: PHARMACOLOGICAL INTERVENTIONS FOR SYMPTOM MANAGEMENT IN ADVANCED DISEASE (*CONTINUED*)

	PHARMACOLOGICAL INTERVENTIONS	
MEDICATION	**DOSE/FREQUENCY (ADULTS ONLY)**	**COST[a]**
	Psyllium (Metamucil) For the treatment of constipation: Capsule: Two capsules PO daily QID prn with 8 ounces of water. If necessary, may increase slowly up to five capsules in a 24-hour period Wafer: Two wafers PO prn with 8 ounces of water. If necessary, may increase slowly to two wafers BID, and then up to TID Powder: 3.4 g PO daily dissolved in 8 ounces of water or juice. If necessary, may increase to BID, and then up to TID Onset of action is 12–72 hours.	<u>0.52 g tablets:</u> 3¢ per tablet $5.70 for 170 tablets
Lubricant	Example of drug in class: *Mineral oil* <u>For the treatment of constipation:</u> Oral dosing: 15 mL PO q 8 hours up to 45 mL daily. Onset of action is typically 6–8 hours. Rectally: 1 bottle (133 mL) rectally—single dose Typically produces results within 5–15 minutes	<u>8-ounce bottle:</u> $7.99 per bottle <u>1 (133 mL) enema bottle:</u> $7 per bottle
Osmotic	Examples of drugs in class: *Lactulose* (Constulose) <u>For the treatment of constipation:</u> Initiate at 15–30 mL PO daily or BID. Maximum of 60 mL per day. May require up to 24–48 for effect. <u>For the treatment of hepatic encephalopathy:</u> Oral dosing: Initiate at 30–45 mL TID to QID. Adjust dose to produce 2–3 soft (not liquid) stools per day. For acute treatment, administer 30 mL q 1–2 hours until soft stools begin. Rectal dosing: Mix 300 mL of lactulose with 700 mL of water or 0.9% NaCl and administer as an enema. Enema should be retained for 30–60 min. Ensure adequate fluid intake when under treatment. Onset of action for oral dosing is 8–24 hours. Onset of action for enema is 1–2 hours.	<u>Oral syrup (10 g/15 mL):</u> 2¢ per mL $17 for 900 mL

APPENDIX D-1: PHARMACOLOGICAL INTERVENTIONS FOR SYMPTOM MANAGEMENT IN ADVANCED DISEASE (*CONTINUED*)

	PHARMACOLOGICAL INTERVENTIONS	
MEDICATION	**DOSE/FREQUENCY (ADULTS ONLY)**	**COST[a]**
	Magnesium hydroxide (Dulcolax, Milk of Magnesia) For the treatment of constipation: Oral suspension: 30 mL PO If necessary, may increase dose to 30 mL PO BID Onset of action is 30 minutes to 24 hours.	24% oral concentrate liquid: $13.62 per 100 mL
	Polyethylene glycol (MiraLax) For the treatment of constipation: Oral powder: 17 g dissolved in 4–8 ounces of liquid daily up to 3 days to produce bowel movement Onset of action is 24–72 hours.	17g per dose powder: $8.50 per 510 g bottle
Stimulant	Examples of drugs in class: *Bisacodyl* (Dulcolax) For the treatment of constipation: Oral dosing: 15 mg PO. If necessary, may increase to 30 mg PO daily. Do not use for longer than 1 week. Onset of action is 6–8 hours.	5 mg tablets: 30¢ per tablet
	Rectal administration: One, 10 mg suppository in a single daily dose Onset of action is 15–60 minutes.	10 mg supp: $2/supp $28.99/16 count
	Docusate (Colace) For the treatment of constipation: Initiate at 50 mg PO daily. If necessary, may slowly increase dose up to 150 mg PO BID Onset of action is 6–72 hours.	50 mg capsules: 60¢ per capsule $6 for 10 capsules
	Sennosides (Senokot) For the treatment of constipation: Initiate at 1 (8.6 mg) tablet PO at hs daily. If necessary, may increase to tablets PO at hs daily, up to 4 tablets PO BID Onset of action is 6–12 hours.	8.5 mg tablet: 24¢ per tablet $12 for 50 tablets
	NITRATES	
Nitroglycerin	For the treatment of acute angina (Nitrostat) Sublingual tab form: 0.3–0.6 mg SL q 5 min Max: Three doses within 15 min Translingual spray form (NitroMist): 1–2 actuations SL q 5 min prn Max: 3 actuations within 15 min ER form (Nitro-Dur): Initiate at 2.5–6.5 mg ER PO TID to QID to a maximum daily dose of 26 mg ER PO QID	2.5 mg tablet: 24¢ per tablet $44.00 for 180 tablets

(continued)

APPENDIX D-1: PHARMACOLOGICAL INTERVENTIONS FOR SYMPTOM MANAGEMENT IN ADVANCED DISEASE (*CONTINUED*)

PHARMACOLOGICAL INTERVENTIONS		
MEDICATION	**DOSE/FREQUENCY (ADULTS ONLY)**	**COST**[a]
PAMORA		
Methylnaltrexone (Relistor)	<u>For the treatment of opioid-induced constipation:</u> Chronic non-cancer pain patients: 450 mg POQ a.m. *or* 12 mg SQ daily Palliative care patients, dosed by weight: <38 kg: 0.15 mg/kg per dose SQ QOD prn; max: 1 dose per 24 hours 38–61 kg: 8 mg SQ QOD prn; max: 1 dose per 24 hours 62–114 kg: 12 mg SQ QOD prn; max: 1 dose per 24 hours >114 kg: 0.15 mg/kg per dose SQ QOD prn; max: 1 dose per 24 hours Dose adjustment is necessary in those with renal or hepatic disease.	• 12 mg/0.6 mL • $3,851.00 for 28 syringes, 0.6 mL each
Naldemedine (Symproic)	<u>For the treatment of opioid-induced constipation:</u> 0.2 mg PO daily Dose adjustment is necessary in those with renal or hepatic disease.	0.2 mg tablet: $13.80 per tablet $414.00 for 30 tablets
Naloxegol (Movantik)	<u>For the treatment of opioid-induced constipation:</u> 25 mg PO/NG q a.m. Administer 1 h before or 2 h after meal Dose adjustment is necessary in those with renal or hepatic disease.	12.5 mg tablet: $12.70 per tablet $383.00 for 30 tablets
PROMOTILITY AGENTS		
Bethanechol (Urecholine)	<u>For the treatment of urinary retention:</u> 25 mg PO QID	5 mg tablet: 81¢ per tablet $72.99 for 90 tablets
Metoclopramide (Reglan)	<u>To treat gastroparesis or GERD:</u> 10–15 mg PO/IM/IV QID; max: 60 mg per day; 12 weeks For elderly patients, start 5 mg PO/IM/IV QID	5 mg tablet: 26¢ per tablet $25.49 for 90 tablets
PSYCHOSTIMULANTS		
Methylphenidate (Concerta)	<u>For the treatment of narcolepsy:</u> Initiate at 5–10 mg PO BID If necessary, may increase by 5–10 mg a day every 7 days to a maximum of 60 mg. This medication is usually administered at 8 a.m. and noon. If the patient needs a third dose late in the afternoon, a dose equal to ½ the morning dose may be added. Last dose should be given before 6 p.m.	2.5 mg tablet: $4 per tablet $203.83 for 50 tablets 10 mg/5 mL oral solution: $384.59 for 300 mL

(continued)

APPENDIX D-1: PHARMACOLOGICAL INTERVENTIONS FOR SYMPTOM MANAGEMENT IN ADVANCED DISEASE (*CONTINUED*)

PHARMACOLOGICAL INTERVENTIONS		
MEDICATION	**DOSE/FREQUENCY (ADULTS ONLY)**	**COST[a]**
Modafinil (Provigil)	For the treatment of narcolepsy: Initiate at 200 mg POQ a.m. Begin with lower dose in geriatric patients. May be increased to 400 mg, but daily doses higher than 200 mg have not been found to be more effective than lower doses	100 mg oral tablet: $20 per tablet $616.99 per 30 tablets
RANK LIGAND INHIBITOR (OSTEOCLAST-TARGETED THERAPY)		
Denosumab (Prolia)	For bone metastasis: 120 mg SQ q 4 weeks	120 mg/1.7 mL: $1,535.38 per mL $2,610.15 for 1.7 mL
SELECTIVE 5-HT3 RECEPTOR ANTAGONISTS		
Ondansetron (Zofran)	For the prevention and treatment of chemotherapy-induced nausea and vomiting: 4–8 mg PO/SQ/IV q 8 hours on day 1 of chemotherapy 12–16 mg PO once or 8–16 IV once (max dose of 16 mg)	4 mg tablet: $3.43 per tablet $102.88 for 30 tablets 2 mg/mL injectable solution: 60¢ per mL $13.67 for 20 mL
VEGF/VEGFR INHIBITORS		
Bevacizumab (Alymsys, Avastin)	For glioblastoma multiforme: 10 mg/kg IV every 2 weeks	25 mg/mL: $210.38 per mL

[a]Cost of medications listed here is considered to be an estimate. Prices may vary according to location, supply, or other variables.

ANC, absolute neutrophil count; CKD, chronic kidney disease; COPD, chronic obstructive pulmonary disease; ER, extended release; GERD, gastroesophageal reflux disease; Hgb, hemoglobin; IV, intravenous; hs, at bedtime; NYHA, New York Heart Association; MAO, monoamine oxidase; ODT, orally disintegrating tablet; PAMORA, peripherally acting mu-opioid receptor antagonists; q, every; SQ, subcutaneous; VEGF, vascular endothelial growth factor; VEGFR, vascular endothelial growth factor receptor; WBC, white blood cell.

Sources: Belk, D. (2021). *The true cost of healthcare.* https://truecostofhealthcare.org; Bodtke, S., & Lingon, K. (2016). *Hospice and palliative medicine handbook: A clinical guide.* www.hpmhandbook.com; Chow, K., Cogan, D., & Mun, S. (2015). Nausea and vomiting. In B. R. Ferrell, N. Coyle, & J. A. Paice (Eds.), *Oxford textbook of palliative nursing* (4th ed., pp. 174–190). Oxford University Press.; Drugs.com. (2021). *Find drugs and conditions.* https://www.drugs.com/; Epocrates. (2021). *Drugs.* https://online.epocrates.com/home; Jackson, V., & Block, S. (2015). *Fast facts concepts #62: Use of psychostimulants in palliative care.* https://www.mypcnow.org/wp-content/uploads/2019/01/FF-61-psychostimulants.-3rd-ed.pdf; Kluger, B. M., Ney, D. E., Bagley, S. J., Mohile, N., Taylor, L. P., Walbert, T., & Jones, C. A. (2020). Top ten tips palliative care clinicians should know when caring for patients with brain cancer. *Journal of Palliative Medicine, 23*(3), 415–421. https://doi.org/10.1089/jpm.2019.0507; O'Donnell, J. M., Beis, R. R., & Shelton, R. C. (2018). Drug therapy of depression and anxiety disorders. In L. L. Brunton, R. Hilal-Dandan, & B. C. Knollmann (Eds.), *Goodman & Gilman's, the pharmacological basis of therapeutics* (pp. 267–302). McGraw-Hill; Prescriber's Digital Reference. (2021). *Doxepin hydrochloride — drug summary.* https://www.pdr.net/drug-summary/Doxepin-Hydrochloride-Capsules—10-mg—25-mg—50-mg—75-mg—100-mg—doxepin-hydrochloride-1965; US Food & Drug Administration. (2016). *FDA drug safety communication: Erythropoiesis-Stimulating Agents (ESAs): Procrit, Epogen and Aranesp.* https://www.fda.gov/drugs/postmarket-drug-safety-information-patients-and-providers/fda-drug-safety-communication-erythropoiesis-stimulating-agents-esas-procrit-epogen-and-aranesp#SA; Vallerand, A. H., & Sanoski, C. A. (2019). *Lactulose.* In Davis's Drug Guide for Nurses (16th ed). F.A. Davis Company. http://www.fadavis.com; Wong, A., & Reddy, S. K. (2016). Pain assessment and management. In S. Yennurajalingam & E. Bruera (Eds.), *Oxford American handbook of hospice and palliative medicine* (pp. 27–68). Oxford University Press.

APPENDIX D-2: NONPHARMACOLOGICAL INTERVENTIONS FOR SYMPTOM MANAGEMENT IN ADVANCED DISEASE

NONPHARMACOLOGICAL INTERVENTIONS		
INTERVENTION	**DOSE/FREQUENCY (ADULTS ONLY)**	**COST**[a]
AROMATHERAPY		
Diffused essential oils	As needed	Prices of essential oils varies by quality and quantity.
Topically applied essential oils (should be combined with carrier oil prior to application)		
HEALING ENERGY MODALITIES		
Reiki	Weekly to biweekly	$25–$80 per 1-hour treatment
MEDITATION		
Mindfulness meditation	As needed	Can be self-managed; guided sessions range from $55–$60 per 1-hour session
MUSIC THERAPY		
Receptive	As needed	$68–$90 per 1-hour session
Recreation		
Improvisation		
Composition/songwriting		
PHYSICAL HEALING MODALITIES		
Acupuncture	Weekly to biweekly	$45–$150 per treatment
Acupressure	As needed	$50–$75 per treatment
Chiropractic care	As needed	$30–$300 per adjustment
Massage	As needed	$60–$80 per session. Many hospice organizations provide massage therapy free of charge to patient.

(continued)

APPENDIX D-2: NONPHARMACOLOGICAL INTERVENTIONS FOR SYMPTOM MANAGEMENT IN ADVANCED DISEASE (CONTINUED)

NONPHARMACOLOGICAL INTERVENTIONS		
INTERVENTION	**DOSE/FREQUENCY (ADULTS ONLY)**	**COST[a]**
PSYCHOTHERAPY		
Cognitive behavioral therapy	As needed	$100–$120 per session
Group therapy	As needed	Often free
Online support groups	As needed	Often free

[a]Cost of therapies listed here is considered to be an estimate. Prices may vary according to location, supply, or other variables.

Sources: American Music Therapy Association. (2019). *2019 AMTA member survey and workforce analysis.* https://www.musictherapy.org/assets/1/7/2019WorkforceAnalysis.pdf; Anxiety and Depression Association of America. (2021). *Low cost treatments.* https://adaa.org/finding-help/treatment/low-cost-treatment; Fan, A. Y., Wang, D. D., Ouyang, H., Tian, H., Wei, H., He, D., Gong, C., Wen, J., Jin, M., He, C., Alemi, S. F., & Rahimi, S. (2019). Acupuncture price in forty-one metropolitan regions in the United States: An out-of-pocket cost analysis based on OkCopay.com. *Journal of Integrative Medicine, 17*(5), 315–320. https://www.sciencedirect.com/journal/journal-of-integrative-medicine; Lindberg, S. (2021). *Best guided meditations.* https://www.verywellmind.com/best-guided-meditations-4843806; Parkinson, M. (2020, July 15). *The four types of interventions in music therapy.* https://wellingtonmusictherapyservices.com/the-four-types-of-interventions-in-music-therapy/; Pembleton, M. (2021). *Guide to chiropractic adjustments: Costs, benefits, and risks.* https://www.forbes.com/health/body/chiropractic-adjustments-costs-and-benefits/#how_often_should_i_get_a_chiropractic_adjustment_section; The International Center for Reiki Healing. (2021). *How much does a treatment usually cost?* https://www.reiki.org/faqs/how-much-does-treatment-usually-cost; UK Reiki Federation. (2021). *How often do I need a reiki session?* https://www.reikifed.co.uk/how-often-do-i-need-a-reiki-session/

APPENDIX D-3: OVERVIEW OF COMMON SYMPTOMS

SYMPTOM	DESCRIPTION	OTHER ASSOCIATED SYMPTOMS	PHARMACOLOGIC INTERVENTIONS (SEE APPENDIX E-1)	NONPHARMACOLOGIC INTERVENTIONS (SEE APPENDIX E-2)
Anemia	Decreased red blood cell count (<13.5 gm/dL in men or <12 gm/dL in women)	Dyspnea, tachycardia, fatigue, angina, muscle pain/weakness, paresthesias, delirium (Hinkle & Cheever, 2018)	Packed red blood cell transfusion (Yennurajalinagam & Bruera, 2016) Erythropoiesis-stimulating agents (Yennurajalinagam & Bruera, 2016) Iron supplementation Daprodustat may be used for anemia associated with chronic kidney disease	Increased iron intake in diet, as directed

(continued)

APPENDIX D-3: OVERVIEW OF COMMON SYMPTOMS (*CONTINUED*)

SYMPTOM	DESCRIPTION	OTHER ASSOCIATED SYMPTOMS	PHARMACOLOGIC INTERVENTIONS (SEE APPENDIX E-1)	NONPHARMACOLOGIC INTERVENTIONS (SEE APPENDIX E-2)
Angina	A symptom of ischemic heart disease. Often paroxysmal and recurrent (Sommers, 2019)	Substernal or precordial chest pain/discomfort (Sommers, 2019)	Beta-blockers Calcium channel blockers Dopamine receptor antagonists Nitrates (Giannopoulos et al., 2016)	Deep breathing exercises Support groups (for chronic angina)
Anxiety (often accompanied by depression)	Subjective feelings of fear/worry	Restlessness, insomnia, depression, akathisia (Yennurajalinagam & Bruera, 2016), perspiration, tachycardia, light-headedness	Anxiolytics Benzodiazepines Antidepressants Neuroleptics (Yennurajalinagam & Bruera, 2016)	Diffused essential oils Reiki Mindfulness Meditation Massage Psychotherapy
Anorexia	Reduced desire for oral intake. May be complicated by oral pain, dysphagia, or odynophagia (Baracos & Watanbe, 2021)	Fatigue, weight loss, cachexia, light-headedness, dehydration	Appetite stimulants Corticosteroids Cannabinoids	Essential oils Acupuncture Small, frequent meals or high-calorie snacks
Ascites	Accumulation of fluid in the peritoneal cavity (Sommers, 2019)	Abdominal discomfort, dyspnea, anorexia, nausea, vomiting, indigestion (Sommers, 2019)	Diuretics	Dietary modification (75 g of protein daily) Supplemental vitamin K (injection) Insertion of peritoneovenous shunt Insertion of PleurX drain
Bone resorption	Breakdown of bone tissue resulting in the release of minerals such as calcium and phosphorus into the blood	Bone pain, inflammation	Bisphosphonates RANK ligand inhibitors	Management of bone pain through: Aromatherapy Mindfulness meditation Healing energy modalities Music therapy

(continued)

APPENDIX D-3: OVERVIEW OF COMMON SYMPTOMS (*CONTINUED*)

SYMPTOM	DESCRIPTION	OTHER ASSOCIATED SYMPTOMS	PHARMACOLOGIC INTERVENTIONS (SEE APPENDIX E-1)	NONPHARMACOLOGIC INTERVENTIONS (SEE APPENDIX E-2)
Brain fog	Mild cognitive impairment involving slower thinking, difficulty focusing and concentrating, forgetfulness, or mental haziness (Ocon, 2013)	Fatigue, anxiety, depression	Psychostimulants	Aromatherapy Mindfulness meditation Healing energy modalities
Constipation	A clinical syndrome defined by the difficult, infrequent passage of small, hard stools. The Rome criteria is used to evaluate constipation. Constipation may result from obstruction (tumor or other cause), nutritional/metabolic imbalances, neurogenic disorders, medications, or immobility (Yennurajalinagam & Bruera, 2016)	Bloating, abdominal discomfort, nausea, indigestion	Laxatives PAMORA Stool softeners	Dietary changes Massage (gentle abdominal)
Delirium	Also called "acute confusional state." Identification of cause is essential as delirium is often reversible (Sommers, 2019; Yennurajalinagam & Bruera, 2016)	Characterized by disorientation, agitation, fear, hallucinations, delusions, anxiety, and paranoia	Pharmacological treatment depends on cause (i.e., pain, anxiety, hypo-oxygenation, etc.)	Aromatherapy Music therapy
Diarrhea	Noninflammatory diarrhea is characterized by a large volume of loose, watery stools. Inflammatory diarrhea is characterized by smaller volumes of bloody stool (Hinkle & Cheever, 2018)	Abdominal cramping, urgency, perianal discomfort, incontinence, nausea. May be a sign of fecal impaction	Identify and treat underlying cause, if possible Antidiarrheals	Removal of cause Dietary changes

(continued)

APPENDIX D-3: OVERVIEW OF COMMON SYMPTOMS (*CONTINUED*)

SYMPTOM	DESCRIPTION	OTHER ASSOCIATED SYMPTOMS	PHARMACOLOGIC INTERVENTIONS (SEE APPENDIX E-1)	NONPHARMACOLOGIC INTERVENTIONS (SEE APPENDIX E-2)
Drooling	Inability to control or swallow oral secretions	Dysphagia, circumoral skin irritation, risk for aspiration	Anticholinergics Injection of botulinum toxin A into salivary glands	Repositioning Suctioning Meticulous skin care
Dysphagia	Difficulty swallowing (Sommers, 2019)	Halitosis, dysphagia, regurgitation, gurgling with swallowing, coughing, persistence of a bad taste in the mouth, respiratory distress, and risk for aspiration (Sommers, 2019)	Treatment is dependent on cause: Promotility agents (GERD) Corticosteroids (inflammation) Antacids (dyspepsia/gas) Antispasmodics (muscle spasm)	Dietary changes: small meals, avoidance of alcohol, tobacco products, and other esophageal irritants, soft foods Repositioning
Dyspnea	Subjective feeling of difficult, labored, or uncomfortable breathing (Yennurajalinagam & Bruera, 2016)	Tachypnea, altered oxygenation, distress, anxiety	Opioids Corticosteroids Bronchodilators Diuretics Anticholinergics (mainly at end of life)	Use of fans/moving air Lower temperature in the room Humidification Aromatherapy
Dysrhythmias	Disturbance in the normal electrical stimulation of the heart. Results in disordered cardiac rhythm, perfusion, and hypoxemia (Sommers, 2019)	Dizziness, fatigue, palpitations, chest pain, hypotension, syncope, and possibly, cardiac arrest (Sommers, 2019)	Adenosine Amiodarone Anticholinergics Anticoagulants Atropine Beta-blockers Calcium channel blockers Epinephrine Lidocaine	Ablation Medical management Cardioversion, as indicated Pacemaker or AICD as indicted Mindfulness meditation or psychotherapy for addressing anxiety related to diagnosis/symptoms

(*continued*)

APPENDIX D-3: OVERVIEW OF COMMON SYMPTOMS (*CONTINUED*)

SYMPTOM	DESCRIPTION	OTHER ASSOCIATED SYMPTOMS	PHARMACOLOGIC INTERVENTIONS (SEE APPENDIX E-1)	NONPHARMACOLOGIC INTERVENTIONS (SEE APPENDIX E-2)
Fatigue	Reduced ability to perform cognitive or physical tasks (Yennurajalinagam & Bruera, 2016)	Pain, depression, anxiety, hypoxia, anemia (Yennurajalinagam & Bruera, 2016)	Psychostimulants	Alternate periods of activity with periods of rest Utilize energy conservation techniques Aromatherapy Exercise (as tolerated)
Fever	Measured body temperature of 100.4°F (38°C) or greater (Centers for Disease Control & Prevention, 2023; Watson & Dyck, 2015)	Irritability, lethargy, chills, myalgias, diaphoresis	Antipyretics Anti-infectives (as needed)	Cool compresses Increase fluids Lightweight clothing Cool room temperature Moving air
Insomnia	Inability to fall asleep or stay asleep. Sleep quality may be poor once asleep	Depression, daytime somnolence, irritability, poor appetite, headache, anxiety, tension, stress (Sommers, 2019)	Benzodiazepines Atypical antidepressants Antihistaminic agents	Proper sleep hygiene (dim lighting, quiet sleep area, no electronics before sleep)
Muscle spasm	Involuntary cramping or contracting of muscle(s)	Pain, anxiety, sleep disturbance, immobility	Analgesics Antispasmodics Benzodiazepines Calcium channel blockers Electrolyte correction (dependent on cause) Muscle relaxants	Alternate activity with periods of rest Aromatherapy Exercise (stretching) Frequent position change Heat therapy Joint splinting Physical healing modalities

(continued)

APPENDIX D-3: OVERVIEW OF COMMON SYMPTOMS (*CONTINUED*)

SYMPTOM	DESCRIPTION	OTHER ASSOCIATED SYMPTOMS	PHARMACOLOGIC INTERVENTIONS (SEE APPENDIX E-1)	NONPHARMACOLOGIC INTERVENTIONS (SEE APPENDIX E-2)
Nausea	Subjective feeling of gastric distress that may lead to vomiting (Yennurajalinagam & Bruera, 2016)	Pain, insomnia, anxiety, depression, anorexia, constipation, diarrhea (Yennurajalinagam & Bruera, 2016)	Antiemetics Antihistaminic agents Benzodiazepines Cannabinoids Corticosteroids Dopamine receptor antagonists Selective 5-HY3 receptor antagonists	Aromatherapy Deep breathing exercises Dietary modifications
Neuropathies	Peripheral nerve damage that results in numbness, tingling, pain, decreased vibration sensation, immobility, and possible injury (Centers for Disease Control & Prevention, 2023; Watson & Dyck, 2015)	Often associated with diabetes, dysproteinemias, and vitamin B12 deficiencies. Can result in progressive functional limitation and pain (Centers for Disease Control & Prevention, 2023; Watson & Dyck, 2015)	Antidepressants Anticonvulsants Anesthetics Opioids	Alternate activity with periods of rest Exercise (as tolerated) Frequent position change Mindfulness meditation Physical healing modalities Psychotherapy (coping strategies)
Pain (see Appendix E)	Subjective experience of an unpleasant physical sensation (Hinkle & Cheever, 2018; Yennurajalinagam & Bruera, 2016)	Chronic illness, acute illness, muscle damage, wounds, malignancy/metastasis, anxiety, depression, anorexia, insomnia, immobility, spiritual distress, tachycardia (Hinkle & Cheever, 2018; Sommers, 2019; Yennurajalinagam & Bruera, 2016)	Antidepressants Non-opioid analgesics Opioids	Exercise (as tolerated) Position change Heat therapy Mindfulness meditation Physical healing modalities Psychotherapy (coping strategies)

(*continued*)

APPENDIX D-3: OVERVIEW OF COMMON SYMPTOMS (*CONTINUED*)

SYMPTOM	DESCRIPTION	OTHER ASSOCIATED SYMPTOMS	PHARMACOLOGIC INTERVENTIONS (SEE APPENDIX E-1)	NONPHARMACOLOGIC INTERVENTIONS (SEE APPENDIX E-2)
Pruritus	Persistent itching of skin (Hinkle & Cheever, 2018)	Skin dryness, flaking, irritation, inflammation, skin damage associated with scratching (Hinkle & Cheever, 2018)	Antihistamines Atypical antidepressants Depending on cause, topical agents such as ointments, barrier creams, or soaks can be trialed (e.g., calamine, menthol, oatmeal bath, antihistamine cream)	Maintain short fingernails Light, loose clothing
Respiratory secretions	Accumulation of respiratory secretions that the patient is unable to clear. When occurring at the end of life, this may be referred to as the "death rattle" (Wright, 2019)	Coughing, throat clearing, increased salivation, dyspnea, hypoxia. At end of life, gradual asthenia, somnolence, and eventually coma (Wright, 2019)	Anticholinergics Antihistaminic agents Expectorants Mucolytics	Repositioning Oropharyngeal suctioning (deep suctioning is not recommended)
Seizures	Result from abnormal electrical impulses within the brain, causing altered movements, consciousness, and/ or behaviors (Wright, 2019)	Medical conditions, disease progression, drug use or interaction	Antiepileptic medications (most commonly used is levetiracetam. If patient is unable to swallow, intranasal midazolam, rectal diazepam, or buccal clonazepam may be used)	Maintain patient's safety Educate caregivers on prompt identification of seizure activity and interventions

AICD, automated implantable cardioverter defibrillator; GERD, gastroesophageal reflux disease; PAMORA, peripherally acting mu-opioid receptor antagonists.

Sources: Hinkle, J. L., & Cheever, K. H. (2018) *Brunner & Siddarth's textbook of medical-surgical nursing* (14th ed., pp. 1377–1427). Wolters Kluwer; Yennurajalinagam, S., & Bruera, E. (2016). *Oxford American handbook of hospice and palliative care.* Oxford University Press; Sommers, M. S. (2019). *Davis's diseases and disorders: A nursing therapeutics manual.* F.A. Davis. https://www.fadavis.com/product/nursing-fundamentals-med-surg-diseases-disorders-nursing-therapeutics-manual-sommers-64; Giannopoulos, A. A., Giannoglou, G. D., & Chatzizisis, Y. S. (2016). Pharmacological approaches of refractory angina. *Pharmacology & Therapeutics, 163,* 118–131. https://www.unmc.edu/intmed/_documents/cardiology/cbbl/2016-9.pdf; Baracos, V., & Watanbe, S. M. (2021). Aetiology, classification, assessment, and treatment of the anorexia-cachexia syndrome. In N. I. Cherny, M. T. Fallon, S. Kaasa, R. K. Portenoy, & D. C. Currow (Eds.), *Oxford textbook of palliative medicine* (6th ed). Oxford University Press; Ocon, A. J. (2013). Caught in the thickness of brain fog: Exploring the cognitive symptoms of chronic fatigue syndrome. *Frontiers in Physiology, 4,* 63. https://www.frontiersin.org/articles/10.3389/fphys.2013.00063/full; Centers for Disease Control and Prevention. (2023). *Definitions of symptoms for reportable illnesses.* https://www.cdc.gov/quarantine/air/reporting-deaths-illness/definitions-symptoms-reportable-illnesses.html; Watson, J. C., & Dyck, P. J. B. (2015, July). Peripheral neuropathy: A practical approach to diagnosis and symptom management. In *Mayo Clinic Proceedings* (Vol. 90, No. 7, pp. 940–951). Elsevier. https://doi.org/10.1016/j.mayocp.2015.05.004; Wright, P. M. (2019). *Certified hospice and palliative nurse (CHPN) exam review: A study guide with review questions.* Springer Publishing Company.

APPENDIX E

PAIN MANAGEMENT

APPENDIX E-1: PAIN ASSESSMENT

P: Palliative and provocative factors	Ask: What makes the pain better or worse?
	• The patient's response to this question helps the nurse to determine whether the pain regimen is effective or need to be modified according to the patient's report.
Q: Quality of the pain	Ask: Please describe what the pain feels like to you.
	• The words the patient uses to describe the pain help the nurse to differentiate what type of pain the patient is experiencing. • **Neuropathic pain** is generally described as burning, tingling, shocking, shooting, radiating, numbness, "pins & needles" • **Visceral pain** is generally described as gnawing, stretching, pressure, crampy, deep, poorly localized • **Somatic pain** is generally described as dull, sore, throbbing
R: Radiation	Ask: Is the pain in one area? Can you point to it? Does it travel or radiate?
	• The response to this question helps to differentiate neuropathic from somatic pain or visceral pain. • Pain that is well-localized is generally somatic. Pain that radiates is usually neuropathic. Visceral pain is often poorly localized.
S: Severity	Ask: Can you tell me how bad the pain is on a scale of 1–10? One means the pain is barely noticeable and 10 means it is the worst pain you have ever felt.
	• The patient's response this question provides a snapshot of how intense the pain is for the patient right now. It also helps the patient and nurse determine if goals are met after intervention.
T: Timing	Ask: Does the pain seem to be better or worse at a certain time of the day? When did it start? How long does it last? Does it ever wake you up?
	• The patient's response to this question helps determine whether the pain is due to muscle fatigue, arthritis, or immobility. It is also useful in planning the timing of interventions to alleveiate the pain.

Source: Adapted from Wright, P. M. (2021). Fast facts for the hospice nurse (2nd ed.). Springer Publishing Company.

APPENDIX E-2: FLACC SCALE

	FLACC BEHAVIORAL PAIN ASSESSMENT SCALE		
	SCORING		
CATEGORIES	**0**	**1**	**2**
Face	No particular expression or smile	Occasional grimace or frown; withdrawn, disinterested	Frequent to constant frown, clenched jaw, quivering chin
Legs	Normal position or relaxed	Uneasy, restless, tense	Kicking or legs drawn up
Activity	Lying quietly, normal position, moves easily	Squirming, shifting back and forth, tense	Arched, rigid, or jerking
Cry	No cry (awake or asleep)	Moans or whimpers, occasional complaint	Crying steadily, screams or sobs; frequent complaints
Consolability	Content, relaxed	Reassured by occasional touching, hugging, or being talked to; distractable	Difficult to console or comfort

How to Use the FLACC

In patients who are awake: Observe for 1 to 5 minutes or longer. Observe legs and body uncovered. Reposition patient or observe activity. Assess body for tenseness and tone. Initiate consoling interventions if needed.

In patients who are asleep: Observe for 5 minutes or longer. Observe body and legs uncovered. If possible, reposition the patient. Touch the body and assess for tenseness and tone.

Face
- Score 0 if the patient has a relaxed face, makes eye contact, shows interest in surroundings.
- Score 1 if the patient has a worried facial expression, with eyebrows lowered, eyes partially closed, cheeks raised, mouth pursed.
- Score 2 if the patient has deep furrows in the forehead, closed eyes, an open mouth, deep lines around the nose and lips.

Legs
- Score 0 if the muscle tone and motion in the limbs are normal.
- Score 1 if patient has increased tone, rigidity, or tension or if there is intermittent flexion or extension of the limbs.
- Score 2 if patient has hypertonicity, the legs are pulled tight, there is exaggerated flexion or extension of the limbs, tremors.

Activity
- Score 0 if the patient moves easily and freely, normal activity or restrictions.
- Score 1 if the patient shifts positions, appears hesitant to move, demonstrates guarding, a tense torso, pressure on a body part.
- Score 2 if the patient is in a fixed position, rocking; demonstrates side-to-side head movement or rubbing of a body part.

Cry
- Score 0 if the patient has no cry or moan, awake, or asleep.
- Score 1 if the patient has occasional moans, cries, whimpers, sighs.
- Score 2 if the patient has frequent or continuous moans, cries, grunts.

Consolability
- Score 0 if the patient is calm and does not require consoling.
- Score 1 if the patient responds to comfort by touching or talking in 30 seconds to 1 minute.
- Score 2 if the patient requires constant comforting or is inconsolable.

(continued)

APPENDIX E-2: FLACC SCALE (*CONTINUED*)

	FLACC BEHAVIORAL PAIN ASSESSMENT SCALE		
	SCORING		
CATEGORIES	**0**	**1**	**2**

Whenever feasible, behavioral measurement of pain should be used in conjunction with self-report. When self-report is not possible, interpretation of pain behaviors and decisions regarding treatment of pain require careful consideration of the context in which the pain behaviors are observed.

Interpreting the behavioral score

Each category is scored on the 0 to 2 scale, which results in a total score of 0 to 10.

0 = Relaxed and comfortable   **4–6** = Moderate pain
1–3 = Mild discomfort   **7–10** = Severe discomfort or pain or both

Source: From Merkel, S. I., Voepel-Lewis, T., Shayevitz, I. R., & Malviya, S. (1997). The FLACC: A behavioral scale for scoring postoperative pain in young children. *Pediatric Nursing, 23*(3), 293–297. (The FLACC scale was developed by Sandra Merkel, MS, RN, Terri Voepel-Lewis, MS, RN, and Shobha Malviya, MD, at C.S. Mott Children's Hospital, University of Michigan Health System, Ann Arbor, MI.)

APPENDIX E-3: FACES PAIN SCALE

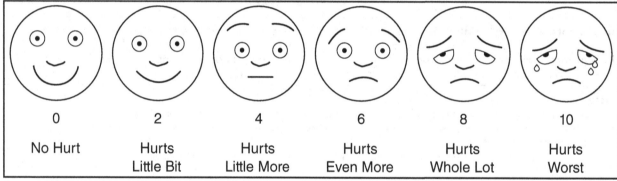

0	2	4	6	8	10
No Hurt	Hurts Little Bit	Hurts Little More	Hurts Even More	Hurts Whole Lot	Hurts Worst

Source: Adapted from Belbury, L. (2020). *Faces pain scale.*

APPENDIX E-4: PAIN ASSESSMENT IN ADVANCED DEMENTIA SCALE FOR ASSESSING PAIN IN ADVANCED DEMENTIA

Instructions: Observe the patient for five minutes before scoring his or her behaviors. Score the behaviors according to the following chart. Definitions of each item are provided on the following page. The patient can be observed under different conditions (e.g., at rest, during a pleasant activity, during caregiving, after the administration of pain medication).

BEHAVIOR	0	1	2	SCORE
Scoring: The total score ranges from 0 to 10 points. A possible interpretation of the scores is: 1–3 = mild pain; 4–6 = moderate pain; 7–10 = severe pain. These ranges are based on a standard 0–10 scale of pain, but have not been substantiated in the literature for this tool.				
Breathing Independent of vocalization	• Normal	• Occasional labored breathing • Short period of hyperventilation	• Noisy labored breathing • Long period of hyperventilation • Cheyne–Stokes respirations	
Negative vocalization	• None	• Occasional moan or groan • Low-level speech with a negative or disapproving quality	• Repeated troubled calling out • Loud moaning or groaning • Crying	
Facial expression	• Smiling or inexpressive	• Sad • Frightened • Frown	• Facial grimacing	
Body language	• Relaxed	• Tense • Distressed pacing • Fidgeting	• Rigid • Fists clenched • Knees pulled up • Pulling or pushing away • Striking out	
Consolability	• No need to console	• Distracted or reassured by voice or touch	• Unable to console, distract, or reassure	
			TOTAL SCORE	

PAIN ASSESSMENT IN ADVANCED DEMENTIA ITEM DEFINITIONS

BREATHING

1. *Normal breathing* is characterized by effortless, quiet, rhythmic (smooth) respirations.

2. *Occasional labored breathing* is characterized by episodic bursts of harsh, difficult, or wearing respirations.

3. *Short period of hyperventilation* is characterized by intervals of rapid, deep breaths lasting a short period of time.

4. *Noisy* labored breathing is characterized by negative-sounding respirations on inspiration or expiration. They may be loud, gurgling, or wheezing. They appear strenuous or wearing.

5. *Long period of hyperventilation* is characterized by an excessive rate and depth of respirations lasting a considerable time.

6. *Cheyne–Stokes respirations* are characterized by rhythmic waxing and waning of breathing from very deep to shallow respirations with periods of apnea (cessation of breathing).

(continued)

APPENDIX E-4: PAIN ASSESSMENT IN ADVANCED DEMENTIA SCALE FOR ASSESSING PAIN IN ADVANCED DEMENTIA (*CONTINUED*)

NEGATIVE VOCALIZATION

1. *None* is characterized by speech or vocalization that has a neutral or pleasant quality.

2. *Occasional moan or groan* is characterized by mournful or murmuring sounds, wails, or laments. Groaning is characterized by louder than usual inarticulate involuntary sounds, often abruptly beginning and ending.

3. *Low-level* speech with a negative or disapproving quality is characterized by muttering, mumbling, whining, grumbling, or swearing in a low volume with a complaining, sarcastic, or caustic tone.

4. *Repeated troubled calling out* is characterized by phrases or words being used over and over in a tone that suggests anxiety, uneasiness, or distress.

5. *Loud moaning or groaning* is characterized by mournful or murmuring sounds, wails, or laments in much louder than usual volume. Loud groaning is characterized by louder than usual inarticulate involuntary sounds, often abruptly beginning and ending.

6. *Crying* is characterized by an utterance of emotion accompanied by tears. There may be sobbing or quiet weeping.

FACIAL EXPRESSION

1. *Smiling or inexpressive.* Smiling is characterized by upturned corners of the mouth, brightening of the eyes, and a look of pleasure or contentment. Inexpressive refers to a neutral, at ease, relaxed, or blank look.

2. *Sad* is characterized by an unhappy, lonesome, sorrowful, or dejected look. There may be tears in the eyes.

3. *Frightened* is characterized by a look of fear, alarm, or heightened anxiety. Eyes appear wide open.

4. *Frown* is characterized by a downward turn of the corners of the mouth. Increased facial wrinkling in the forehead and around the mouth may appear.

5. *Facial grimacing* is characterized by a distorted, distressed look. The brow is more wrinkled, as is the area around the mouth. Eyes may be squeezed shut.

BODY LANGUAGE

1. *Relaxed* is characterized by a calm, restful, mellow appearance. The person seems to be taking it easy.

2. *Tense* is characterized by a strained, apprehensive, or worried appearance. The jaw may be clenched. (Exclude any contractures.)

3. *Distressed pacing* is characterized by activity that seems unsettled. There may be a fearful, worried, or disturbed element present. The rate may be faster or slower.

4. *Fidgeting* is characterized by restless movement. Squirming about or wiggling in the chair may occur. The person might be hitching a chair across the room. Repetitive touching, tugging, or rubbing body parts can also be observed.

5. *Rigid* is characterized by stiffening of the body. The arms and/or legs are tight and inflexible. The trunk may appear straight and unyielding. (Exclude any contractures.)

6. *Fists clenched* is characterized by tightly closed hands. They may be opened and closed repeatedly or held tightly shut.

7. *Knees pulled up* is characterized by flexing the legs and drawing the knees up toward the chest. An overall troubled appearance. (Exclude any contractures.)

8. *Pulling or pushing away* is characterized by resistiveness upon approach or to care. The person is trying to escape by yanking or wrenching themselves free or shoving you away.

9. *Striking out* is characterized by hitting, kicking, grabbing, punching, biting, or other form of personal assault.

CONSOLABILITY

1. *No need to console* is characterized by a sense of well-being. The person appears content.

2. *Distracted or reassured by voice or touch* is characterized by a disruption in the behavior when the person is spoken to or touched. The behavior stops during the period of interaction, with no indication that the person is at all distressed.

3. *Unable to console, distract, or reassure* is characterized by the inability to soothe the person or stop a behavior with words or actions. No amount of comforting, verbal or physical, will alleviate the behavior.

Source: Warden, V., Hurley, A. C., & Volicer, L. (2003). Development and psychometric evaluation of the Pain Assessment in Advanced Dementia (PAINAD) scale. *Journal of the American Medical Directors Association, 4*(1), 9–15.

APPENDIX E-5: NONOPIOID PAIN INTERVENTIONS

DRUG	DOSE AND SCHEDULE (PATIENTS OVER 50 KG)	DOSE AND SCHEDULE (PATIENTS UNDER 50 KG)	KEY POINTS
Acetaminophen	Orally: 500–1,000 mg q 4 hours Rectally: 325–650 mg q 4–6 hours IV: 1,000 mg over 15 minutes	Orally: 10–15 mg/kg q 4 hours Rectally: 15–20 mg/kg q 4 hours IV: 15 mg/kg q 6 hours	Maximum daily dose of 4,000 mg. In patients under 50 kg, maximum daily dose of IV acetaminophen is 75 mg Reduce dose by 50% for patients who have impaired liver function
Aspirin	Oral: 325–650 mg q 4 hours for pain or fever Rectally: 300–600 mg q 4 hours	Orally: 10–15 mg/kg q 4 hours Rectally: 15–20 mg/kg q 4 hours	Maximum daily dose of 4,000 mg Nonselective COX-2 inhibitor Robust antiplatelet properties May cause gastric, renal, and CNS toxicity Nausea, vomiting, diaphoresis, and tinnitus occur at toxic doses
Celecoxib	Orally: 100–200 mg daily; may be increased to BID	No data available	Selective COX-2 inhibitor Risk for renal and cardiac toxicities No effect on platelets
Choline magnesium trisalicylate	Orally: 500–750 mg q 8 hours	Orally: 25 mg/kg q 8 hours.	Maximum daily dose of 3,000 mg Less antiplatelet action than other NSAIDs Minimal GI toxicity
Ibuprofen	Orally: 200–400 mg q 6 hours	Orally: 10 mg/kg q 6–8 hours	Maximum daily dose of 2,400 mg Potential toxicities similar to aspirin Patients taking aspirin for cardiac protection should not use ibuprofen Use with caution in geriatric patients Patients who have peptic ulcer disease, chronic kidney disease, or congestive heart failure should not use ibuprofen
Indomethacin	Orally: 25–50 mg BID; may increase to TID	0.5–1 mg/kg q 8 hours	Maximum daily dose of 150–200 mg Risk for serious renal and cardiac toxicities

(continued)

APPENDIX E-5: NONOPIOID PAIN INTERVENTIONS (*CONTINUED*)

DRUG	DOSE AND SCHEDULE (PATIENTS OVER 50 KG)	DOSE AND SCHEDULE (PATIENTS UNDER 50 KG)	KEY POINTS
Ketorolac	IV/IM: 30–60 mg initial dose. Bolus of 15–30 mg may be given IV or SQ q 6 hours. Continuous IV/SQ infusion may be used for only 3–5 days, then discontinued	IV/IM: 0.25–1 mg/kg q 6 hours. Use for only 3–5 days, then discontinue	Significant GI and renal toxicities May precipitate renal failure in patients who are severely dehydrated May prolong bleeding time
Naproxen	Orally or rectally: 500–750 mg q 8 hours	Orally or rectally: 5 mg/kg q 8 hours	Maximum daily dose of 1,000 mg Lowest risk for cardiac toxicity

CNS, central nervous system; COX, cyclooxygenase; GI, gastrointestinal; IM, intramuscular; IV, intravenous; NSAIDs, nonsteroidal anti-inflammatory drugs; PRN, as needed; SQ, subcutaneous.

Sources: U.S. Federal Drug Administration. (2016). *Indomethacin capsules, USP.* https://www.accessdata.fda.gov/drugsatfda_docs/label/2016/018829s022lbl.pdf; Paice, J. A. (2015). Pain at the end of life. In B. R. Ferrell, N. Coyle, & J. A. Paice (Eds.), *Oxford textbook of palliative nursing* (pp. 135–153). Oxford University Press; Smith, E. L., & Castor, T. (2015). Pain management in geriatric patients. In K. A. Sackheim (Ed), *Pain management and palliative care* (pp. 245–263). Springer Publishing Company; Coyle, N., & Layman-Goldstein, M. (2007). Pharmacologic management of adult cancer pain. *Cancer Network, 21*(2). http://www.cancernetwork.com/palliative-and-supportive-care/pharmacologic-management-adult-cancer-pain

APPENDIX E-6: OPIOID PAIN INTERVENTIONS

DRUG	DRUG ACTION	APPROXIMATE EQUIANALGESIC ORAL DOSE	APPROXIMATE EQUIANALGESIC PARENTERAL DOSE	RECOMMENDED STARTING DOSE (PATIENT >50 KG)	RECOMMENDED STARTING DOSE (PATIENT <50 KG)	KEY POINTS
Morphine	μ receptor agonist, weak κ receptor agonist	30 mg	10 mg	**Oral:** 15 mg q 3–4 hours **Parenteral:** 5 mg q 3–4 hours	**Oral:** 0.3 mg/kg q 3–4 hours **Parenteral:** 5 mg q 3–4 hours	Morphine is the standard by which all opioids are measured. Constipation, nausea, and sedation are the most common side effects. Risk for respiratory depression Common side effects such as nausea and sedation usually dissipate within a few days. Patients do not build a tolerance to the constipating effects of morphine (or other opioids) **Availability:** parenteral, oral, suppository. Long-acting and short-acting forms available
Codeine	μ and κ receptor agonist	150 mg	50 mg	**Oral:** 30 mg q 3–4 hours **Parenteral:** 30 mg q 2 h (IM/IV)	**Oral:** 0.5 mg/kg q 3–4 hours **Parenteral:** not recommended	Roughly 10% of the Caucasian population lacks the enzyme that converts codeine to morphine, making it ineffective for them Often combined with acetaminophen or guaifenesin **Availability:** parenteral, oral, suppository

(continued)

APPENDIX E-6: OPIOID PAIN INTERVENTIONS (CONTINUED)

DRUG	DRUG ACTION	APPROXIMATE EQUIANALGESIC ORAL DOSE	APPROXIMATE EQUIANALGESIC PARENTERAL DOSE	RECOMMENDED STARTING DOSE (PATIENT >50 KG)	RECOMMENDED STARTING DOSE (PATIENT <50 KG)	KEY POINTS
Fentanyl	μ receptor agonist Weak κ and δ agonist	Noninjectable fentanyl products are for patients tolerant to opioid only. Do not convert mcg for mcg among fentanyl products (i.e., transdermal patch, transmucosal lozenge, nasal spray, etc.)				Fentanyl 100 mcg patch ≈4 mg IV morphine/hour. Fentanyl is lipid-soluble; absorption is decreased in patients who are cachexic. Breakthrough pain medication should be used in conjunction with long-acting transdermal patch. **Availability:** parenteral, oral, transdermal, nebulized, transmucosal
Hydrocodone	μ and κ receptor agonist	30 mg	Not available	**Oral:** 5 mg q 3–4 hours **Parenteral:** not available	**Oral:** 0.1 mg/kg q 3–4 hours **Parenteral:** not available	Only available in combination with other drugs such as acetaminophen that limits usefulness in end-of-life and palliative care settings. Hydrocodone is a synthesized form of codeine. Used to treat moderate to severe pain and as a cough suppressant. Equipotent to codeine. **Availability:** oral

DRUG	DRUG ACTION	APPROXIMATE EQUIANALGESIC ORAL DOSE	APPROXIMATE EQUIANALGESIC PARENTERAL DOSE	RECOMMENDED STARTING DOSE (PATIENT >50 KG)	RECOMMENDED STARTING DOSE (PATIENT <50 KG)	KEY POINTS
Hydromorphone	μ receptor agonist, weak κ and δ agonist	6 mg	1.5 mg	**Oral:** 2 mg q 3–4 hours **Parenteral:** 0.5 mg q 3–4 hours	**Oral:** 0.03 mg/kg q 3–4 hours **Parenteral:** 0.005 mg/kg q 3–4 hours	Faster onset than morphine and more potent Increased blood plasma levels with renal disease. Removed with dialysis **Availability:** parenteral, oral, suppository. Long-acting formulation available
Levorphanol	μ-opioid receptor agonist with some effect at κ- and δ-receptors	4 mg	2 mg	**Oral:** 4 mg q 6–8 hours **Parenteral:** 2 mg q 6–8 hours	**Oral:** 0.04 mg/kg q 6–8 hours **Parenteral:** 0.02 mg/kg q 6–8 hours	Causes less N/V than morphine Longer half-life than morphine; may lead to accumulation with repeated administration **Availability:** parenteral and oral
Methadone	μ-opioid receptor agonist with some effect at κ- and δ-receptors; NMDA-receptor antagonist	10 mg	10 mg	**Oral:** 5 mg q 12 hours **Parenteral:** not recommended	**Oral:** 0.1 mg/kg q 12 hours **Parenteral:** not recommended	Risk for toxicity due to accumulation, including respiratory depression and sedation related to long half-life of drug Less costly than many other opioid medications Myoclonus may occur with parenteral use PRN dosing not recommended. Should not be used for breakthrough pain

(continued)

APPENDIX E-6: OPIOID PAIN INTERVENTIONS (CONTINUED)

DRUG	DRUG ACTION	APPROXIMATE EQUIANALGESIC ORAL DOSE	APPROXIMATE EQUIANALGESIC PARENTERAL DOSE	RECOMMENDED STARTING DOSE (PATIENT >50 KG)	RECOMMENDED STARTING DOSE (PATIENT <50 KG)	KEY POINTS
Oxycodone	μ-opioid receptor agonist, strong effect at κ agonist and some effect at δ-receptors	20 mg	Not available	**Oral:** 5 mg q 3–4 hours **Parenteral:** not available	**Oral:** 1 mg/kg q 3–4 hours **Parenteral:** not available	Onset of action 5–10 min Less nausea and vomiting than morphine Extensively metabolized by the liver; use caution in patients with hepatic disease Often combined with acetaminophen **Availability:** oral, suppository. Extended-release form available
Tramadol	Partial μ-receptor agonist	100 mg	Not recommended	**Oral:** 50–100 mg q 3–4 hours **Parenteral:** 50–100 mg q 3–4 hours	Not recommended	Synthetic codeine analogue; less effective for severe or chronic pain Adverse effects are nausea, vomiting, dizziness, and constipation. *Lowers seizure threshold* **Availability:** parenteral, oral, suppository. Extended-release form available

NMDA, N-methyl-D-aspartate; N/V, nausea and vomiting.

Sources: Paice, J. A. (2015). Pain at the end of life. In B. R. Ferrell, N. Coyle, & J. A. Paice (Eds.), *Oxford textbook of palliative nursing* (pp. 135–153). Oxford University Press; P. L. Detail-Document. (2012). Equianalgesic dosing of opioids for pain management. *Pharmacist's Letter/Prescriber's Letter.* https://www.nhms.org/sites/default/files/Pdfs/Opioid-Comparison-Chart-Prescriber-Letter-2012.pdf; Smith, H. S., & Peppin, J. F. (2016). Toward a systematic approach to opioid rotation. *Journal of Pain Research, 14*(7), 589–608. https://www.ncbi.nlm.nih.gov/pmc/articles/PMC4207581/pdf/jpr-7-589.pdf; Yaksh, T., & Wallace, M. (2018). Opioids, analgesia, and pain management. In L. L. Brunton, R. Hilal-Dandan, & B. C. Knollman (Eds.), *Goodman & Gillman's: The pharmacological basis of therapeutics* (13th ed., pp. 355–420). McGraw-Hill Education.

APPENDIX E-7: OPIOID EQUIANALGESIC DOSING GUIDELINES

OPIOID	APPROXIMATE EQUIANALGESIC DOSE (ORAL AND TRANSDERMAL)
Morphine (reference)	30 mg
Codeine	200 mg
Fentanyl transdermal	12.5 mcg/hour
Hydrocodone	30 mg
Hydromorphone	7.5 mg
Oxycodone	20 mg
Oxymorphone	10 mg

Source: Indian Health Service. (n.d.). *Safe opioid prescribing.* https://www.ihs.gov/painmanagement/treatmentplanning/safeopioidprescribing/

APPENDIX E-8: ADJUVANT PAIN INTERVENTIONS

TYPE OF PAIN	DRUG CLASS	DRUG EXAMPLES AND STARTING DOSES	KEY POINTS
Bone pain or pain from bony metastasis Vertebral compression fractures Arthritis pain Joint pain	Biphosphonates	Pamidronate 60–90 mg IV over 2 hours every 2–4 weeks	May also consider radiofrequency ablation or radiopharmaceuticals (i.e., strontium chloride-89, samariaum-153) for metastatic bone pain Monitor for dyspepsia and "steroid psychosis," and glucose intolerance if using corticosteroids
	Corticosteroids	Dexamethasone 2–20 mg PO/SQ daily. May give up to 100 mg IV bolus for pain crisis Prednisone 15–30 mg PO TID	
	NSAIDs	Diclofenac 1.3% patch BID Ibuprofen 400–800 mg PO q6 hours (with food) Ketorolac 30 mg PO/SC/IV q 6 hours	

(continued)

APPENDIX E-8: ADJUVANT PAIN INTERVENTIONS (*CONTINUED*)

TYPE OF PAIN	DRUG CLASS	DRUG EXAMPLES AND STARTING DOSES	KEY POINTS
Somatic pain (described as sharp and well-localized; the patient can point to the source of the pain)	Antispasmodics	Baclofen 10–20 mg q 6 hours Tizanidine 2 mg PO TID Dantrolene 25 mg PO daily × 7 days, then 25 mg PO TID × 7 days, then 50 mg PO TID × 7 days, then 100 mg PO QID (max). Discontinue if no response after 45 days	For patients experiencing proximal muscle weakness, consider hydrotherapy or physical therapy (at home), if patient is able to tolerate this therapy. Provide assistive devices in the home for safety and to promote independence. Baclofen is the only drug that is FDA-approved for muscle spasticity. Baclofen may cause muscle weakness and/or cognitive changes. Skeletal muscle relaxants and antispasmodics enhance the efficacy of NSAIDs for treating muscle injury or spasm. Skeletal muscle relaxants are relatively contraindicated in patients who have liver or renal disease. Benzodiazepines are FDA-approved for spasticity, but the somnolence caused by combining these drugs with opioids prohibits injudicious use.
	NSAIDs	Diclofenac 1.3% patch BID Ibuprofen 400–800 mg PO q 6 hours (with food) Ketorolac 30 mg PO/SC/IV q 6 hours	
	Skeletal muscle relaxants	Carisoprodol 250–350 mg TID and at HS Metaxalone 800 mg PO TID–QID (on empty stomach) Chlorzoxazone 250–500 mg PO TID–QID (max 750/dose) Cyclobenzaprine 5–10 mg PO TID up to 3 weeks Orphenadrine 100 mg PO BID for musculoskeletal pain; 100 mg PO at HS for leg cramps Methocarbamol start with 1,500 mg PO QID × 2–3 days, then reduce to 1,000 mg PO QID; 1,000 mg IV × 1 for muscle spasm	

(*continued*)

APPENDIX E-8: ADJUVANT PAIN INTERVENTIONS (*CONTINUED*)

TYPE OF PAIN	DRUG CLASS	DRUG EXAMPLES AND STARTING DOSES	KEY POINTS
Neuropathic pain (described as shooting, burning, tingling, or as pins and needles)	Anticonvulsants	Gabapentin 100–300 mg PO TID Carbamazepine 200 mg PO q 12 hours (monitor blood levels) Clozapine 0.5 mg PO BID Lamotrigine 100–200 mg PO q 12 hours Phenytoin 300–400 mg PO daily (monitor blood levels) Pregabalin 25–50 mg PO q 8 hours Topiramate 100–200 mg PO q 12 hours	Monitor patients for side effects of medications such as nausea, vomiting, sedation, dizziness, or anticholinergic effects (antidepressants and anticonvulsants). Neuropathic pain often requires a multimodal approach to pain management. If pain is severe and refractory at the end of life, sedation may be considered. Use of topical lidocaine should be considered when even light touch or clothing is painful on the skin. Neuropathic pain related to postherpetic neuralgia may be treated using a lidocaine patch. The patch should not be used on broken skin. Importantly, antiviral medications should be used during active herpes zoster or simplex outbreaks in conjunction with analgesics and co-analgesics.
	Antidepressants	Desipramine 10–25 mg PO at HS Duloxetine 30–60 mg PO daily Nortriptyline 10–50 mg PO at HS Trazodone 25–150 mg PO at HS Venlafaxine XR 37.5 mg PO daily	
	Anesthetics	Ketamine 10–15 mg PO q 6 hours or IV dose of 5–10 mg × 1, which may be repeated in 15–30 minutes. Starting infusion dose is 0.2 mg/kg/h. May increase by 0.1 mg/kg/h q 6 hours. Lidocaine 1–5 mg/kg hourly IV or SC Mexiletine 150 mg BID–TID	

(continued)

APPENDIX E-8: ADJUVANT PAIN INTERVENTIONS (*CONTINUED*)

TYPE OF PAIN	DRUG CLASS	DRUG EXAMPLES AND STARTING DOSES	KEY POINTS
Visceral pain (described as achy, dull, spasmic, crampy, or gnawing. This type of pain often radiates away from the site of injury) This type of pain may be related to ischemia, organ damage, obstruction, or bladder spasms, among other causes.	Anticholinergics	B&O suppositories 30 or 60 mg up to QID Dicyclomine 10–20 mg PO up to TID PRN Glycopyrrolate 0.2–0.4 mg PO/SC every 2–4 hours and titrate Hyoscyamine 0.125 mg PO/SL q 4–8 hours Scopolamine 1–2 TD patch(es) q 3 days. For acute bowel obstruction: 10 mcg/h SC/IV continuous infusion or 0.1 mg SC every 6 h. Titrate every 24 h.	Anticholinergics are used to reduce secretions in cases of painful bowel obstruction. Octreotide has been found to be effective and to have minimal adverse effects, but may be cost-prohibitive. B&O suppositories are useful for patients who have bladder or rectal spasms. Consider pretreating rectal area with lidocaine or hydrocortisone prior to administration in patients with rectal cancer. Use of benzodiazepines with opioids increases the risk of opioid side effects, particularly respiratory depression. Metoclopramide may decrease the risk for aspiration in patients fed via NG tube. However, it should be used cautiously in patients who have CHF due increased risk for fluid overload.
	Antisecretory agent	Octreotide 100 mcg SC/IV q 8 hours	
	Benzodiazepines	Lorazepam 0.5–1 mg PO/SC q 4 hours	
	Prokinetic agent	Metoclopramide 5–10 mg PO/SC q 4 hours	
	Corticosteroids	Dexamethasone 2–20 mg PO/SC daily. May give up to 100 mg IV bolus for pain crisis Prednisone 15–30 mg PO TID	

B&O, belladonna and opium; CHF, congestive heart failure; FDA, Federal Drug Administration; IV, intravenous; NG, nasogastric; NSAIDs, nonsteroidal anti-inflammatory drugs; SQ, subcutaneous.

Sources: Abrahm, J. L. (2014). *A physician's guide to pain and symptom management in cancer patients* (3rd ed.). Johns Hopkins University Press; Bodtke, S., & Ligon, K. (2016). *Hospice and palliative medicine handbook: A clinical guide.* http://www.hpmhandbook.com/; Milgrom, D. P., Lad, N. L., Koniaris, L. G., & Zimmers, T. A. (2017). Bone pain and muscle weakness in cancer patients. *Current Osteoporosis Reports, 15*(2), 76–87. https://doi.org/10.1007/s11914-017-0354-3; Paice, J. A. (2015). Pain at the end of life. In B. R. Ferrell, N. Coyle, & J. A. Paice (Eds.), *Oxford textbook of palliative nursing* (pp. 135–153). Oxford University Press; Peng, X., Wang, P. Li, S., Zhang, G., & Hu, S. (2015). Randomized clinical trial comparing octreotide and scopolamine butylbromide in symptom control of patients with inoperable bowel obstruction due to advanced ovarian cancer. *Journal of Surgical Oncology, 13*(5), 1–6. https://doi.org/10.1186/s12957-015-0455-3; Roland, E. & von Gunten, C. F. (2009). Current concepts in malignant bowel obstruction management. *Current Oncology Reports, 11*(4), 298–303. https://link.springer.com/journal/11912; Saulino, M., Anderson, D. J., Doble, J., Farid, R., Gul, F., Konrad, P., & Boster, A. L. (2016). Best practices for intrathecal baclofen therapy: Troubleshooting. *Neuromodulation: Technology at the Neural Interface, 19*(6), 632–641. https://doi.org/10.1111/ner.12467; Warusevitane, A., Karunatilake, D., Sim, J., Lally, F., & Roffe, C. (2015). Safety and effect of metoclopramide to prevent pneumonia in patients with stroke fed via nasogastric tubes trial. *Stroke, 46*(2), 454–460. https://doi.org/10.1161/STROKEAHA.114.006639

PRESSURE WOUND PREVENTION AND ASSESSMENT PATHWAY

APPENDIX F-1: PRESSURE WOUND PREVENTION AND ASSESSMENT PATHWAY

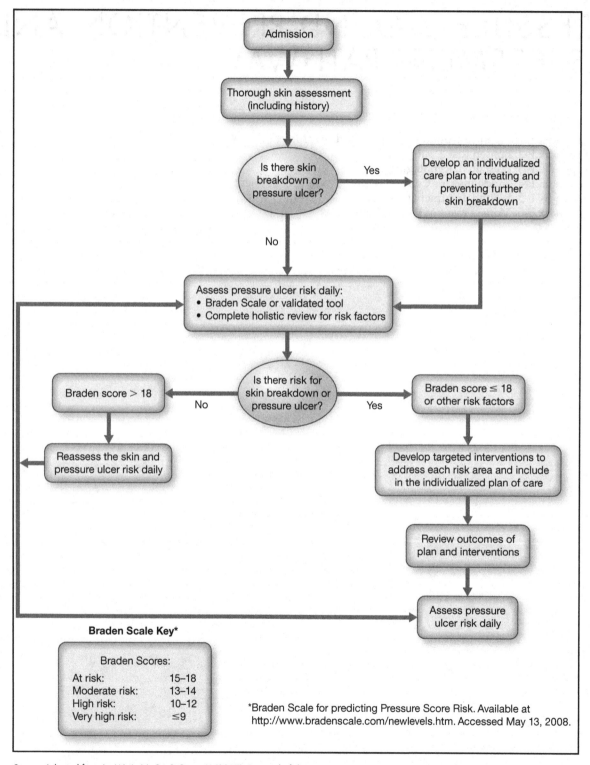

Braden Scale Key*

Braden Scores:

At risk:	15–18
Moderate risk:	13–14
High risk:	10–12
Very high risk:	≤9

*Braden Scale for predicting Pressure Score Risk. Available at http://www.bradenscale.com/newlevels.htm. Accessed May 13, 2008.

Source: Adapted from Ju, W. A. N. G., & Gong, Y. (2017). Potential of decision support in preventing pressure ulcers in hospitals. *Context Sensitive Health Informatics: Redesigning Healthcare Work, 241,* 15.

APPENDIX F-2: BRADEN RISK SCALE

BRADEN SCALE – For Predicting Pressure Sore Risk

SEVERE RISK: Total score 9 **HIGH RISK:** Total score 10-12			**DATE OF ASSESS ➡**	
MODERATE RISK: Total score 13-14 **MILD RISK:** Total score 15-18				

RISK FACTOR	SCORE/DESCRIPTION				1	2	3	4
SENSORY PERCEPTION Ability to respond meaningfully to pressure-related discomfort	**1. COMPLETELY LIMITED** – Unresponsive (does not moan, flinch, or grasp) to painful stimuli, due to diminished level of consciousness or sedation, **OR** limited ability to feel pain over most of body surface.	**2. VERY LIMITED** – Responds only to painful stimuli. Cannot communicate discomfort except by moaning or restlessness, **OR** has a sensory impairment which limits the ability to feel pain or discomfort over ½ of body.	**3. SLIGHTLY LIMITED** – Responds to verbal commands but cannot always communicate discomfort or need to be turned, **OR** has some sensory impairment which limits ability to feel pain or discomfort in 1 or 2 extremities.	**4. NO IMPAIRMENT** – Responds to verbal commands. Has no sensory deficit which would limit ability to feel or voice pain or discomfort.				
MOISTURE Degree to which skin is exposed to moisture	**1. CONSTANTLY MOIST** – Skin is kept moist almost constantly by perspiration, urine, etc. Dampness is detected every time patient is moved or turned.	**2. OFTEN MOIST** – Skin is often but not always moist. Linen must be changed at least once a shift.	**3. OCCASIONALLY MOIST** – Skin is occasionally moist, requiring an extra linen change approximately once a day.	**4. RARELY MOIST** – Skin is usually dry; linen only requires changing at routine intervals.				
ACTIVITY Degree of physical activity	**1. BEDFAST** – Confined to bed.	**2. CHAIRFAST** – Ability to walk severely limited or nonexistent. Cannot bear own weight and/or must be assisted into chair or wheelchair.	**3. WALKS OCCASIONALLY** – Walks occasionally during day, but for very short distances, with or without assistance. Spends majority of each shift in bed or chair.	**4. WALKS FREQUENTLY** – Walks outside the room at least twice a day and inside room at least once every 2 hours during waking hours.				
MOBILITY Ability to change and control body position	**1. COMPLETELY IMMOBILE** – Does not make even slight changes in body or extremity position without assistance.	**2. VERY LIMITED** – Makes occasional slight changes in body or extremity position but unable to make frequent or significant changes independently.	**3. SLIGHTLY LIMITED** – Makes frequent though slight changes in body or extremity position independently.	**4. NO LIMITATIONS** – Makes major and frequent changes in position without assistance.				
NUTRITION Usual food intake pattern [1]NPO: Nothing by mouth. [2]IV: Intravenously. [3]TPN: Total parenteral nutrition.	**1. VERY POOR** – Never eats a complete meal. Rarely eats more than 1/3 of any food offered. Eats 2 servings or less of protein (meat or dairy products) per day. Takes fluids poorly. Does not take a liquid dietary supplement, **OR** is NPO[1] and/or maintained on clear liquids or IV[2] for more than 5 days.	**2. PROBABLY INADEQUATE** – Rarely eats a complete meal and generally eats only about ½ of any food offered. Protein intake includes only 3 servings of meat or dairy products per day. Occasionally will take a dietary supplement **OR** receives less than optimum amount of liquid diet or tube feeding.	**3. ADEQUATE** – Eats over half of most meals. Eats a total of 4 servings of protein (meat, dairy products) each day. Occasionally refuses a meal, but will usually take a supplement if offered, **OR** is on a tube feeding or TPN[3] regimen, which probably meets most of nutritional needs.	**4. EXCELLENT** – Eats most of every meal. Never refuses a meal. Usually eats a total of 4 or more servings of meat and dairy products. Occasionally eats between meals. Does not require supplementation.				
FRICTION AND SHEAR	**1. PROBLEM** – Requires moderate to maximum assistance in moving. Complete lifting without sliding against sheets is impossible. Frequently slides down in bed or chair, requiring frequent repositioning with maximum assistance. Spasticity, contractures, or agitation leads to almost constant friction.	**2. POTENTIAL PROBLEM** – Moves feebly or requires minimum assistance. During a move, skin probably slides to some extent against sheets, chair, restraints, or other devices. Maintains relatively good position in chair or bed most of the time but occasionally slides down.	**3. NO APPARENT PROBLEM** – Moves in bed and in chair independently and has sufficient muscle strength to lift up completely during move. Maintains good position in bed or chair at all times.					
TOTAL SCORE	Total score of 12 or less represents HIGH RISK							

ASSESS	DATE	EVALUATOR SIGNATURE/TITLE	ASSESS.	DATE	EVALUATOR SIGNATURE/TITLE
1	/ /		3	/ /	
2	/ /		4	/ /	

NAME-Last	First	Middle	Attending Physician	Record No.	Room/Bed

Source: www.bradenscale.com. Reprinted with permission.

APPENDIX F-3: PRESSURE ULCER STAGING

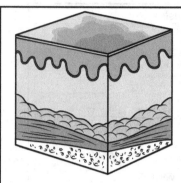

Stage I
Nonblanchable erythema of localized area of skin, usually over a bony prominence. Skin is intact and red in color (darker skin may show blue or purple tones).

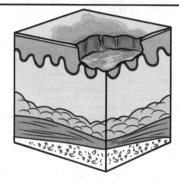

Stage II
Partial-thickness loss of the epidermis and some of the dermis. Looks like a shallow open ulcer or a superficial erosion with a pink-red wound bed and has no slough.

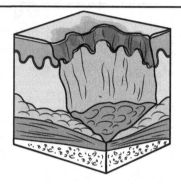

Stage III
Full-thickness loss of the skin and necrosis of subcutaneous tissue. Subcutaneous fat may be visible, but tendon, muscle, or bone is not exposed. Ulcer may include undermining and tunneling and have some slough or necrotic tissue.

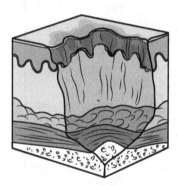

Stage IV
Full-thickness loss of skin including the epidermis, dermis, and subcutaneous tissue. Muscle, bone, or tendon may be exposed. Slough, undermining, and tunneling may be present.

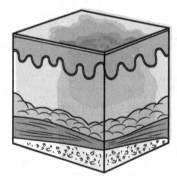

Suspect Deep Tissue Injury
Localized area of discolored skin that is purple or maroon in color. It is nonblanching with and intact epidermis, and skin feels "boggy."

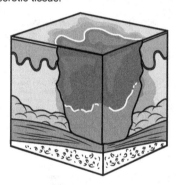

Unstageable
Ulcer has full-thickness tissue loss covered by either an eschar or extensive necrotic tissue (tan, yellow-green, brown), which must be cleared away before the true depth can be determined.

Source: Adapted from Wright, P. M. (Ed.). (2019). *Certified hospice and palliative nurse (CHPN) exam review: A study guide with review questions.* Springer Publishing Company.

APPENDIX F-4: GUIDELINES FOR COMPREHENSIVE WOUND ASSESSMENT

COMPONENTS OF A COMPREHENSIVE WOUND ASSESSMENT

ASSESSMENT AREA	SPECIFIC DOCUMENTATION

Wound bed	**Wound type, age, and location**
	• Pressure injury, lower extremity ulcer (venous, arterial, neuropathic), traumatic wound (skin tear, laceration), malignant wound; superficial, partial thickness, or full thickness
	• Acute versus chronic wound
	• Use correct anatomic location (e.g., right lateral malleolus)
	Wound size
	• Document length × width × depth in centimeters
	  ▪ Length: measure head to toe
	  ▪ Width: measure side to side
	  ▪ Depth: measure deepest depth (only if the wound bed is visible)
	Wound bed tissue
	• Use: slough (devitalized tissue, yellow/brown/grey), eschar (necrotic tissue, black), granulation tissue (red, healthy tissue), epithelial tissue (pale pink, epithelial cells)
	• Describe in percentages (e.g., 40% slough and 60% granulation tissue)
	Exudate type
	• Serous: thin, watery exudate
	• Serosanguineous: thin, red exudate
	• Sanguineous: bloody exudate
	• Purulent: pus-like exudate
	Exudate amount
	• None: dry wound bed
	• Scant: wound is moist but no exudate is present on dressing
	• Small: wound bed is moist and <25% of the dressing has exudate present
	• Moderate: wound bed is wet and 25%–75% of the dressing has exudate present
	• Large/copious: wound bed is wet and ≥75% of the dressing has exudate present
	Odor
	• Describe odor: foul, pungent, absent, strong, sweet
	Signs/symptoms of infection
	• Superficial (NERDS) versus deeper or possible systemic (STONES)
	Pain
	• Document current pain assessment and non-pharmacological and pharmacological interventions. See treatment grids for additional pain management recommendations. Base interventions on the type of pain:
	  ▪ Noncyclic acute (associated with a onetime procedure), cyclic acute (associated with recurring procedures), or chronic wound pain (can be nociceptive or neuropathic in nature)

Wound edge	**Tunneling/undermining** • Measure depth in centimeters, describe location using clock system: head 12 o'clock, toes 6 o'clock **Defining characteristics** • Defined/undefined, attached/detached, rolled (epibole), dry, macerated, shape (regular, irregular)
Periwound tissue	• Describe the appearance of the surrounding tissue: intact, denuded, edematous, firm, indurated, pale, reddened

(continued)

APPENDIX F-4: GUIDELINES FOR COMPREHENSIVE WOUND ASSESSMENT (*CONTINUED*)

COMPONENTS OF A COMPREHENSIVE WOUND ASSESSMENT	
ASSESSMENT AREA	**SPECIFIC DOCUMENTATION**

Holistic patient	• **Preventive measures:** describe preventive measures currently in place: dietary modifications, support surface, turning/repositioning schedule, heel suspension, incontinence care, barrier creams, laboratory monitoring
	• **Comorbidities/contributing factors:** patient prognosis or preference, diagnoses, limitations to repositioning/off-loading pressure, nutritional status, infection, mobility status, medications
	• **Goals of care:** prescription, preservation, palliation, prevention, patient preference
	• **Outcome of care**
	  ▪ Consider if the orders are appropriate for present wound condition and are improving quality of life
	  ▪ Document evidence of healing or deterioration—PUSH displays healing graphically for pressure injuries if healing is a goal of care
	  ▪ Document impact on quality of life and any interventions to improve symptoms
	  ▪ Document notification of physician/patient/responsible party and any new orders received
	• **Education:** document the education provided to the patient

PUSH, pressure ulcer scale for healing.

Source: Brinker, J., Protus, B, M., & Kimbrel, J. M. (2018). *Wound care at end of life: A guide for hospice professionals* (2nd ed.). Optum Hospice Pharmacy Services.

APPENDIX F-5: WOUND TREATMENT GUIDELINES

WOUND TREATMENT GRID: PRESSURE INJURIES STAGES 1 AND 2		
WOUND NEED	**INTERVENTION**	**COMMENTS**
Cleanse	• **Clean wound bed:** pour normal saline or wound cleanser • **Infection:** irrigate with wound cleanser or antiseptic[a]	• Irrigate with 4–15 psi: piston syringe (4.2 psi), squeeze bottle with irrigation cap (4.5 psi), or 35 mL syringe and 18-gauge needle (8 psi)
Debridement	• Necrotic tissue should not be present in a Stage 1 or 2 pressure injury	• Review staging if slough/eschar are present
Exudate	Stage 1 (select based on contributing factors): • **Moisture:** barrier cream, liquid barrier film • **Pressure:** foam • **Shear:** hydrocolloid, transparent film, foam Stage 2 (select based on exudate level): • **None/minimal exudate:** transparent film, hydrocolloid, PMD[a] • **Moderate exudate:** foam, calcium alginate, PMD[a] • **Heavy exudate:** PMD,[a] GFD[a] (Hydrofiber)	• Consider using barrier ointment/cream if area is difficult to apply dressing • Protect periwound: apply skin barrier film or barrier cream/ointment • Hydrocolloid and transparent film contraindicated in infection • PMDs[a] can be used on all exudate levels—moisten with saline if wound bed is dry
Infection	• **None/minimal exudate:** hydrogel with silver, honey • **Moderate exudate:** silver alginate, honey alginate, silver foam • **Heavy exudate:** GFD[a] (Hydrofiber) with silver, cadexomer iodine, GV/MB PU foam[a]	May treat infection empirically: • MRSA: cadexomer iodine, mupirocin,[a] silver • Pseudomonas: cadexomer iodine, acetic acid • VRE: GV/MB PU foam,[a] silver • MSSA: cadexomer iodine, chlorhexidine, GV/MB PU foam,[a] mupirocin,[a] silver
Malodor	• **Cleansers[a]:** hypochlorous acid (Vashe), sodium hypochlorite (Dakin's 0.25%), acetic acid (0.25%–0.5%) • **Dressings:** cadexomer iodine, honey, charcoal, metronidazole (Flagyl) to wound bed, essential oils (wintergreen or lavender) on dressing • **Environmental strategies:** kitty litter, vanilla extract, coffee grounds, dryer sheets placed in the room	• Wound cleansing aids odor control • Change dressing more often to manage odor (e.g., hydrocolloid every 24–48 hours) • Hydrocolloid dressings tend to create odor (doesn't mean infection is present)
Dead space	N/A	N/A
Pruritus	• Not usually associated with wound; assess surrounding skin and consider wound care product being used	• Evaluate for contact dermatitis, hypersensitivity, or yeast dermatitis

(continued)

APPENDIX F-5: WOUND TREATMENT GUIDELINES (*CONTINUED*)

WOUND TREATMENT GRID: PRESSURE INJURIES STAGES 1 AND 2		
WOUND NEED	**INTERVENTION**	**COMMENTS**
Bleeding	• **Dressing strategies:** calcium alginate (silver alginate is not hemostatic), nonadherent dressing, or coagulants (gelatin sponge, thrombin) • **Topical/local strategies:** sclerosing agent (silver nitrate), antifibrinolytic agent (tranexamic acid), astringents (alum solution, sucralfate), vasoconstrictive agents (topical oxymetazoline [Afrin], topical epinephrine)	• Atraumatic removal of dressings—irrigate with normal saline to remove dressings • Ask: Is the wound infected? Is patient on warfarin? Is transfusion appropriate? • Consider checking: platelet count, PT/INR, vitamin K deficiency • Use topical vasoconstrictors only when bleeding is minimal, oozing, or seeping
Support surface	• Pressure-redistributing cushion for wheelchair • Select a support surface	• Float heels—support surfaces are NOT used to prevent pressure injuries to heels
Pain	**Nonpharmacological interventions:** • **Procedural:** moisture-balanced, nonadherent, long-wear dressings; warm saline irrigation to remove dressings; time-outs; patient participation • **Complementary therapies:** music, relaxation, aromatherapy, visualization, meditation **Pharmacological interventions:** • **Topically:** 2% lidocaine, EMLA cream, morphine gel • **Systemically:** scheduled and pre-procedural opioid, tricyclic antidepressant, anticonvulsant	• Rule out infection or wound deterioration • Consider placing: hydrocolloid, foam, calcium alginate, PMD,[a] soft silicone, or hydrogel • EMLA cream is applied to periwound tissue 60 minutes before the procedure • Morphine gel is only applied to open/inflamed wounds

WOUND TREATMENT GRID: PRESSURE INJURIES STAGES 3 AND 4		
WOUND NEED	**INTERVENTION**	**COMMENTS**
Cleanse	• **Clean wound bed:** pour normal saline or wound cleanser • **Infection/necrosis:** irrigate with wound cleanser or antiseptic[a]	• Irrigate with 4–15 psi: piston syringe (4.2 psi), squeeze bottle with irrigation cap (4.5 psi), or 35 mL syringe and 18 gauge needle (8 psi)
Debridement	• **Dry:** hydrocolloid, hydrogel, transparent film • **Moist:** hydrocolloid, calcium alginate, GFD[a] (Hydrofiber) • **Infected:** silver alginate, Dakin's BID, NaCl IG[a]	• Stable eschar of heels, toes, or fingers should NOT be debrided—if present, paint perimeter with povidone-iodine (Betadine) daily • Apply Dakin's soaked gauze BID for debridement
Exudate	• **None/minimal exudate:** hydrogel, PMD[a] • **Moderate exudate:** foam, calcium alginate, PMD[a] • **Heavy exudate:** PMD[a], GFD[a] (Hydrofiber), specialty absorptive	• Pain/bleeding: PMD[a] or contact layer (PMDs[a] can be used on all exudate levels—moisten with saline if wound bed is dry) • Protect periwound: skin barrier film/barrier cream

(continued)

APPENDIX F-5: WOUND TREATMENT GUIDELINES (*CONTINUED*)

WOUND TREATMENT GRID: PRESSURE INJURIES STAGES 3 AND 4		
WOUND NEED	**INTERVENTION**	**COMMENTS**
Infection	• **None/minimal exudate:** hydrogel with silver, honey • **Moderate exudate:** silver alginate, honey alginate, silver foam • **Heavy exudate:** GFD[a] (Hydrofiber) with silver, cadexomer iodine, GV/MB PU foam[a]	May treat infection empirically: • MRSA: cadexomer iodine, mupirocin,[a] silver • Pseudomonas: cadexomer iodine, acetic acid • VRE: GV/MB PU foam,[a] silver • MSSA: cadexomer iodine, chlorhexidine, GV/MB PU foam,[a] mupirocin,[a] silver
Malodor	• **Cleansers[a]:** hypochlorous acid (Vashe), sodium hypochlorite (Dakin's 0.25%), acetic acid • **Dressings:** cadexomer iodine, honey, charcoal, metronidazole (Flagyl) to wound bed; essential oils • **Environmental strategies:** kitty litter, vanilla extract, coffee grounds, or dryer sheets placed in the room	• Wound cleansing aids odor control • Change dressing more often to manage odor (e.g., hydrocolloid every 24–48 hours) • Hydrocolloid dressings tend to create odor (doesn't mean infection is present) • Essential oils: wintergreen or lavender on dressing
Dead space	• **None/minimal exudate:** hydrogel, PMD[a] • **Moderate exudate:** foam, calcium alginate, PMD[a] • **Heavy exudate:** foam, GFD[a] (Hydrofiber), PMD[a]	• Loosely fill any dead space • Products are available in different forms, such as roping to pack tunneling
Pruritus	• Not usually associated with wound, assess surrounding skin, rule out wound care product	• Evaluate for contact dermatitis, hypersensitivity, or yeast dermatitis
Bleeding	• **Dressing strategies:** calcium alginate (silver alginate is not hemostatic), nonadherent dressing, or coagulants (gelatin sponge, thrombin) • **Topical/local strategies:** sclerosing agent (silver nitrate), antifibrinolytic agent (tranexamic acid), astringents (alum solution, sucralfate), vasoconstrictive agents (topical oxymetazoline [Afrin], topical epinephrine)	• Atraumatic removal of dressings—irrigate with normal saline to remove dressings • Ask: Is the wound infected? Is patient on warfarin? Is transfusion appropriate? • Consider checking: platelet count, PT/INR, vitamin K deficiency • Use topical vasoconstrictors only when bleeding is minimal, oozing, or seeping
Support surface	• Pressure-redistributing cushion for wheelchair • Select a support surface using table on page 39	• Float heels—support surfaces are not used to prevent pressure injuries to heels

(continued)

APPENDIX F-5: WOUND TREATMENT GUIDELINES (*CONTINUED*)

WOUND TREATMENT GRID: PRESSURE INJURIES STAGES 3 AND 4		
WOUND NEED	**INTERVENTION**	**COMMENTS**
Pain	**Non-pharmacological interventions:** • **Procedural:** moisture-balanced, nonadherent, long-wear dressings; warm saline irrigation to remove dressings; time-outs; patient participation • **Complementary therapies**: music, relaxation, aromatherapy, visualization, meditation **Pharmacological Interventions:** • **Topically:** 2% lidocaine; EMLA, morphine gel • **Systemically:** scheduled and pre-procedural opioid; tricyclic antidepressant; anticonvulsant	• Rule out infection or wound deterioration • Consider placing: hydrocolloid, foam, calcium alginate, PMD,[a] soft silicone, or hydrogel • EMLA cream is applied to periwound tissue 60 minutes before the procedure • Morphine gel is only applied to open/inflamed wounds

Note: Use of a topical antibiotic is not recommended due to the potential for adverse reactions and antimicrobial resistance.

[a]Rinse wound bed with normal saline after using antiseptic cleanser to minimize toxic effects.

GFD, Gelling fiber dressing; GV/MB PU foam, gentian violet/methylene blue (Hydrofera Blue Ready); MRSA, methicillin-resistant Staphylococcus aureus; MSSA, methicillin-resistant Staphylococcus; NaCl IG, sodium chloride impregnated gauze (Mesalt); PMD, polymeric membrane dressing (PolyMem); PT/INR, prothrombin time/international normalized ratio; VRE, vancomycin-resistant enterococci.

Source: Brinker, J., Protus, B, M., & Kimbrel, J. M. (2018). *Wound care at end of life: A guide for hospice professionals* (2nd ed.). Optum Hospice Pharmacy Services. Used with permission

APPENDIX F-6: MANAGEMENT OF WOUND SYMPTOMS

WOUND SYMPTOM	INTERVENTION
Pain	Reduce number of dressing changes, if possible. Medicate patient prior to dressing changes. Note onset time of pain medication and plan dressing change accordingly. Apply 2% topical lidocaine gel or low-dose morphine gel to wound bed.
Odor	Topical metronidazole, activated charcoal, silver dressings, iodine, honey dressings, debridement Place pan of clean cat litter under patient's bed to absorb odor. May also place coffee beans or essential oils near the patient
Exudate	Dress wound in layers with nonadherent dressing at base. Use highly absorbent and conforming layers over base dressing. Alginate and foam dressings are recommended for wounds with heavy exudate
Hemorrhage	Apply pressure to wound. Topical application of epinephrine 1:1,000 solution to wound followed by application of epinephrine-soaked gauze for several minutes Afrin may be sprayed on wound (this is an off-label use). Gently cleanse wound with warmed normal saline.
Superficial infection	Apply topical antimicrobials such as gentamicin sulfate, metronidazole, mupirocin 2% cream, or polymyxin B sulfate. Silver delivery products are commonly used but little evidence supports efficacy.

Source: Brinker, J., Protus, B, M., & Kimbrel, J. M. (2018). *Wound care at end of life: A guide for hospice professionals* (2nd ed.). Optum Hospice Pharmacy Services. Used with permission.

INDEX

Printed in the United States
by Baker & Taylor Publisher Services